Lippincott Williams & Wilkins'

ADMINISTRATIVE

Medical Assisting

THIRD EDITION

Lippincott Williams & Wilkins'

ADMINISTRATIVE
Medical Assisting

THIRD EDITION

Laura Southard Durham, BS, CMA

Medical Assisting Technologies Program Coordinator (Retired)
Forsyth Technical Community College
Winston-Salem, North Carolina

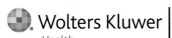 Wolters Kluwer | Lippincott Williams & Wilkins
Health

Philadelphia • Baltimore • New York • London
Buenos Aires • Hong Kong • Sydney • Tokyo

Acquisitions Editor: Kelley Squazzo
Senior Product Manager: Amy Millholen
Design Coordinator: Stephen Druding
Marketing Manager: Shauna Kelley
Compositor: SPi Global
Printer: C & C Offset Printing Co.

Library of Congress Cataloging-in-Publication Data
Durham, Laura Southard.
   Lippincott Williams & Wilkins' administrative medical assisting / Laura Southard Durham. — 3rd ed.
     p. ; cm.
   Lippincott Williams and Wilkins' administrative medical assisting
   Administrative medical assisting
   Includes index.
   ISBN 978-1-4511-1579-6
  I. Title. II. Title: Lippincott Williams and Wilkins' administrative medical assisting. III. Title: Administrative medical assisting.
   [DNLM: 1. Medical Secretaries—organization & administration. 2. Practice Management, Medical. 3. Office Management. 4. Physicians' Offices—organization & administration. W 80]
   651'.961—dc23
                                2012006658

DISCLAIMER

Care has been taken to confirm the accuracy of the information present and to describe generally accepted practices. However, the authors, editors, and publisher are not responsible for errors or omissions or for any consequences from application of the information in this book and make no warranty, expressed or implied, with respect to the currency, completeness, or accuracy of the contents of the publication. Application of this information in a particular situation remains the professional responsibility of the practitioner; the clinical treatments described and recommended may not be considered absolute and universal recommendations.

The authors, editors, and publisher have exerted every effort to ensure that drug selection and dosage set forth in this text are in accordance with the current recommendations and practice at the time of publication. However, in view of ongoing research, changes in government regulations, and the constant flow of information relating to drug therapy and drug reactions, the reader is urged to check the package insert for each drug for any change in indications and dosage and for added warnings and precautions. This is particularly important when the recommended agent is a new or infrequently employed drug.

Some drugs and medical devices presented in this publication have Food and Drug Administration (FDA) clearance for limited use in restricted research settings. It is the responsibility of the health care provider to ascertain the FDA status of each drug or device planned for use in their clinical practice.

The publishers have made every effort to trace the copyright holders for borrowed material. If they have inadvertently overlooked any, they will be pleased to make the necessary arrangements at the first opportunity.

To purchase additional copies of this book, call our customer service department at **(800) 638-3030** or fax orders to **(301) 223-2320**. International customers should call **(301) 223-2300**.

Visit Lippincott Williams & Wilkins on the Internet: *http://www.lww.com*. Lippincott Williams & Wilkins customer service representatives are available from 8:30 am to 5:00 pm, EST.

                                              13
1 2 3 4 5 6 7 8 9 10

CCS0412

This third edition is dedicated to my granddaughter, Gracie Ruth Melton, who is the best granddaughter in the world. Family is what keeps me grounded and moving forward, and I thank God for her every single day of my life.

LAURA SOUTHARD DURHAM

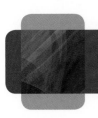

About the Author

Laura Southard Durham

Laura Southard Durham has been a Certified Medical Assistant (CMA) since 1983. She holds a Bachelor of Science degree in Business Administration from Averett University. She has more than 30 years' experience working in the medical field, starting out as a unit secretary in a hospital and continuing in a variety of medical specialties as a CMA and a medical transcriptionist. Laura's true love is teaching. She served as program director of the medical assisting programs in two colleges. She recently retired from Forsyth Technical Community College, where she served as program coordinator for 14 years. She now enjoys writing, public speaking, and consulting in all things medical assisting. Laura is very active in her professional organization, AAMA, on the state and local levels, having served as president of her local chapter and the North Carolina Society of Medical Assistants. She is the newsletter editor of her local chapter. In September of 2010, she was awarded the prestigious Golden Apple Award, given by AAMA each year to one outstanding medical assisting educator in the country. She is known by her students as Mama Durham, but has a daughter Amanda, and a granddaughter Gracie who call her Mom and Nana. In her 17-year career as a medical assisting educator, she boasts over 400 graduates who have gone on to become professional and competent medical assistants. Many of them are members and leaders in their local chapters and state societies of AAMA. She calls these graduates her children and enjoys watching them succeed in their careers and in their lives. Laura believes humor is important in life and in the classroom and is known by her students to make learning fun.

Reviewers

Lenora Binegar, AAS
Medical Program Advisor
Department of Health
Washington County Career Center
Marietta, Ohio

Mindy Brown
Medical Assisting Instructor
Pima Medical Institute
Colorado Springs, Colorado

Patricia Bucho, AS
Instructor
Department of Allied Health
Long Beach City College
Long Beach, California

Estelle Coffino, BS, MPA
Administrator/Chair of Allied Health Programs
Department of Allied Health
The College of Westchester
White Plains, New York

Brandi DeLeon, RT(R), RMA, BS
Medical Insurance Coding Specialist
Fortis Institute
Mulberry, Florida

Jane W. Dumas, MSN, CCMA, CPT, CET
Allied Health Department Chair, MA Program
    Director
Department of Allied Health
Remington College, Cleveland West Campus
Cleveland, Ohio

Donna Guisado, RDA, MSLM
Corporate Director of Education & Compliance
North-West College
West Covina, California

Forrest Heredia, CPC-I
Administrative Assistant Instructor
Medical Administrative Assistant Department
Pima Medical Institute
Tucson, Arizona

Heather Kies, MHA, CMA (AAMA)
Program Director of Medical Assisting
Department of Health & Natural Sciences
Goodwin College
East Hartford, Connecticut

Paul Lucas, AS
Program Director of Medical Assisting
Department of Medical Assisting
Brown Mackie College
Fort Wayne, Indiana

Dona Marotta, CMA (AAMA), BS
Program Director
Department of Medical Assisting
Alegent Health School of Medical Assisting
Omaha, Nebraska

Joyce Minton, MS, EdS
Medical Assisting Director
Department of Advanced Health Technologies
Wilkes Community College
Wilkesboro, North Carolina

Jean L. Mosley, BS, CMA (AAMA)
Medical Assisting Program Director, Instructor
Department of Medical Assisting
Surry Community College
Dobson, North Carolina

Brigitte Niedzwiecki, BSN, MSN
Medical Assistant Program Director, Instructor
Department of Medical Assisting
Chippewa Valley Technical College
Eau Claire, Wisconsin

Wanda Sciambi-Wines, LPN, CMA
National Director of Medical Programs
Department of Education (Corporate Level)
Education Affiliates
Baltimore, Maryland

Sharon Skonieczki, MS, BS, CMA (AAMA)
Program Director
Department of Medical Assisting
Elmira Business Institute
Elmira, New York

Carrie Smith
Instructor
Pima Medical Institute
Tucson, Arizona

Patti Zint, MA, HCA
Program Director
Department of Medical Assisting and Health Care
    Administration
Carrington College
Phoenix, Arizona

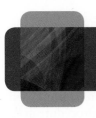

Preface

Health care is changing; however, your role as the most versatile health care member is an important part of the successful physician practice and will continue to be integral as health care changes. Although the skills you perform may vary among medical offices, your education and training in the exciting field of medical assisting will prepare you for a variety of administrative skills, making you an essential part of the health care team.

Lippincott Williams & Wilkins' Administrative Medical Assisting, Third Edition, will provide you with the information and skills necessary to perform competently and with confidence. This edition has been updated to include the most current (2008) American Association of Medical Assistants (AAMA) curriculum standards for medical assistants in all three domains: cognitive, psychomotor, and affective. These standards are required for Commission on Accreditation of Allied Health Education Programs (CAAHEP)-accredited programs. This edition also includes the content and skills required by the American Medical Technologists (AMT) for Accrediting Bureau of Health Education Schools (ABHES)-accredited programs. These standards and competencies define your roles and responsibilities as a professional medical assistant and this edition of the textbook and ancillary materials continue to support your education and training to fulfill these role responsibilities.

Organization of the Text

As with previous editions, great care and concern were taken to organize this book in a logical and reader-friendly presentation. Icons have been added to indicate content that is part of the cognitive, psychomotor, and affective learning domains. The third edition is divided into three sections:

- Part I, Introduction to Medical Assisting, consists of Unit One. Chapter 1 provides you with a brief history of the medical profession and the practice of medical assisting. Legal and ethical issues governing the medical community and your practice are discussed in Chapter 2. Chapter 3 helps you sharpen your communication skills, and Chapter 4 gives you the tools to deliver effective patient education.
- Part II, The Administrative Medical Assistant, consists of Unit Two (Chapters 5 through 10) and Unit

Three (Chapters 11 through 15). Unit Two helps you master basic administrative skills and the basics of office management and basic disaster preparedness, whereas Unit Three explores financial management of the medical office.
- Part III, Career Strategies, helps you make a smooth transition from the classroom environment to the workforce.

Features

Instructors should find the time invested to "link" the text and ancillary materials with the most current CAAHEP and ABHES standards useful. Our goal is to make this textbook the most student-friendly resource available in the medical assisting field.

A variety of key chapter features are included to spark interest and promote comprehension, including:

- Chapter outline
- Learning outcomes specific to CAAHEP and ABHES standards
- Key terms
- Key points highlighted throughout the text
- Icons to indicate content that is part of the cognitive, psychomotor, and affective learning domains—NEW!
- Step-by-step procedure boxes
- Spanish terminology boxes
- Critical thinking challenges
- Checkpoint questions
- Unique information boxes, tables, and displays
- Video icons next to topics and procedures for which there is a skills video available in the online student resources—NEW!
- Full-color illustrations
- Media Menu, containing information on videos and Internet resources

This textbook is fully supported with a robust teaching and learning package, each element of which is designed to help you and your instructor get the most out of the textbook. The resource package includes the following:

- A code in each text to access CareTracker, a web-based electronic medical record (EMR) and practice management (PM) software. This fully integrated EMR and PM gives students the experience of documenting and tracking patient encounters from check in to check out for a real-world experience. Case Studies provided on thePoint walk students through the software helping them build proficiency and confidence in an EMR/PM environment and helping instructors meet the CAAHEP and ABHES EHR competency.

- A complete instructor's resource kit accompanying the textbook includes a test generator, image bank, PowerPoint slides, lesson plans, answer keys for the text checkpoint questions and Study Guide, CAAHEP and ABHES competencies mapping spreadsheets linking the text and ancillary content to the competencies, and more.
- Online student resources, including certification exam preparation review questions, games and review activities, competency evaluation forms, work products, videos, key terms audio glossary, and Spanish-English audio glossary.
- A separate student Study Guide is available for purchase to enhance learning and comprehension, with competency evaluation forms for each procedure in the textbook; critical thinking exercises; self-assessment exercises, such as matching and multiple choice; and study and work products.

As a former medical assisting instructor, I hope this book exceeds your expectations. May your career in medical assisting be challenging and fulfilling!

Laura Southard Durham, BS, CMA

User's Guide

This User's Guide shows you how to the put the features of *Lippincott Williams & Wilkins' Administrative Medical Assisting, Third Edition* to work for you.

Chapter Opening Elements

Each chapter begins with the following elements, which will help orient you to the material:

Chapter Outline

This serves as your "roadmap" to the chapter content.

Learning Outcomes

The Learning Outcomes list the skills learned, including the CAAHEP and ABHES Competencies specific to the chapter.

Key Terms

The key terms that are defined in the chapter are listed for quick reference.

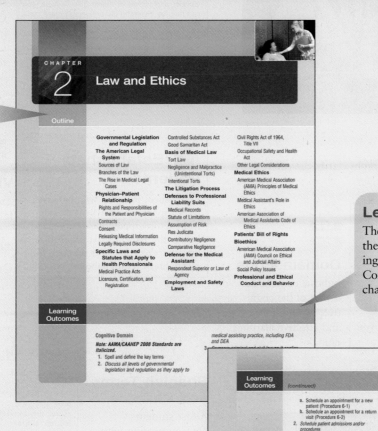

Special Features

Unique chapter features will aid readers' comprehension and retention of information—and spark interest in students and faculty:

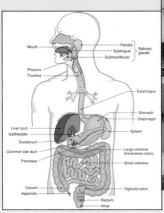

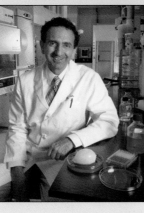

Stunning Art Program

Full-color illustrations and photographs clarify clinical concepts for the learner.

COG **History of Medicine**

Tremendous achievements in the general health, comfort

PSY **Self Boundaries**

What kind of person are you? Are you a friendly

8. **AFF** Explain how you would handle the following situation.

COG
AFF
PSY

Domain Icons

Indicate content that is part of the cognitive, psychomotor, and affective learning domains.

 PSY PROCEDURE 6-2: | **Making an Appointment for an Established Patient**

Purpose: To secure an allotted time for a patient who is returning to your office as an established patient
Equipment: Appointment book or computer with appointment software, appointment card

Steps	Reasons
1. Determine what will be done at the return visit. Check your appointment book or computer system before offering an appointment.	If a specific examination, test, or scan is to be performed, you will want to avoid scheduling two patients for the same examination at the same time.
2. Offer the patient a specific time and date. Avoid asking the patient when he or she would like to return, as this can cause indecision.	Give the patient a choice, and if neither time is convenient, offer another specific time and date. Giving a patient a choice is good practice. "Mrs. Chang, we can see you next Tuesday, the 15th, at 3:30 p.m. or Wednesday, the 16th, at 9:00 a.m."
3. Write the patient's name and telephone number in the appointment book or enter it in computer.	Writing the phone number in the appointment book or making a notation in the computer will the give you a quick reference if you need to call the patient to change the appointment.
4. Transfer the pertinent information to an appointment card and give it to the patient. Repeat aloud appointment the appointment day, date, and time to the patient as you hand over the card (see Fig. 6-4).	Repeating the information reinforces the patient's memory and helps ensure that the will be kept.
5. Double-check your book or computer to be sure you have not made an error.	Errors in appointments waste the patient's, staff's, and physician's time.
6. Whether in person or on the phone, end your conversation with a pleasant word and a smile.	A smile always feels good to a patient who may be apprehensive about needing to return to the doctor.
7. Explain how you would respond to a patient who insists on coming for a return appointment at a time when their doctor is in	Explain that the doctors have certain hours that they see patients, but he/she is welcome to see another provider in the practice.

Procedure Boxes

Break procedures down into steps, demonstrating how to perform essential skills properly. Needed equipment and supplies are listed. Reasons are given for the steps, ensuring greater understanding.

 PATIENT EDUCATION
THE HEALTH CARE SYSTEM

As a medical assistant, you play a key role in teaching patients not only about their health, but also about the health care system. Some patients become confused and are overwhelmed by the number and variety of health care workers. You can help by providing the answers to these common questions:

- What is a multidisciplinary team?
- Who will conduct the examination (physician, physician's assistant, or nurse practitioner)?
- What is a medical assistant?
- What do medical assistants do?
- What kind of training is required for medical assistants?

Patient Education Boxes

Contain in-depth information on topics the student needs to know in order to educate patients.

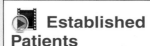 ## Established Patients

Established patients will be given return appointments when necessary. Most return appointments are made before the patient leaves the office. Procedure 6-2 describes the steps for scheduling a return appointment.

Video Icons

Are located next to topics for which there is a skills video available in the online student resources.

---

español español

Spanish Terms and Phrases

Assist students communicating with Spanish-speaking patients.

SPANISH TERMINOLOGY

¿Usted entiende la información que acaba de recibir?
  Do you understand the information I have given?
¿Usted nos autoriza a llevar a cabo este procedimiento médico?
  Do you give us permission to perform this procedure?
¿Firme aquí, por favor.
  Please sign here.

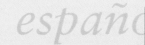 **AFF** WHAT IF?

A patient is hearing impaired, and you cannot communicate with him to explain the procedure you are about to perform. What should you do?
  If the patient does not understand the procedure, he or she is not *informed*. Legally, you have not met your responsibilities to obtain informed consent if the patient does not understand the information you are trying to convey (see Legal Tip box; also see Chapter 2 for more information about informed consent).
  Most community colleges offer courses in sign language. The let

What If Boxes

Present a variety of real-life scenarios that students must be prepared to handle in the medical office. Each situation is clearly defined and explained.

Special Features *(continued)*

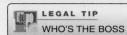

CHECKPOINT QUESTION

2. What governmental agency monitors medical care finances?

Checkpoint Questions

Review questions appear throughout the chapter to ensure student comprehension of the material learned in the section.

Legal Tip Boxes

Contain important legal information to help the aspiring medical assistant understand the legal implications associated with the profession.

LEGAL TIP

WHO'S THE BOSS

Although a nurse's training involves inpatient or hospital care, some physicians choose to employ nurses in their offices. In some states, nurses working in physician offices are not allowed to supervise or delegate their authority to medical assistants. However, nurses and medical assistants work side by side in many instances because the medical assistant works under the supervision of the physician, not the nurse. For example, in the North Carolina law regarding this issue, the legislation refers to medical assistants as "unlicensed health care personnel." Medical

ETHICAL TIP

Who is Who?

It is important that medical assistants represent themselves honestly. Physicians often innocently refer to every employee as "the nurse." It is more accurate to say my assistant, my certfied medical assistant, my registered medical assistant, or my clinical assistant. There are documented court cases involving misrepresentation of one's education and credentials. Protect yourself by referring to yourself appropriately to patients and co-workers. Do not identify yourself as "Dr. Smith's nurse." When

Ethical Tip Boxes

Offer guidelines to help the student learn and abide by the ethical standards set forth by the AAMA.

MEDIA MENU

- **Student Resources on thePoint**
  - **CMA/RMA Certification Exam Review**
- **Internet Resources**

  Accrediting Bureau of Health Education Schools
  http://www.abhes.org

  American Board of Medical Specialties
  http://www.abms.org

  American Health Information Management Association

Media Menus

Located at the end of every chapter, the Media Menu contains information on video clips, animations, and Internet resources that are available to the student.

Chapter Closing Elements

Chapter Summary

Reviews key points from the chapter.

Chapter Summary

- Medical history reveals 150 years of progress, with the most amazing strides made in the 20th century. New technologies continue to expand the possibilities of health care.
- Changes in the American health care system brought the necessity for highly trained professionals.
- The health care team works together to deliver quality patient care and remain financially sound.
- Professionalism is highly desired by employers. Medical assistants must understand their scope of practice.

- A graduate of an accredited medical assisting program can pursue certification or registration, which brings increasing marketability in the health care arena.
- By ensuring that educational levels are constantly enhanced and by continuing to grow professionally, the medical assistant graduate will prepare for the challenge of a lifelong career that is both fascinating and rewarding.

Warm Ups for Critical Thinking

1. Visit the Web site dedicated to regenerative medicine, http://regenerativemedicine.net and determine the goals and accomplishments related to the field of regenerative medicine.
2. Review the list of characteristics for medical assistants. Which characteristics do you already have? How will you acquire the others? Are there additional characteristics that you have that will make you a good medical assistant?
3. Look at the list of physician specialties. Which type of physician would you want to work for and why? Which physician specialties would you least want to work with? Explain your response.

4. Visit www.aama... ...omedtech.org and determine which lo... ...member of. How would membe... ...career as a medical assistant?
5. How does certification or registration as a medical assistant impact scope of practice?
6. What is the importance of having adaptive coping mechanisms in place? Give an example of a situation in which such tools would be helpful.
7. How would you answer the question, "Legally, who is responsible for the actions of certified medical assistants or registered medical assistants as they perform their skills?"

24

Warm Ups for Critical Thinking

Real-life scenarios that require the student to develop, create, write, or search for more information.

Additional Learning Resources

This powerful learning tool also includes:

• the**Point** Companion Site for Students comes with new review activities and games, videos, certification preparation question bank, competency evaluation forms, an English-to-Spanish audio glossary and key terms glossary, and student work products. The student companion site can be accessed at: http://thepoint.lww.com/durhamadmin3e

• Instructor Resources on thePoint include lesson plans, image bank, test generator, PowerPoint lecture slides, answer keys, CAAHEP and ABHES competencies mapping spreadsheets linking the text and ancillary content to the competencies, and more.

Available for purchase separately:

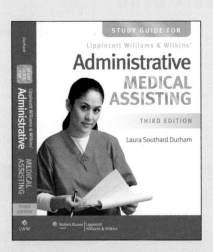

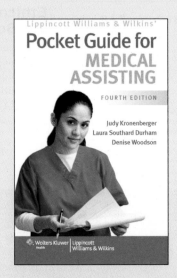

• *Study Guide for Lippincott Williams & Wilkins' Administrative Medical Assisting* comes with procedure skill sheets, case studies for critical thinking, and a variety of question types to meet the needs of different learning styles and to reinforce content and knowledge.

• *Lippincott Williams & Wilkins' Pocket Guide for Medical Assisting* gives step-by-step coverage of medical assisting procedures in both administrative and clinical settings. The small size makes it perfect for clinical and office use.

Acknowledgments

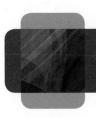

This book would never have been successfully completed without the assistance, persistence, and hard work of many people. At the risk of leaving out others at Lippincott Williams & Wilkins (LWW) who made this book possible (I apologize in advance!), I would like to thank Kelley Squazzo, the Acquisitions Editor, who was there from the beginning to offer support, insight, and guidance whenever needed. A special thank you should also go to Julie Stegman, (Senior Publisher, Health Professions), John Larkin (Product Manager), Rachel Stark (Editorial Assistant), Eric Branger (Product Director), and Kelly Horvath (Copyeditor) for making this book and ancillary materials a reality and supporting the education of medical assistants.

In particular, I owe a huge thank you to Amy Millholen, Senior Product Manager at LWW, for keeping me focused and the project organized to ensure that the chapter content remained student-centered. I could not have done it without you, Amy! To all the other staff at LWW who helped in this edition of the book but who may not be mentioned specifically, I offer my most sincere gratitude and thanks!

I would like to acknowledge the many contributions of my daughter, Amanda Melton, who provided technical and moral support throughout this project. I would also like to thank Brenda Allen at Orthopedic Specialists of the Carolinas for her expertise and encouragement.

The author and staff at LWW thank the administration, staff, and students at Forsyth Technical Community College in Winston-Salem, NC, who provided the location, faces, and skills for the photo and video shoots.

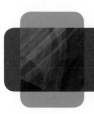

List of Procedures

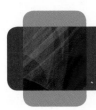

Contents

PART III
Career Strategies

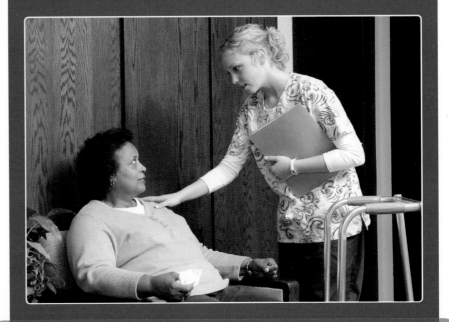

Introduction to Medical Assisting

Understanding the Profession

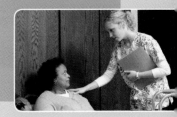

Welcome! The world of medicine is an exciting and challenging frontier. This unit consists of four chapters that will introduce you to the field of medicine and medical assisting, offer vital help in communication skills, and provide you with information to enable you to educate your patients. In the first chapter, you will learn how medicine has evolved through the years from the era of superstition and magical cures to the age of modern technology, in which professionalism is expected from allied health professionals. The second chapter introduces you to legal and ethical responsibilities that affect medical professionals. Sometimes, the advances in medicine challenge our laws and ethics. Chapter 3 covers communication skills, and Chapter 4 introduces you to the concepts of patient education. This unit will help you to understand the bond between medicine, professionalism, law, and ethics, and to communication with patients and co-workers. Let the exploration begin!

CHAPTER 1

Medicine and Medical Assisting

Outline

History of Medicine
Modern Medical History
Strides in the Prevention of
Disease Transmission
Possibilities in Surgery
Women in Medicine
Important Discoveries
Recent Medical History
**The American Health Care
System**
The Medical Office
Medical Specialties

The Medical Assisting Profession
What is a Medical Assistant?
Duties of a Medical Assistant
Professionalism
Scope of Practice and Standards
of Care
Self Boundaries in the Health Care
Environment
Members of the Health Care Team
Health Care Providers
The Nursing Profession
Allied Health Professionals
The History of Medical Assisting

Medical Assisting Education
Medical Assisting Program
Accreditation
Medical Assisting Credentials
Certified Medical Assistant
Registered Medical Assistant
Certified Clinical Medical
Assistant
National Certified Medical
Assistant
**Medical Assisting and Related
Allied Health Associations**
Association Membership
Employment Opportunities

Learning Outcomes

Cognitive Domain

***Note: AAMA/CAAHEP 2008 Standards are
italicized.***

1. Spell and define the key terms
2. Summarize a brief history of modern medicine
3. Explain the system of health care in the United States
4. Discuss the typical medical office

5. List medical specialties a medical assistant may encounter
6. List settings in which medical assistants may be employed
7. List the duties of a medical assistant
8. Describe the desired characteristics of a medical assistant
9. *Discuss legal scope of practice for medical assistants*

10. Compare and contrast physician and medical assistant roles in terms of standard of care
11. Recognize the role of patient advocacy in the practice of medical assisting
12. Identify the role of self boundaries in the health care environment
13. Differentiate between adaptive and nonadaptive coping mechanisms
14. Identify members of the health care team
15. Explain the pathways of education for medical assistants
16. Discuss the importance of program accreditation
17. Name and describe the two nationally recognized accrediting agencies for medical assisting education programs
18. Explain the benefits and avenues of certification for the medical assistant
19. *Discuss licensure and certification as it applies to health care providers*
20. List the benefits of membership in a professional organization
21. *Identify the effect personal ethics may have on professional performance*
22. *Compare personal, professional, and organizational ethics*
23. *Discuss all levels of governmental legislation and regulation as they apply to medical assisting practice, including FDA and DEA regulations*

Psychomotor Domain

Note: AAMA/CAAHEP 2008 Standards are italicized.
1. *Perform within scope of practice*
2. *Practice within the standard of care for a medical assistant*
3. *Develop a plan for separation of personal and professional ethics*
4. *Respond to issues of confidentiality*
5. *Document accurately in the patient record*

Affective Domain

Note: AAMA/CAAHEP 2008 Standards are italicized.
1. *Demonstrate awareness of the consequences of not working within the legal scope of practice*
2. *Apply ethical behaviors, including honesty and integrity in performance of medical assisting practice*
3. *Examine the impact personal ethics and morals may have on the individual's practice*

ABHES Competencies

1. Comprehend the current employment outlook for the medical assistant
2. Compare and contrast the allied health professions and understand their relation to medical assisting
3. Understand medical assistant credentialing requirements and the process to obtain the credential. Comprehend the importance of credentialing
4. Have knowledge of the general responsibilities of the medical assistant
5. Define scope of practice for the medical assistant, and comprehend the conditions for practice within the state that the medical assistant is employed
6. Demonstrate professionalism by:
   a. Exhibiting dependability, punctuality, and a positive work ethic
   b. Exhibiting a positive attitude and a sense of responsibility
   c. Maintaining confidentiality at all times
   d. Being cognizant of ethical boundaries
   e. Exhibiting initiative
   f. Adapting to change
   g. Expressing a responsible attitude
   h. Being courteous and diplomatic
   i. Conducting work within scope of education, training, and ability
7. Comply with federal, state, and local health laws and regulations
8. Analyze the effect of hereditary, cultural, and environmental influences

Key Terms

accreditation
administrative
certification
clinical
concierge medicine

continuing education units (CEUs)
inpatient
laboratory
medical assistant

multidisciplinary
multiskilled health professional
outpatient
practicum

recertification
scope of practice
self boundaries
specialty

Welcome to the field of medicine and to the medical assisting profession! You have selected a fascinating and challenging career, one of the fastest growing specialties in the medical field. The need for the **multiskilled health professional**—an individual with versatile training in the health care field—will continue to grow within the foreseeable future, and you are now a part of this exciting career direction.

To help you understand the significance of the medical knowledge and skills you will receive during your course of study, we begin by taking a chronological look at the history of medicine and then explore the profession of medical assisting.

COG History of Medicine

Tremendous achievements in the general health, comfort, and well-being of patients have been made just within the past 100 to 150 years, with the greatest advances occurring in the 20th century. The 21st century has brought continued advancement in cancer research, the human genome project, and the eradication of more diseases. It is difficult to imagine health care without antibiotics, x-ray machines, or anesthesia, but these developments are fairly new to medicine. For example, penicillin was not produced in large quantities until World War II, and surgery was performed without anesthesia until the mid 1800s. The possibility of cures for some of the devastating diseases humans face gets closer with every research project, and there are many being conducted. Chances are good that the next great medical discovery will result from stem cell and cord blood research.

COG Modern Medical History

The Renaissance was a period of enlightenment in all areas of art, science, and education, and it fostered great strides in medicine. The advent of the printing press and the establishment of great universities made the practice of medicine more accessible to larger numbers of practitioners. Great minds collaborated to advance medical and scientific theories and perform experiments that led to discoveries of enormous benefit in the fight against disease.

During this period, Andreas Vesalius (1514–1564) became known as the "Father of Modern Anatomy." He corrected many of Galen's errors and wrote the first relatively correct anatomy textbook. Soon afterward, William Harvey identified the pumping action of the heart. He described circulation as a continuous circuit pumped by the heart to carry blood through the body. Harvey studied the action of the heart using dogs, not humans.

The microscope was invented in the mid 1660s by a Dutch lens maker, Anton von Leeuwenhoek. He was the first person to observe bacteria under a lens, although he had no idea of the significance of the microorganisms

to human health. His instrument also allowed him to accurately describe a red blood cell.

John Hunter (1728–1793) became known as the "Father of Scientific Surgery." He developed many surgical techniques that are still used today. Hunter also developed and inserted the first artificial feeding tube into a patient in 1778 and was the first to classify teeth in a scientific manner.

In 1796, Edward Jenner, a physician in England, overheard a young milkmaid explain that she could not catch smallpox because she had already had the very mild cowpox caught while milking her cows. Several weeks later, Jenner inoculated a small boy with smallpox crusts. The boy did not contract the disease, and the prevention for smallpox was discovered. Jenner's discovery of the smallpox vaccine led to more emphasis on prevention of disease rather than on cures.

Also during the early 1800s, the importance of the mind as a part of the health care process was becoming a recognized field of medicine. The first extensive work and writing on mental health was published in 1812 by Benjamin Rush, titled *Medical Inquiries and Observations upon Diseases of the Mind*. He advocated humane treatment of the mentally ill at a time when most were imprisoned, chained, starved, exhibited like animals, or simply killed. Rush's influence began the separate field of study into the working of the mind that became modern psychiatry.

Strides in the Prevention of Disease Transmission

The mid 1880s saw a surge in the study of disease transmission. Louis Pasteur (1822–1895) became famous for his work with bacteria. Pasteur discovered that wine turned sour because of the presence of bacteria. He found that, when the bacteria were eliminated, the wine lasted longer. Pasteur's discovery that bacteria in liquids could be eliminated by heat led to the process known as pasteurization. This finding led to using heat to sterilize surgical instruments. Pasteur has been called the "Father of Bacteriology" for this accomplishment. Pasteur also focused on preventing the transmission of anthrax and discovered the rabies vaccine and was honored with the title "Father of Preventive Medicine" for this work.

In the mid 1880s, Ignaz Semmelweis, a Hungarian physician, noticed that women whose babies were born at home with a midwife in attendance had childbed fever less often than those who delivered in well-respected hospitals with prestigious physicians at the bedside. He was ridiculed by the medical establishment and was fired from his position when he required medical personnel to wash their hands in a solution of chlorinated lime before performing obstetric examinations. He was right, of course, and handwashing is still the most important factor in the fight against disease transmission.

At about the same time, Joseph Lister began to apply antiseptics to wounds to prevent infection. The concept was not clearly understood, but before Lister's practices, as many patients died of infection as died of the primitive surgical techniques of the early part of the century.

In 1928, Sir Alexander Fleming, a bacteriologist, accidentally discovered penicillin when his assistant forgot to wash the Petri dishes Fleming had used for experiments. When he noticed the circles of nongrowth around areas of a certain mold, he was able to extract the prototype for one of our most potent weapons against disease. He won the Nobel Prize in 1945 for this accomplishment.

Possibilities in Surgery

Modern anesthesia was discovered in 1842 by Crawford Williamson Long. The effects of nitrous oxide were known by the mid 1700s, but Long discovered its therapeutic use by accident when he observed a group of chemistry students inhaling it for amusement. Before this time, anesthesia consisted of large doses of alcohol or opium, leather straps for patient restraint, or the unconsciousness resulting from pain. Ether and chloroform came into use at about this time.

Women in Medicine

The 1800s brought the first notable records of the contributions of women to the medical field. Florence Nightingale (1820–1910) was the founder of modern nursing. She set standards and developed educational requirements for nurses.

Elizabeth Blackwell (1821–1910) became the first woman to complete medical school in the United States when she graduated from Geneva Medical College in New York. In 1869, Blackwell established her own medical school in Europe for women only, opening the door for a rapidly expanding role for women in the medical field.

Clara Barton (1821–1912) founded the American Red Cross in 1881 and was its first president. She identified the need for psychological as well as physical support for wounded soldiers in the Civil War.

Marie Curie (1867–1934), a brilliant science student, married Pierre Curie, and together they discovered polonium and radium. Their discovery revolutionized the principles of energy and radioactivity. Marie and Pierre Curie shared the Nobel Prize for chemistry in 1903. Marie continued the research after Pierre's death and again won the Nobel Prize for physics in 1911.

Important Discoveries

X-rays were discovered in 1895 by Wilhelm Konrad Roentgen when he observed that a previously unknown ray generated by a cathode tube could pass through soft tissue and outline underlying structures. Medical diagnosis was revolutionized, earning Roentgen a Nobel Prize in 1901 for his discovery. The therapeutic uses of x-rays were recognized much later.

Jonas Edward Salk and Albert Sabin discovered the vaccines for polio in the 1950s, which led to near eradication of one of the 20th century's greatest killers.

 CHECKPOINT QUESTION

1. How was penicillin discovered?

COG Recent Medical History

Throughout the next three decades, public health protection improved and advancements continued. Government legislation mandated clean water, and citizens reaped the benefits of preventive medicine and education about health issues.

In the 1980s, advancements in radiology gave doctors ways to see inside a patient with such accuracy that patients no longer had to have exploratory surgery. With computed tomography (CT) scans, radiologists can see tumors, cysts, inflammation, and so on, with cross-sectional slices of the patient's body. Magnetic resonance imaging (MRI) uses a strong magnetic field to realign ions to form an image on a screen. MRI is used to detect internal bleeding, tumors, cysts, and so on. Positron emission tomography (PET) has further revolutionized radiology. A "map" of the body shows the tissues in which the molecular probe has become concentrated and can be interpreted by nuclear medicine physicians or radiologists in the context of the patient's diagnosis and treatment plan. PET scans are increasingly read alongside CT scans or MRI scans, the combination giving both anatomic and metabolic information (what the structure is and what it is doing). PET is used in clinical oncology, showing tumors and determining areas where cancer has spread or metastasized. Researchers are using these scans in studying the human brain and the heart.

In July 1998, Ryuzo Yanagimachi of the University of Hawaii announced the cloning of mice when 7 of 22 mice were cloned from the cell of a single mouse. In December 1998, researchers from Kinki University in Nara, Japan, cloned 8 calves from a single cell.

In 2006, the final human genome papers were published. After years of work, a team of scientists from both the public and private sectors completed the identification and mapping of human genes. Mapping the sequence of the letters of the human genome that represent the handbook of a human being is a breakthrough that will revolutionize the practice of medicine by paving the way for new drugs and therapies. The achievement is one of the most significant scientific landmarks of all time. Many medicines that can be tailored to an individual's genetic makeup are on the market or in development. New discoveries will continue to expand the parameters of medicine as further research in recombinant DNA, transplantation, immunizations, diagnostic procedures, and so forth push back the boundaries of health care and make today's therapies seem as primitive as those we have just covered. You will be present during this fascinating evolution of health care.

Regenerative medicine is an area of research that has seen real progress in accelerating the healing process to fully restore the health of damaged tissues and organs. The goal of regenerative medicine is to one day be capable of maintaining the body in such a way that there will be no need to replace whole organs. These innovative medical therapies are showing great promise over traditional medical treatments. Stem cell procedures have restored sight to the blind, for example, in an Italian study published June 23, 2010, by the *New England Journal of Medicine* of three patients with alkali burns of the eyes. Figure 1-1 shows a printer used for printing skin cells.

Scientists at Wake Forest Institute for Regenerative Medicine in Winston-Salem, NC, were the first in the world to successfully implant a laboratory-grown organ into humans, and, today, are working to grow more than 22 different organs and tissues in the laboratory. A series of child and teenage patients have received urinary bladders grown from their own cells. In addition, they are working to develop cell therapies that can help restore organ function. Figure 1-2 shows a bladder made in the laboratory from the patient's own cells.

Within the next decade, expect to see immunization against or cures for many of the illnesses that continue to plague us. And when we need a new kidney, we can make one in the laboratory!

Your role as a **medical assistant,** the ultimate multiskilled health care professional, will expand as

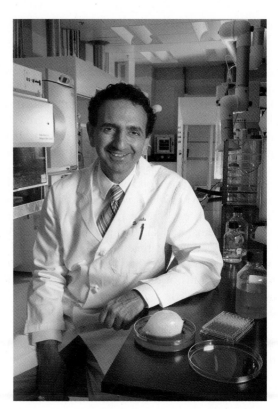

Figure 1-2 Dr. Anthony Atala of Wake Forest University Institute for Regenerative Medicine and other scientists can now make a human bladder from the patient's own cells. Photo: Courtesy of WFU Institute for Regenerative Medicine.

the need for highly trained, versatile medical personnel keeps pace with the ever-changing practice of medicine. Today, heart bypass surgeries and organ transplants are performed routinely. Researchers continue to search for the cures for cancer, acquired immunodeficiency syndrome, and many other ailments. Scientists are learning more about mutating organisms and ways to fight them. As a medical assistant, you will witness the progress made as you play a key role in caring for patients.

COG The American Health Care System

The American health care system is complex and has seen many changes in the past few decades. Twenty years ago, a patient had medical insurance that paid a percentage of his or her medical bills. In today's world of managed care, which is discussed in the chapter on health insurance, many patients are a part of a group of covered members of an HMO (health maintenance organization). With this change came new ways of treating patients. The doctor–patient relationship was one of trust and privacy. In a managed care system, patients are treated as outlined by the insurance companies. The purpose of this change was to control health care costs. The government

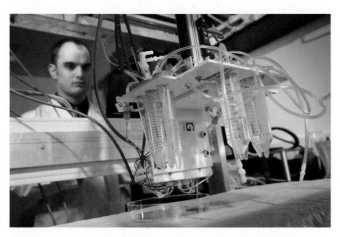

Figure 1-1 Using a modified version of ink jet printing, scientists at the Wake Forest Institute for Regenerative Medicine are working on a project to print skin cells directly onto burns. Each cell type is placed in a vial, rather than in cartridges, and is then "printed" directly on the wound. Photo: Courtesy of WFU Institute for Regenerative Medicine.

monitors medical finances and controls the Medicare and Medicaid systems through the Centers for Medicare and Medicaid Services (CMS). This government agency was formerly called the Health Care Financing Administration (HFCA). It has been estimated that, by 2013, 60% of patients being seen in the medical office will be over 65 years of age and will be covered under the Medicare system of insurance for the elderly. As technology advanced the capabilities of medical facilities to operate electronically, the government responded with The Health Insurance Portability and Accountability Act of 1996 (HIPAA), which was passed to simplify the **administrative** process of transmitting insurance claims, receiving payments, and sharing private health information. HIPAA is discussed throughout the text and covered thoroughly in Chapter 8. The need to adhere to the rules and regulations of the government drives the management practices of the **outpatient** medical facility. The allied health care arena has grown quickly. New professions have been added to the health care team, and each one is an important part of a patient's total care. As an allied health student, you have an exciting course of study ahead of you. Soon you will find yourself among a caring and conscientious group of health care professionals.

COG The Medical Office

Today's medical office is quite different from the office of the past, where patients were treated by their family physician, insurance was filed, and reimbursement was based on a percentage of the cost. Large corporations and hospitals now own many medical clinics, and physicians are their employees. Billing, collections, insurance processing, laboratory procedures, and other tasks performed in the medical office may be outsourced or handled in a central office for the corporation. Medical practices now have the capability to maintain a patient's record without a single piece of paper. Office employees need a general understanding of the many regulations of insurance carriers. Every employee must be computer literate and should understand the legal aspects of the medical office. Although there are many medical specialties, the skills and basic functions of any medical office will be similar. With the new technology and the need for constant monitoring of regulations and changes, the medical office employee is now expected to acquire a formal education and certification.

The typical medical office employs one or more physicians. To assist with examining and treating patients, the physician may employ physician assistants and/or nurse practitioners. These are the providers, and they need support staff. The goal of any medical practice is to provide quality care while maintaining sound financial practices within the laws and ethics of the medical profession. To achieve this goal, the physician needs a solid team. The administrative staff handles the financial

aspects of the practice, and the clinical staff assists the providers with patient care. Both aspects of the office must run smoothly to reach the ultimate goal of the practice. The makeup of the team may differ among specialties. For example, an orthopedist may have an x-ray technologist on staff, or an obstetrician may have an on-site sonographer to perform ultrasounds on mothers to be. Regardless of the mix of the team, the medical assistant is an integral part.

Concierge medicine is a new type of medicine cropping up across the country. It involves a relationship between a patient and a primary care physician in which the patient pays an annual fee or retainer. This may or may not be in addition to other charges. In exchange for the retainer, doctors provide enhanced care. Just as a concierge in a five-star hotel caters to the customer's needs, a physician practicing concierge medicine may see only seven to eight patients a day, attending to their particular health care needs.

The day-to-day operation of a medical office requires all the skills you learn in your curriculum. The patient's health care encounter can be pleasant or unpleasant, depending on the skills and the attitude of the team.

 PATIENT EDUCATION

THE HEALTH CARE SYSTEM

As a medical assistant, you play a key role in teaching patients not only about their health, but also about the health care system. Some patients become confused and are overwhelmed by the number and variety of health care workers. You can help by providing the answers to these common questions:

- What is a multidisciplinary team?
- Who will conduct the examination (physician, physician's assistant, or nurse practitioner)?
- What is a medical assistant?
- What do medical assistants do?
- What kind of training is required for medical assistants?
- What does credentialing mean for a medical assistant?

When patients understand the health care field and know what to expect, they recover more quickly and are more comfortable asking questions about their health.

 CHECKPOINT QUESTION

2. What governmental agency monitors medical care finances?

COG Medical Specialties

After completion of medical school, physicians choose a **specialty**. Some prefer treating patients of all ages and will choose family medicine or internal medicine. Others choose surgery and further specialize in fields like cosmetic surgery or vascular surgery. Table 1-1 lists the most common surgical specialties. Table 1-2 lists specialists who may employ medical assistants.

 CHECKPOINT QUESTION

3. What is the specialty that treats newborn babies?

COG The Medical Assisting Profession

What is a Medical Assistant?

According to the Commission on Accreditation of Allied Health Education Programs (CAAHEP), medical assistants are multiskilled allied health professionals specifically educated to work in ambulatory settings performing administrative and clinical duties. The practice of medical assisting directly influences the public's health and well-being, and requires mastery of a complex body of knowledge and specialized skills requiring both formal education and practical experience that serve as standards for entry into the profession.

Administrative tasks usually focus on office procedures. **Clinical** tasks generally involve direct patient care. Salaries depend on experience, size of practice or corporation, and geographic region. Hours and working conditions for medical assistants vary according to state laws regarding the medical assisting profession and the scope of the specialty of employer and job responsibilities. **Scope of practice** is defined as the procedures, actions, and processes that are permitted for a particular health care profession. State laws and regulations describe the particular requirements for education and training and define the scope of training for health care practitioners.

Because a medical assistant is not licensed, your scope of practice will depend on your physician-employer's delegation of duties according to state law regarding patient care (see Figure 1-4). For signs that you are crossing the line, see Box 1-1.

Duties of a Medical Assistant

The duties of a medical assistant are divided into three categories: general, administrative and clinical, which includes **laboratory** duties. The ratio of administrative to clinical duties varies with your job description. For example, if you work in a family practice office, you may do mostly clinical work; a psychiatric practice will probably require primarily administrative duties.

Administrative Duties

Performing administrative tasks correctly and in a timely manner will make the office more efficient and productive. Conversely, an office that is not managed correctly can result in loss of business, poor patient service, and loss of revenue. Following is a partial list of standard administrative duties:

- Managing and maintaining the waiting room, office, and examining rooms
- Handling telephone calls
- Using written and oral communication
- Maintaining medical records
- Bookkeeping
- Scheduling appointments
- Ensuring good public relations
- Maintaining office supplies
- Screening sales representatives
- Filing insurance forms

TABLE 1-1	Common Surgical Specialties
Surgical Specialty	**Description**
Cardiovascular	Repairs physical dysfunctions of the cardiovascular system
Cosmetic, reconstructive	Restores, repairs, or reconstructs body parts
General	Performs repairs on a variety of body parts
Maxillofacial	Repairs disorders of the face and mouth (a branch of dentistry)
Neurosurgery	Repairs disorders of the nervous system including brain and back surgery
Orthopedic	Corrects deformities and treats disorders of the musculoskeletal system
Thoracic	Repairs organs within the rib cage
Trauma	Limited to correcting traumatic wounds
Vascular	Repairs disorders of blood vessels, usually excluding the heart

TABLE 1-2   Specialists Who Employ Medical Assistants

Specialty	Description
Allergist	Performs tests to determine the basis of allergic reactions to eliminate or counteract the offending allergen
Anesthesiologist	Determines the most appropriate anesthesia during surgery for the patient's situation
Cardiologist	Diagnoses and treats disorders of the cardiovascular system, including the heart, arteries, and veins
Chiropractor	Manipulates the musculoskeletal system and spine to relieve symptoms
Dermatologist	Diagnoses and treats skin disorders; may provide cosmetic treatments
Emergency physician	Usually works in emergency or trauma centers
Endocrinologist	Diagnoses and treats disorders of the endocrine system and its hormone-secreting glands, e.g., diabetes and dwarfism
Epidemiologist	Specializes in epidemics caused by infectious agents; studies toxic agents, air pollution, and other health-related phenomena; and works with sexually transmitted disease control
Family practitioner	Serves a variety of patient age levels, seeing patients for everything from ear infections to school physicals
Gastroenterologist	Diagnoses and treats disorders of the stomach and intestine
Gerontologist	Limits practice to disorders of the aging population and its unique challenges
Gynecologist	Diagnoses and treats disorders of the female reproductive system and may also be an obstetrician or limit the practice to gynecology, including surgery
Hematologist	Diagnoses and treats disorders of the blood and blood-forming organs
Immunologist	Concentrates on the body's immune system and disease incidence, transmission, and prevention
Internist	Limits practice to diagnosis and treatment of disorders of internal organs with medical (drug therapy and lifestyle changes) rather than surgical means
Neonatologist	Limits practice to the care and treatment of infants to about 6 weeks of age
Nephrologist	Diagnoses and treats disorders of the kidneys
Neurologist	Limits practice to the nonsurgical care and treatment of brain and spinal cord disorders
Obstetrician	Limits practice to care and treatment for pregnancy, the postpartum period, and fertility issues
Oncologist	Diagnoses and treats tumors, both benign (noncancerous) and malignant (cancerous)
Ophthalmologist	Diagnoses and treats disorders of the eyes, including surgery (an optometrist monitors and measures patients for corrective lenses, and an optician makes the lenses or dispenses contact lenses)
Orthopedist	Diagnoses and treats disorders of the musculoskeletal system, including surgery and care for fractures
Otorhinolaryngologist	Diagnoses and treats disorders of the ear, nose, and throat
Pathologist	Analyzes tissue samples or specimens from surgery, diagnoses abnormalities, and performs autopsies
Pediatrician	Limits practice to childhood disorders or may be further specialized to early childhood or adolescent period
Podiatrist	Diagnoses and treats disorders of the feet and provides routine care for diabetic patients who may have poor circulation and require extra care
Proctologist	Limits practice to disorders of the colon, rectum, and anus
Psychiatrist	Diagnoses and treats mental disorders
Pulmonologist	Diagnoses and treats disorders of the respiratory system
Radiologist	Interprets x-rays and imaging studies and performs radiation therapy
Rheumatologist	Diagnoses and treats arthritis, gout, and other joint disorders
Surgeon	Performs surgical procedures (see Table 1-1, Common Surgical Specialties)
Urologist	Diagnoses and treats disorders of the urinary system, including the kidneys and bladder, and disorders of the male reproductive system

- Processing the payroll
- Arranging patient hospitalizations
- Sorting and filing mail
- Instructing new patients regarding office hours and procedures
- Applying computer concepts to office practices
- Implementing ICD-9 and CPT coding for insurance claims
- Completing medical reports from dictation

Clinical Duties

Clinical responsibilities vary among employers. As mentioned, state laws regarding the scope of practice for medical assistants also differ. In some states, medical assistants are not allowed to perform invasive procedures, such as injections or laboratory testing. Remember, states leave the responsibility for the medical assistant's actions with the physician-employer. Both the American Association of Medical Assistants (AAMA) and American Medical Technologists (AMT) have outlined the duties of a medical assistant. Following is a partial list of clinical duties:

- Preparing patients for examinations and treatments
- Assisting other health care providers with procedures
- Preparing and sterilizing instruments
- Completing electrocardiograms

- Applying Holter monitors
- Obtaining medical histories
- Administering medications and immunizations
- Obtaining vital signs (blood pressure, pulse, temperature, respirations)
- Obtaining height and weight measurements
- Documenting in the medical record
- Performing eye and ear irrigations
- Recognizing and treating medical emergencies
- Initiating and implementing patient education

Laboratory Duties

A medical assistant may perform the following types of laboratory duties in the medical office.

- Low-complexity laboratory tests as determined by the Clinical Laboratory Improvement Amendments (CLIA) of 1988
- Collecting and processing laboratory specimens

 CHECKPOINT QUESTION

4. What are five administrative duties and five clinical or laboratory duties performed by a medical assistant?

AFF The Professional Medical Assistant

Experts say that professionalism is the one quality all employers seek. An allied health care career holds excitement, variety, and prestige. But with that comes a responsibility to the patients you serve. This requires professionalism and a strong work ethic. Work ethic refers to the commitment to your job and is a reflection that you place your job at high importance in your life. Table 1-3 focuses on the actions of an employee with a strong work ethic.

One sign of professionalism and seriousness of purpose is membership in a professional organization. The benefits of membership will be invaluable to you and your future. Participation in a professional organization keeps you abreast of changes and issues facing your profession. If you are a student member, continue as an active member. If not, consider joining. Many employers will pay dues and other expenses for professional activities. Information about joining these organizations can be found at their Web sites (see Media Menu).

Medical assistants play a key role in creating and maintaining a professional image for their employers. Medical assistants must always appear neat and well groomed. Clothing should be clean, pressed, and in good condition. Footwear should be neat, comfortable, and professional. If sneakers are approved by your supervisor, they should be all white. Only minimal makeup and jewelry should be worn. Tatoos and

TABLE **1-3**	Do You Have a Strong Work Ethic?
Always do the right thing	Your physician-employer has been in the papers lately for charges of tax evasion. Everywhere you go, people want to talk about it. You do *not* discuss it with anyone, saying, "Dr. Miller is my employer, and I am loyal to him."
Always try to exceed expectations	You are asked to head a committee to determine patient satisfaction. You complete the task with enthusiasm and see it as a chance to shine.
Be a team player	A co-worker's mother is in the hospital, and your co-worker needs to take a few days off. You were scheduled to be off, but you step in to cover for her knowing that patient care will be affected if both of you are out of the office.
Be self-motivated	The physician has seen his last patient. It's time to go home, but the autoclave needs to be emptied. You stay the few extra minutes it takes to put the sterilized items away.
Be committed to the organization	You overhear two patients complaining about their wait time. You offer your apologies and tell them you will pass on their concerns. You do just that and suggest that the problem of waiting times be discussed at the next staff meeting. Patient satisfaction is your goal because you are committed to the practice.

piercings should not be visible. You should wear a watch with a second hand. Fingernails should be clean and at a functional length. If polish is worn, it should be pale or clear (Figure 1-3).

Medical assistants must be dependable and punctual (see Table 1-3). Tardiness and frequent absences are not acceptable. If you are not at work, someone must fill in for you. Medical assistants must be flexible and adaptable to

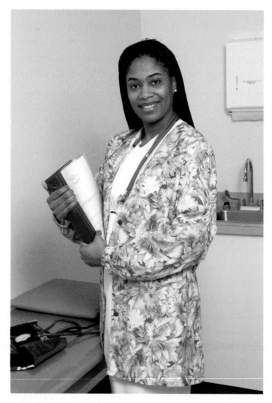

Figure 1-3 Medical assistants play a key role in creating and maintaining a professional image for their employers.

meet the constantly changing needs of the office. Weekend and holiday hours may be required in some specialties. You must be a team player and go the extra mile to make sure patients are receiving excellent care.

Additional characteristics vital to the profession include the following:

- Excellent written and oral communications skills. You will be required to interact with patients and other health care workers on a professional basis. Only the best spelling and grammar skills are acceptable. (Communication skills are covered in appropriate sections of this text.)
- Maturity. Remaining calm in an emergency or during stressful situations and being able to calm others is a key skill. You must also be able to accept constructive criticism without resentment.
- Accuracy. The physician must be able to trust you to pay close attention to detail because the health and well-being of the patients are at stake. Careless errors could cause harm to the patient and result in legal action against the physician.
- Honesty. If errors are made, they must be admitted, and corrective procedures must be initiated immediately. Covering up errors or blaming others is dishonest. So are using office property for personal business, making telephone calls during work time, and falsifying time records. Such practices can ruin your career and are to be strictly avoided.
- Ability to respect patient confidentiality. Few issues in health care can damage your career as profoundly as divulging confidential patient information.
- Empathy. The ability to care deeply for the health and welfare of your patients is the heart of medical assisting.
- Courtesy. Every patient who enters the office must be treated with respect and gracious manners.

- Good interpersonal skills. Tempers may flare in stressful situations; learn to keep yours in check and work well with all levels of interaction.
- Ability to project a positive self-image. If you are confident in your abilities as a professional, this attitude will reflect in all of your relationships.
- Ability to work as a team player. The patient's return to health is the most important objective of the office. Each staff member must work toward this goal.
- Initiative and responsibility. You must be able to move from one task to another quickly and without direct supervision. The entire team expects each of its members to perform assigned responsibilities.
- Tact and diplomacy. The right word at the right moment can calm and soothe anger, depression, and fear and relieve a potentially unsettling situation.
- High moral and ethical standards. Project for your profession the highest level of professionalism.
- Demonstration of adaptive coping mechanisms. The health care arena is constantly changing, and you must be able to see the positive in change.

 CHECKPOINT QUESTION

5. What are eight characteristics that a professional medical assistant should have?

COG Scope of Practice and Standards of Care

Health professionals operate under a scope of practice—the specific activities allowed by state licensing boards and laws or by the practice itself. The term "scope of practice" refers to all medical professions, and staying within that scope is an important of part of your work ethic. Figure 1-4 shows a decision-making tool for clinical professionals.

A handful of states specify scope of practice for medical assistants. However, in most of those states, medical assistants are barred from providing any type of direct patient care or procedure without the presence of a licensed medical professional on site, typically a doctor, physician assistant, or nurse practitioner.

In states with no scope of practice, your duties as a medical assistant depend on those assigned by the physician, physician's assistant, or nurse practitioner who oversees you. A medical assistant's scope of practice is based on his or her education. The educational program that a medical assistant completes will determine what knowledge and skills the medical assistant possesses. Tasks that require medical judgment or interpretation are reserved for providers. In some cases, however, a provider will establish a specific protocol for certain patient encounters. For example, a patient's request for a refill on a narcotic medication may be handled by a medical assistant through the use of a flow chart.

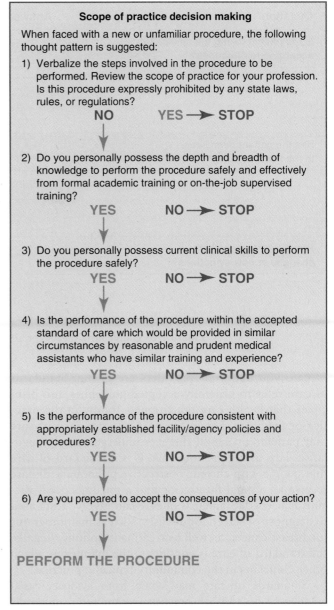

Figure 1-4 Scope of Practice Decision Making Tree. (Adapted from the Washington State Department of Health, Nursing Care Quality Assurance Commission, "Scope of Practice Decision Tree.")

Figure 1-5 shows a typical tool used for such physician-delegated tasks.

The medical professional who oversees you is held personally responsible for your actions and can be sued for any actions you take that cross over into the practice of medicine or that may potentially harm a patient. The medical professional could even lose his or her license. Even something as seemingly innocent as telling a patient over the phone not to worry about a symptom could be construed as "practicing medicine without a license."

In addition to practicing within the scope of your education, you must also be mindful of the standard

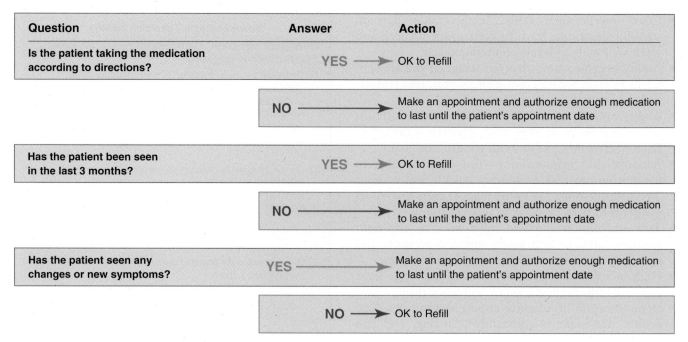

Question	Answer	Action
Is the patient taking the medication according to directions?	YES	OK to Refill
	NO	Make an appointment and authorize enough medication to last until the patient's appointment date
Has the patient been seen in the last 3 months?	YES	OK to Refill
	NO	Make an appointment and authorize enough medication to last until the patient's appointment date
Has the patient seen any changes or new symptoms?	YES	Make an appointment and authorize enough medication to last until the patient's appointment date
	NO	OK to Refill

Figure 1-5 Sample flow sheet representing established protocol set by physician.

of care you and your providers are giving. Standards of care refer to generally accepted guidelines and principles that health care practitioners follow in the practice of medicine. For instance, it is a standard of care that patients on blood thinners undergo blood coagulation labs at regular intervals. It is a standard of care that people with chronic obstructive pulmonary disease receive an annual flu vaccine and a pneumococcal vaccine as needed. Standards of care can involve tests used to diagnose or screen for diseases, such as mammograms for breast cancer, as well as treatment options. Legally, the standard of care is considered the manner in which other clinicians in the community typically practice.

Standards of care may come from evidence-based guidelines, decades of practice, community standards, and licensing and regulatory agencies, such as The Joint Commission and the Centers for Medicare and Medicaid Services. Hospitals and insurance organizations also set standards of care when they release practice guidelines, as do large medical organizations, such as the American Heart Association and the American Diabetes Association.

As a medical assistant, you must also adhere to accepted standards of care for any clinical services you provide. For instance, if you give an injection incorrectly, resulting in a problem for the patient, then the technique you used may be questioned as to whether it met the agreed-upon standard of care.

PSY Self Boundaries

What kind of person are you? Are you a friendly, outgoing person who immediately bonds with everyone you meet and has no problem sharing personal information? Or, are you more reserved, polite but private, maintaining strict boundaries between your personal and professional lives?

The answer is important because, when you work in the medical field, it is critical that you maintain what are called **self boundaries**. This means setting limits on the relationships between yourself and your patients. Those limits, or boundaries, help delineate the personal from the professional and enable you to avoid inappropriate behavior with patients or even being perceived as displaying such inappropriate behavior.

Self boundaries are particularly important in a health care setting because trust and confidentiality are so important. If you relax your self boundaries and become friends with a patient, then you will, most likely, learn confidential information about his or her medical condition or other aspects of his or her life that you may inadvertently share. Conversely, sharing information about yourself with a patient begins to move that relationship from the professional to the personal, which is often inappropriate. You may already know some of your patients in your personal life. The What If box addresses such situations.

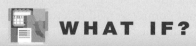

WHAT IF?

You work in a busy family practice. You know several of the patients you serve because you are all members of a small community. How do you stay within your boundaries?

(continued)

This can be an uncomfortable and touchy situation. Even though it is understood that you will not share information acquired in the course of your duties, no one wants to assist with the pap smear of his or her son's teacher. When such a situation arises, it is appropriate to ask the patient if she would prefer to have another medical assistant step in and assist the physician. If this is not possible, try to make the patient as comfortable as possible by making conversation to distract her. Remember, humor can be a valuable tool if used appropriately. Follow the lead of the patient. Many patients will understand that this is your job, and they will trust that you will be the professional you were trained to be. Maintaining a professional demeanor will help you stay within your boundaries.

BOX 1-2

SIGNS THAT YOU'RE CROSSING SELF-BOUNDARY LIMITS

- Thinking about a patient when you're not at work
- Seeing the patient outside of work and/or sharing personal information
- Inappropriately touching the patient or the patient inappropriately touching you
- Keeping secrets with the patient
- Not sharing important aspects of the patient's behavior with the medical professionals in the office

To prevent boundary violations:

- Do not accept gifts from patients
- Do not share personal information with patients
- Do not develop personal relationships with patients
- Do not accept invitations to personal parties or other social events from patients

---

Another way to think about self boundaries is to recall the rule many of us learned at a young age: Never talk about sex, politics, or money unless you know the other person *very* well. So, for instance, if you take a patient's blood pressure on election day and notice that she is wearing an "I voted" sticker, it is inappropriate to ask who she voted for or to share information about your own vote.

Other boundary violations can occur if you misuse the power you have as a member of the health care team or betray a patient's trust in any way. For instance, if you handle the billing for your office, and a patient calls to tell you that her husband just lost his job and she needs to delay payment, sharing that information with anyone other than your manager is a violation of the patient's trust.

Boundary violations also include not respecting the patient's religious, cultural, and social beliefs and values; neglecting the patient; and abusing the patient financially, verbally, emotionally, and physically. One of the worst boundary violations is crossing the sexual line. This could be as seemingly benign as remaining in the examining room as the patient undresses or as overt as inappropriately touching a patient or developing a sexual relationship with him or her. Box 1-2 outlines signs that you are crossing the self-boundary limits and offers suggestions for preventing boundary violations.

 CHECKPOINT QUESTION

6. Why is it important to set self boundaries?

Adaptive and Maladaptive Coping Mechanisms

There is no doubt that the workplace—any workplace—is stressful. But a health care setting has stresses beyond the normal issues of workload, coworker interactions, and authoritarian supervisors. You're also dealing with sick, cranky patients and their commonly serious illnesses. How you cope with the stress and the situations that arise as a result will make a major difference in your professional success. For instance, suppose your office just installed a new electronic records management system. You not only have to learn the new system, you have to change nearly every aspect of how you work. Plus, you have to manually enter patient background information currently residing in paper files.

People with an adaptive coping mechanism would view the new system as an exciting learning opportunity, one that will add to their professional skills. They volunteer for extra training, view the need to enter the background information into the system as an opportunity to identify gaps in patient information, and restructure their workflow to reduce wasted time and identify opportunities for improvement.

Conversely, those with a maladaptive coping mechanism complain to their coworkers and patients about the extra work, convince themselves that the new system takes more time and effort, and do the bare minimum to maintain their jobs.

Now suppose that the transition to the new system is challenging, with the glitches and delays that are common with all new computer systems. At the end of one particularly difficult day, you feel drained. When you go home, do you go for a brisk walk to clear your head and stretch tight muscles? Or, do you get a spoon and devour a half-gallon of butter pecan ice cream?

Obviously, the first choice is the more adaptive coping mechanism. Too often, people deal with stress by turning to food, alcohol, drugs, or other maladaptive behavior. Instead, consider:

- Taking a candlelit bubble bath
- Meeting a friend for dinner
- Writing in a journal
- Going bowling
- Cleaning out a closet

Other aspects of adaptive coping behavior include:

- **Identifying ways to modify the stressor.** Maybe you cannot get rid of the new electronic records system, but you can ask for additional training.
- **Reframing the situation.** Instead of viewing the new system as cumbersome and time consuming, focus on how it will positively impact the office in a few months, when everyone is familiar with it, and patient medical information is just a few clicks away.
- **Creating boundaries.** Stay away from those in the office who are being negative about the new system; negativity is contagious.

When you develop tools to use when you must adapt in the workplace, you become a positive and valued member of the team.

COG Members of the Health Care Team

As a medical assistant, you will work with a variety of health care workers. Today's health care team must be **multidisciplinary.** A multidisciplinary team is a group of specialized professionals who are brought together to meet the needs of the patient. Some patients will need the assistance of many individuals, whereas other patients may only need one or two members of the team. The team may be broken into three groups: health care providers, nurses, and allied health care professionals.

Health Care Providers

Physicians

Physicians generally are the team leaders. They are responsible for diagnosing and treating the patient. Minimum education for a physician consists of a 4-year undergraduate degree, often consisting of premedical studies, and 4 years of medical school, followed by a residency program usually concentrating on a certain specialty. The residency program can vary from 2 to 6 years based on the field of study. Physicians must pass a licensure examination for the state in which they wish to practice. A physician who chooses a specialty must pass an examination in that area of study and become board certified by the American Board of Medical Specialties (ABMS). The title "doctor" refers to a medical doctor (M.D.) but is also used to designate those who have received a doctoral degree in any discipline. For example, a podiatrist uses the title "Dr." He or she holds a doctorate degree in podiatric medicine or, a DPM. One who reaches the highest degree of education in his or her field receives a Ph.D. (Doctorate of Philosopy). Psychologists, educators, and others may hold doctoral degrees but are not medical doctors. In all instances, this title necessitates a degree of respect for the knowledge and hard work the recipient has shown.

Physician Assistants

Physician assistants (PAs) are specially trained and usually licensed. They work closely with a physician and may perform many of the tasks traditionally done by physicians. What a physician assistant does varies with training, experience, and state law. Their scope of practice corresponds to the supervising physician's practice. In general, a physician assistant will see many of the same types of patients as the physician. The cases handled by physicians are generally the more complicated medical cases or those cases that require care that is not a routine part of the PA's scope of work. Close consultation between the patient, the PA, and the physician is done for unusual or hard to manage cases. Forty-nine states, the District of Columbia, and Guam have enacted laws that allow PAs to prescribe medications. Their educational levels vary from several months to 2 years, depending on the program and the individual's background in medicine. Most PA programs require a Bachelor's degree and 2 to 4 years of experience in the medical field.

National certification is available through the American Association of Physician Assistants. A physician assistant may also choose to become certified by the National Commission on Certification of PAs (NCCPA) and become a PA-C. This requires the PA to acquire 100 hours of continuing medical education every 2 years and take a recertification exam every 6 years.

Nurse Practitioners

Nurse practitioners (NPs) are trained to diagnose patients and treat illnesses. In most states, NPs can write prescriptions, operate their own offices, and admit patients to hospitals. In other states, NPs work more closely with a physician. NPs are experienced RNs and, in most cases, have a master's degree in nursing with the addition of specialized training as an NP. In some states, NPs are regulated by the Board of Nursing. In five states, they are regulated by the Board of Nursing and the Board of Medicine. There has been a recent collaborative effort by the American Academy of Nurse Practitioners (AANP) to identify the Nurse Practitioners' Primary Care Competencies, which include adult, family, gerontology, pediatrics, and women's health.

The Nursing Profession

Nurses are trained to work with physicians and implement various patient care needs in the **inpatient** or hospital setting. Their job descriptions vary according to their experiences, specialties, and certifications. There are several levels of education in nursing. A Bachelor of Science (BS) degree in nursing requires 4 years of college. A Licensed Practical Nurse (LPN) must complete a 1-year program. A nurse with an Associate in Applied Science (AAS) degree in nursing attends 2 years of college and becomes a Registered Nurse (RN). The nursing profession also monitors the education and provides the means for certification of the Certified Nursing Assistant (CNA I and CNA II). CNAs offer personal care and assist in nursing tasks. CNA programs usually last 4 to 6 weeks.

LEGAL TIP
WHO'S THE BOSS

Although a nurse's training involves inpatient or hospital care, some physicians choose to employ nurses in their offices. In some states, nurses working in physician offices are not allowed to supervise or delegate their authority to medical assistants. However, nurses and medical assistants work side by side in many instances because the medical assistant works under the supervision of the physician, not the nurse. For example, in the North Carolina law regarding this issue, the legislation refers to medical assistants as "unlicensed health care personnel." Medical assistants are certified, not licensed. There is a difference. **Certification**, by definition, indicates a higher level of competence. The legal issues involving licensure and certification are discussed in Chapter 2.

ETHICAL TIP

Who is Who?

It is important that medical assistants represent themselves honestly. Physicians often innocently refer to every employee as "the nurse." It is more accurate to say my assistant, my certfied medical assistant, my registered medical assistant, or my clinical assistant. There are documented court cases involving misrepresentation of one's education and credentials. Protect yourself by referring to yourself appropriately to patients and co-workers. Do not identify yourself as "Dr. Smith's nurse." When patients refer to you as a nurse, you should correct them. The more your credentials are heard by patients and co-workers, the more understood and recognized they will be. You should be proud of your profession and your credentials. Let it be known.

Allied Health Professionals

Allied health care professionals make up a large section of the health care team. Box 1-3 lists and describes some of these team members. The educational requirements and responsibilities vary greatly among these professionals. One thing they all have in common is the support of a professional organization. Medical assistants fall into this category.

BOX 1-3
ALLIED HEALTH CARE PROFESSIONALS

Cardiovascular technologist—Assists in diagnostic process and treatment stage of all related heart and vascular problems

Dental assistant—Works under the supervision of dentists by doing a wide range of tasks in the dental office, ranging from patient care to administrative duties to laboratory functions

Dental hygienist—Trained and licensed to work with a dentist by providing preventive care

Electrocardiograph technician—Assists with the performance of diagnostic procedures for cardiac electrical activity

Electroencephalograph technician—Assists with the diagnostic procedures for brain wave activity

Electroneurodiagnostic technologist—Assists in the recording and study of the electrical activity of the brain and nervous system using a variety of techniques and instruments

Emergency medical technician—Trained in techniques of administering emergency care en route to trauma centers

Health information technologist—Trained in managing medical records, health care coding, and HIPAA regulations

Laboratory technician—Trained in performance of laboratory diagnostic procedures

Medical assistant—Trained in administrative, clinical, and laboratory skills for the medical facility

Medical coder—Assigns appropriate codes to report medical services to third-party payers for reimbursement

Medical office assistant—Trained in the administrative area of the outpatient medical facility

Medical transcriptionist—Trained in administrative skills; produces printed records of dictated medical information

Nuclear medical technician—Specializes in diagnostic procedures using radionuclides (electromagnetic radiation); works in a radiology department

(continued)

BOX 1-3   *(continued)*

Nutritionist—Addresses dietary needs associated with illness; assists and trains patients with special diets for weight control and supplementation needed for patients undergoing cancer treatment, etc.

Occupational therapist—Evaluates and plans programs to relieve physical and mental barriers that interfere with activities

Paramedic—Trained in advanced rescue and emergency procedures

Pharmacist—Prepares and dispenses medications by the physician's order

Phlebotomist—Collects blood specimens for laboratory procedures by performing venipuncture

Physical therapist—Plans and conducts rehabilitation to improve strength and mobility

Polysomnographer—Performs sleep diagnostics that are required for the diagnosis of sleep disorders

Psychologist—Trained in methods of psychological assessment and treatment

Radiographer—Works with a radiologist or physician to operate x-ray equipment for diagnosis and treatment. Radiography technologists may specialize in computed tomography/magnetic resonance imaging, nuclear medicine, mammography, etc.

Respiratory therapist—Trained to preserve or improve respiratory function

Risk manager—Identifies and corrects high-risk situations within the health care field

Sonographer—Uses high frequency sound waves to image internal structures in the human body including abdominal organs, pelvic organs, small parts and the vascular system

Speech therapist—Treats and prevents speech and language disorders

Surgical technician—Assists in the care of the surgical patient in the operating room and to function as a member of the surgical team

COG The History of Medical Assisting

Medical assisting as a separate profession dates from the 1930s. In 1934, Dr. M. Mandl recognized the need for medical professionals who possessed the skills required in an office environment and opened the first school for medical assistants in New York City. Although medical assistants were employed before 1934, no formal schooling was available. Office assistants were trained on the job to perform clinical procedures, or nurses were trained to perform administrative procedures. The need

for a highly trained professional with a background in administrative and clinical skills led to the formation of an alternative field of allied health care. In 1956, the AAMA, a professional organization for medical assistants, was founded during a meeting of medical assistants in Milwaukee, Wisconsin. The constitution and bylaws adopted by the group were commended by the American Medical Association (AMA), the professional association of licensed physicians. In 1959, Illinois recognized the AAMA as a not-for-profit educational organization. The national office was established in Chicago, with state and local chapters throughout the United States. In 1963, a certification examination for CMA was conducted that would set the standards required for medical assistant education. The first AAMA examinations were given in Kansas, California, and Florida. In the next two decades, the profession grew rapidly. The AMA collaborated in the development of the curriculum and **accreditation** of educational programs. In 1974, the U.S. Department of Health, Education, and Welfare recognized the AAMA Curriculum Review Board in conjunction with the American Medical Association's Council on Medical Education as an official accrediting agency for medical assisting programs in public and private schools.

In 1991, the Board of Trustees of the AAMA approved the current definition of medical assisting: Medical assisting is an allied health profession whose practitioners function as members of the health care delivery team and perform administrative and clinical procedures. Medical assistants continue to be vigilant for threats to their right to practice their profession. Each state mandates the actions of allied health professionals. It is the responsibility of medical assistants to be familiar with the laws of the state in which they are working. Membership in the AAMA exceeds 20,000 medical assistants, with more than 300 local chapters in 43 states. A complete history of the AAMA is available at www.aama-ntl.org. Box 1-4 outlines important changes made by the House of Delegates of the AAMA.

CHECKPOINT QUESTION

7. What prompted the establishment of a school for medical assistants?

COG Medical Assisting Education

A medical assisting curriculum prepares individuals for entry into the medical assisting profession. Medical assisting programs are found in postsecondary schools, such as private business schools and technical colleges, 2-year colleges, and community colleges. Programs vary in length. Programs of 6 months to a year offer a certificate of graduation or a diploma, and 2-year programs award the graduate an associate degree. The

AAMA HOUSE OF DELEGATE CHANGES

- In 1995, the American Association of Medical Assistants (AAMA) House of Delegates approved changing the eligibility pathway for candidates of the AAMA certification examination as follows: "Any candidate for the AAMA CMA Certification Exam must be a graduate of a CAAHEP-accredited medical assisting program." Before June 1998, medical assistants who had been employed by a physician for 1 year full time or 2 years part time were eligible to sit for the CMA Certification Examination.
- In 2001, AAMA made the decision to grant graduates of medical assisting programs accredited by the Accrediting Bureau of Health Education Schools immediate eligibility to sit for the certified medical assistant (CMA) examination beginning in January 2002.
- In January 2003, all CMAs employed or seeking employment were required to have current certification to use the CMA credentials in connection with employment.
- Effective January 2007, CMAs recertifying by continuing education method must attain 30 credits that are AAMA approved, with 10 recertification points in each content category: general, administrative, and clinical. Prior to 2007, 20 of the 60 continuing education units required had to be AAMA approved with 15 recertification points in each content category.
- In 2007, Certified Medical Assistant® became a trademark.
- In 2008, the CMA credentials changed to CMA (AAMA) in order to differentiate from other credentials being offered in the marketplace.
- In 2008, the Curriculum Review Board of the AAMA Endowment was officially changed to the Medical Assisting Education Review Board (MAERB).

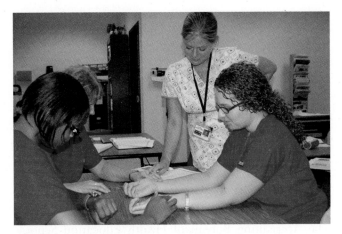

Figure 1-6 Students practice competencies taught in their medical assisting classes. Their scope of practice is determined by their training.

offered in the last module or semester during which the student works in the field gaining hands-on experience. It varies in length from 160 to 240 hours. Students are not paid but are awarded credit toward the degree (see Chapter 46 for more detailed information). Some schools offer job placement services.

After you finish school, your education should not stop. You should continue to take courses on various related topics. These may include new computer programs, new clinical procedures, new laws and regulations, or pharmaceutical updates. Some employers pay for conferences. In some situations, conference costs may be listed as a tax deduction when filing your income tax.

Medical Assisting Program Accreditation

Accreditation is a nongovernmental professional peer review process that provides technical assistance and evaluates educational programs for quality based on pre-established academic and administrative standards. Medical assisting program accreditation is based on a school's adherence to the essentials of a sound education and services for students. The skills that medical assistants need to be successful in a job are taught and documented in a competency-based format. Entry level competency is acquired and documented in a competency-based format that includes the specific skill to be mastered, the conditions under which you are to perform the skill (including equipment and supplies needed), and the standard of performance for the skill.

The Commission on Accreditation of Allied Health Education Programs

The Commission on Accreditation of Allied Health Education Programs (CAAHEP), in collaboration with the Medical Assisting Education Review Board (MAERB), accredits medical assisting programs in both public and

2-year curriculum usually includes general studies such as English, mathematics, and computer skills, in addition to the core courses, such as medical terminology and insurance coding. The curriculum in every accredited program must include the skills determined by the accrediting agency. Figure 1-6 shows students learning to take a patient's pulse rate. Specific requirements for an accredited program are discussed later.

Accredited programs must include a practicum. A **practicum** or **externship** is an educational course

private postsecondary institutions throughout the United States. According to the CAAHEP Web site, CAAHEP is the largest programmatic accreditor in the health sciences field. In collaboration with its Committees on Accreditation, specifically the MAERB, CAAHEP reviews and accredits over 2,000 educational programs in 22 health science occupations. Its mission is to assure quality health professions education to serve the public interest. CAAHEP processes, actions, and strategies are guided by integrity, collaboration, accountability, and consensus.

The Accrediting Bureau of Health Education Schools

The Accrediting Bureau of Health Education Schools (ABHES) accredits private postsecondary medical assisting programs. ABHES is nationally recognized by the U.S. Secretary of Education as a private, nonprofit, independent accrediting agency. ABHES enhances the quality of education and training and promotes institutional and programmatic accountability through systematic and consistent program evaluation. Its mission is to assure the quality of the programs it accredits and assist in the improvement of the programs. This quality determination is accomplished by rigorous and systematic evaluation based on valid standards.

The goals of ABHES focus on three key areas: recognition, resources, and service; all of which it believes are essential and paramount to achieving its mission.

 CHECKPOINT QUESTION

8. What are the two accrediting agencies for medical assisting education programs?

COG Medical Assisting Credentials

Today, busy physician offices prefer to employ medical assistants who demonstrate competence through evidence of a credential such as certification. However, the types of medical assistant credentials available vary and not all credentials or their requirements for obtainment are alike. This section outlines the most common credentials, including recertification information if known.

Certified Medical Assistant (American Association of Medical Assistants)

The CMA (AAMA) is the only credential sponsored by the American Association of Medical Assistants. Currently, only students who graduate from a CAAHEP (Commission on Accreditation of Allied Health Education Programs) or ABHES (Accrediting Bureau of Health Education Schools) accredited medical assistant program may sit for this certification examination. The

exam was first offered in 1963 and has the distinction of having the National Board of Medical Examiners as test consultants. To maintain the credential, 60 continuing education units (CEUs) must be obtained every 5 years in three categories.

Registered Medical Assistant (American Medical Technologist)

The RMA (AMT) credential is awarded by the American Medical Technologists, who also sponsors several allied health professions in addition to medical assistants. In addition to graduates from ABHES or CAAHEP accredited programs, others who may sit for the RMA exam include anyone who completes a medical assistant program in a post-secondary school or college that is regionally or nationally accredited and approved by the U.S. Department of Education, anyone who completes a formal training program that is part of the U.S. Armed Forces, anyone who has not received formal training but who has been employed in the profession of medical assisting for a minimum of 5 years, or anyone who has passed a medical assistant certification examination offered by another certification agency approved by the AMT Board of Directors.

To recertify, RMAs who received the credential prior to January 1, 2006 are encouraged to remain current, however recertification is not required. Those who became certified after January 2006 are required to obtain 30 points every 3 years through a Certification Continuation Program (CCP).

Certified Clinical Medical Assistant (National Healthcareer Association)

The CCMA exam was first offered in 1989. Like the AMT, the NHA certifies several allied health professions.

To sit for this examination, the applicant must be at least 18 years of age, have a high school diploma (or equivalent), have successfully complete an allied health training program within the past year, *or* have 1 year of experience as a medical assistant. Ten continuing education hours are required from the NHA every 2 years to maintain this credential and if certification expires, 10 CE credits, payment of the 2-year recertification fee, and a reinstatement fee are required.

National Certified Medical Assistant (National Center for Competency Testing)

The NCMA credential is offered by the NCCT, which also offers exams for several allied health professions. Eligibility to sit for this examination includes a high school diploma or equivalent and either completion of an NCCT approved medical assisting program within the last 10 years or 2 qualifying years (4,160 hours) of full-time employment (or equivalent part-time employment) within the last 10 years as a medical assistant.

 CHECKPOINT QUESTION

9. What is required to maintain current status as a certified medical assistant?

COG Medical Assisting and Related Allied Health Associations

Association Membership

You are not required to join a national organization to work as a medical assistant or to be eligible to take the certification examination. The associations have many benefits, however, for members. These benefits include the following:

- Access to educational seminars
- Access to continuing education units
- Subscription to the professional journals that alert you to new procedures and trends in medicine
- Access to the annual conventions
- Group insurance plans
- Networking opportunities

For further information on these organizations, visit the Web sites listed at the end of the chapter. Contact your local chapter or speak with your instructor for the procedure for applying for membership. You can download applications and requirements from the AAMA Web site (http://www.aama-ntl.org/) and the AMT Web site (http://americanmedtech.org).

American Association of Medical Assistants

The purpose of the AAMA is to promote the professional identity and stature of its members and the medical assisting profession through education and credentialing. *CMA Today,* which is published and distributed to members of the organization, includes articles of interest to the medical assistant to keep knowledge and skills current. Readers may take post-tests at the end of articles and receive CEUs. Approved continuing education opportunities are available through the national organization, and free transcripts of acquired AAMA approved CEUs are available online to members. Professional benefits, such as insurance, are also made available to AAMA members. Active members are CMAs; associate members are medical assistants who are not yet CMAs; and affiliate members are those interested in medical assisting. Students are encouraged to join and stay active in AAMA. Student members receive a reduced dues rate while in school and for 1 year following graduation. Figure 1-7 displays the logo for AAMA-sponsored Medical Assisting Recognition week, which falls on the third full week of October each year.

American Medical Technologists

The AMT and its governing body are set up similarly to the AAMA, with local, state, and national affiliations, opportunities for continuing education, professional benefits, and a professional journal. Members include medical technologists, medical laboratory technicians,

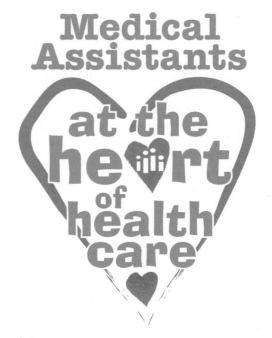

Figure 1-7 Logo for the American Association of Medical Assistants–sponsored Medical Assisting Recognition Week. Used with permission from AAMA.

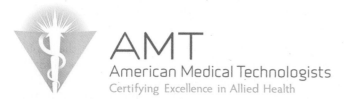

Figure 1-8 Insignia of American Medical Technologists. Used with permission from AMT.

medical assistants, dental assistants, office laboratory technicians, phlebotomy technicians, laboratory consultants, and allied health instructors. To join AMT, you need to be certified or registered by meeting educational, professional experience, and examination requirements. Figure 1-8 displays the insignia of the AMT.

Professional Coder Associations

The American Academy of Professional Coders (AAPC) was founded in 1988 to provide education and professional certification to physician-based medical coders and to elevate the standards of medical coding by providing student training, certification, ongoing education, and networking and job opportunities. Services to members include discounts on services and products and networking opportunities. AAPC certifications encompass the physician office (CPC®), the hospital outpatient facility (CPC-H®), payer perspective coding (CPC-P®), interventional radiology cardiovascular coding (CIRCC™), and medical coding auditor (CPMA™).

American Health Information Management Association

The American Health Information Management Association (AHIMA) is a national professional organization dedicated to supporting the medical records or health information specialists. According to their Web site, health information management (HIM) is the body of knowledge and practice that ensures the availability of health information to facilitate real-time health care delivery and critical health-related decision making for multiple purposes across diverse organizations, settings, and disciplines. AHIMA administers the examination and awards the certified coding specialist (CCS) and certified coding specialists–physician-based (CCS-P) through testing at a specified time and place.

CHECKPOINT QUESTION

10. List six benefits of membership in a professional organization.

Employment Opportunities

The medical assisting profession has found its place in the allied health arena. In many areas, credentialed medical assistants are in great demand. Salaries are going up, and employers appreciate the value of the skills a medical assistant possesses. Health care costs are a concern, and health care management consultants tout medical assistants as cost-effective employees in health care today. Because of the flexible, multiskilled nature of their education, medical assistants can work in a variety of health care settings. Medical assistants work under the direct supervision of a licensed health care provider. They perform many functions. Following are examples of the ambulatory settings where a medical assistant may work with a variety of responsibilities:

- Physicians' offices
- Chiropractors' offices
- Podiatrists' offices
- Physical therapy facilities
- Laboratories
- Imaging centers
- Research facilities
- Walk-in clinics
- Ambulatory surgical centers

CHECKPOINT QUESTION

11. Why is it important that medical assistants are multiskilled?

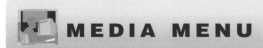

MEDIA MENU

- **Student Resources on thePoint**
  - **CMA/RMA Certification Exam Review**
- **Internet Resources**

  Accrediting Bureau of Health Education Schools
  http://www.abhes.org

  American Board of Medical Specialties
  http://www.abms.org

  American Health Information Management Association
  http://www.ahima.org

  American Medical Technologists
  http://americanmedtech.org

  Council on Accreditation of Allied Health Education Programs
  http://www.caahep.org

  American Association of Professional Coders
  http://www.aapc.com

  Regenerative Medicine Overview
  http://regenerativemedicine.net

Chapter Summary

- Medical history reveals 150 years of progress, with the most amazing strides made in the 20th century. New technologies continue to expand the possibilities of health care.
- Changes in the American health care system brought the necessity for highly trained professionals.
- The health care team works together to deliver quality patient care and remain financially sound.
- Professionalism is highly desired by employers. Medical assistants must understand their scope of practice.
- A graduate of an accredited medical assisting program can pursue certification or registration, which brings increasing marketability in the health care arena.
- By ensuring that educational levels are constantly enhanced and by continuing to grow professionally, the medical assistant graduate will prepare for the challenge of a lifelong career that is both fascinating and rewarding.

Warm Ups for Critical Thinking

1. Visit the Web site dedicated to regenerative medicine, http://regenerativemedicine.net and determine the goals and accomplishments related to the field of regenerative medicine.
2. Review the list of characteristics for medical assistants. Which characteristics do you already have? How will you acquire the others? Are there additional characteristics that you have that will make you a good medical assistant?
3. Look at the list of physician specialties. Which type of physician would you want to work for and why? Which physician specialties would you least want to work with? Explain your response.
4. Visit www.aama-ntl.org and americanmedtech.org and determine which local chapter you would be a member of. How would membership benefit your career as a medical assistant?
5. How does certification or registration as a medical assistant impact scope of practice?
6. What is the importance of having adaptive coping mechanisms in place? Give an example of a situation in which such tools would be helpful.
7. How would you answer the question, "Legally, who is responsible for the actions of certified medical assistants or registered medical assistants as they perform their skills?"

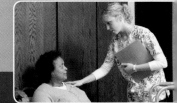

CHAPTER 2

Law and Ethics

Learning Outcomes

Cognitive Domain

Note: AAMA/CAAHEP 2008 Standards are italicized.

1. Spell and define the key terms
2. *Discuss all levels of governmental legislation and regulation as they apply to medical assisting practice, including FDA and DEA*
3. *Compare criminal and civil law as it applies to the practicing medical assistant*
4. *Provide an example of tort law as it would apply to a medical assistant*

5. List the elements and types of contractual agreements and describe the difference in implied and express contracts

6. List four items that must be included in a contract termination or withdrawal letter

7. List six items that must be included in an informed consent form and explain who may sign consent forms

8. List five legally required disclosures that must be reported to specified authorities

9. Describe the four elements that must be proven in a medical legal suit

10. Describe four possible defenses against litigation for the medical professional

11. Explain the theory of respondeat superior, or law of agency, and how it applies to the medical assistant

12. Outline the laws regarding employment and safety issues in the medical office

13. *Identify how the Americans with Disabilities Act (ADA) applies to the medical assisting profession*

14. *Differentiate between legal, ethical, and moral issues affecting health care*

15. *Explain how the following impact the medical assistant's practice and give examples*
    a. *Negligence*
    b. *Malpractice*
    c. *Statute of limitations*
    d. *Good Samaritan Act*
    e. *Uniform Anatomical Gift Act*
    f. *Living will/advanced directives*
    g. *Medical durable power of attorney*

16. List the seven American Medical Association principles of ethics

17. List the five ethical principles of ethical and moral conduct outlined by the American Association of Medical Assistants

18. *Recognize the role of patient advocacy in the practice of medical assisting*

19. Describe the purpose of the Self-Determination Act

20. *Explore the issue of confidentiality as it applies to the medical assistant*

21. *Describe the implications of HIPAA for the medical assistant in various medical settings*

22. *Summarize the Patients' Bill of Rights*

23. *Discuss licensure and certification as it applies to health care providers*

24. *Describe liability, professional, personal injury, and third party insurance*

Psychomotor Domain

Note: AAMA/CAAHEP 2008 Standards are italicized.

1. Monitor federal and state health care legislation (Procedure 2-1)

2. *Incorporate the Patients' Bill of Rights into personal practice and medical office policies and procedures*

3. *Apply local, state, and federal health care legislation and regulation appropriate to the medical assisting practice setting*

Affective Domain

Note: AAMA/CAAHEP 2008 Standards are italicized.

1. *Demonstrate sensitivity to patient rights*

2. *Recognize the importance of local, state, and federal legislation and regulations in the practice setting*

ABHES Competencies

1. Comply with federal, state, and local health laws and regulations

2. Institute federal and state guidelines when releasing medical records or information

3. Follow established policies when initiating or terminating medical treatment

4. Understand the importance of maintaining liability coverage once employed in the industry

Key Terms

abandonment	assault	bioethics	breach
advance directive	battery	blood-borne pathogens	certification
appeal	bench trial		civil law

common law	deposition	implied contracts	precedents
comparative negligence	durable power of attorney	informed consent	protocol
confidentiality	duress	intentional tort	registered
consent	emancipated minor	legally required disclosures	res ipsa loquitur
contract	ethics		res judicata
contributory negligence	expert witness	libel	respondeat superior
damages	express consent	licensure	slander
defamation of character	express contracts	litigation	stare decisis
defendant	fee splitting	locum tenens	statute of limitations
	fraud	malpractice	tort
	implied consent	negligence	
		plaintiff	

During your career as a medical assistant, you will be involved in many medical situations with potential legal implications. You must uphold ethical standards to ensure the patient's well-being. Ethics deals with the concept of right and wrong. Laws are written to carry out these concepts. Physicians may be sued for a variety of reasons, including significant clinical errors (e.g., removing the wrong limb, ordering a toxic dose of medication), claims of improperly touching a patient without consent, or failure to properly diagnose or treat a disease. Medicare **fraud** (concealing the truth) and falsifying medical records can also result in a lawsuit. Medical assistants and other health care workers are included in many of the suits brought to court. You may help to prevent many of these claims against your physician and protect yourself by complying with medical laws, keeping abreast of medical trends, and acting in an ethical manner by maintaining a high level of professionalism at all times.

COG Governmental and Legislative Regulation

Health care in America is monitored and controlled by the federal government. There are three branches of the federal government. The executive branch is headed by the President of the United States. The legislative branch comprises the Senate and the House of Representatives and makes most laws. The legislative branch is made up of representatives from each state. Laws passed by congress are then approved by the President. The judicial branch includes the court system.

The federal government is made up of executive departments that regulate such areas as agriculture, commerce, defense, education, energy, transportation, homeland security, labor, etc. The executive department that regulates health care is the Department of Health and Human Services (HHS). Within the HHS is the Food and Drug Administration (FDA). The FDA regulates the manufacture and distribution of drugs, including drug quality and safety. The Drug Enforcement Agency (DEA) is a branch of the Department of Justice (DOJ) and regulates the sale and use of drugs. Providers who prescribe and/or dispense drugs are required to register with the DEA and are assigned a DEA number. Of course, each state has laws as well. Is is important to understand the federal and state laws that govern your actions as a medical assistant. The various federal and state regulations associated with the practice of medical assisting are discussed throughout this textbook.

COG The American Legal System

Our legal system is in place to ensure the rights of all citizens. We depend on the legal system to protect us from the wrongdoings of others. Many potential medical suits prove to be unwarranted and never make it into the court system, but even in the best physician–patient relationships, **litigation** (lawsuits) between patients and physicians may occur. Litigation may result from a single medication error or a mistake that costs a person's life. It is essential that you have a basic understanding of the American legal system to protect yourself, your patients, and your physician-employer by following the legal guidelines. You must know your legal duties and understand the legal nature of the physician–patient relationship and your role and responsibilities as the physician's agent.

Sources of Law

Laws are rules of conduct that are enforced by appointed authorities. The foundation of our legal system is our rights outlined in the Constitution and the laws established by our Founding Fathers. These traditional laws are known as **common law**.

Common law is based on the theory of **stare decisis**. This term means "the previous decision stands." Judges usually follow these **precedents** (previous court decisions) but sometimes overrule a previous decision, establishing new precedent. Statutes are another source of law. Federal, state, or local legislators make laws or statutes, the police enforce them, and the court system ensures justice. Statutes pertaining to Medicare, Medicaid, and the Food and Drug Administration are common examples in the medical profession.

The third type of law is administrative. These laws are passed by governmental agencies, such as the Internal Revenue Service.

Branches of the Law

The two main branches of the legal system are public law and private or **civil law**.

Public Law

Public law is the branch of law that focuses on issues between the government and its citizens. It can be divided into four subgroups:

1. Criminal law is concerned with issues of citizen welfare and safety. Examples include arson, burglary, murder, and rape. A medical assistant must stay within the boundaries of the profession. Treating patients without the physician's orders could result in a charge of practicing medicine without a license—an act covered under criminal law.
2. Constitutional law is commonly called the law of the land. The United States government has a constitution, and each state has a constitution of its own, laws, and regulations. State laws may be more restrictive than federal laws but may not be more lenient. Two examples of constitutional law are laws on abortion and civil rights.
3. Administrative law is the regulations set forth by governmental agencies. This category includes laws pertaining to the Food and Drug Administration, the Internal Revenue Service, and the Board of Medical Examiners.
4. International law pertains to treaties between countries. Related issues include trade agreements, extradition, boundaries, and international waters.

Private or Civil Law

Private or civil law is the branch of the law that focuses on issues between private citizens. The medical profession is primarily concerned with private law. The subcategories that pertain to the medical profession are contract, commercial, and tort law. Contract and commercial laws concern the rights and obligations of those who enter into contracts, as in a physician–patient relationship. **Tort** law governs the righting of wrongs or

injuries suffered by someone because of another person's wrongdoing or misdeeds resulting from a **breach** of legal duty. Tort law is the basis of most lawsuits against physicians and health care workers. Other civil law branches include property, inheritance, and corporation law.

 CHECKPOINT QUESTION

1. Which branch of law covers a medical assistant charged with practicing medicine without a license?

COG **The Rise in Medical Legal Cases**

Malpractice refers to an action by a professional health care worker that harms a patient. A rise in the amounts of settlement awards has had a negative impact on the cost and coverage of malpractice insurance. With this rise, some physicians have actually changed the scope of their practice to reduce their costs. For example, an obstetrician may choose to limit practice to the care of nonpregnant women to avoid the high cost of malpractice insurance for physicians who deliver babies. In an attempt to protect professionals, legislation designed to limit the amount a jury can award has been introduced in Congress. Legal issues involving the medical field are referred to as medicolegal, which combines the words medical and legal.

A government task force found four primary reasons for the rise in malpractice claims:

1. *Scientific advances.* As new and improved medical technology becomes available, the risks and potential for complications of these procedures escalate, making physicians more vulnerable to litigation.
2. *Unrealistic expectations.* Some patients expect miracle cures and file lawsuits because recovery was not as they hoped or expected, even if the physician is not at fault.
3. *Economic factors.* Some patients view lawsuits as a means to obtain quick cash. (In fact, the number of lawsuits filed has increased during economic recesions.)
4. *Poor communication.* Studies show that when patients do not feel a bond with their physician, they are more likely to sue. Attention to customer service helps develop a good rapport between patients, the provider, and the staff.

Physician–Patient Relationship

Rights and Responsibilities of the Physician

In any contractual relationship, both parties have certain rights and responsibilities. Physicians have the right to limit their practice to a certain specialty or a certain

RESPONSIBILITIES OF THE PATIENT AND THE PHYSICIAN

Responsibilities of the Patient

- Provide the physician with accurate data about the duration and nature of symptoms
- Provide a complete and accurate medical history to the physician
- Follow the physician's instructions for diet, exercise, medications, and appointments
- Compensate the physician for services rendered

Responsibilities of the Physician

- Respect the patient's confidential information
- Provide reasonable skill, experience, and knowledge in treating the patient
- Continue treating the patient until the contract has been withdrawn or as long as the condition requires treatment
- Inform patients of their condition, treatments, and prognosis
- Give complete and accurate information
- Provide competent coverage during time away from practice
- Obtain informed consent before performing procedures (informed consent is a statement of approval from the patient for the physician to perform a given procedure after the patient has been educated about the risks and benefits of the procedure)
- Caution against unneeded or undesirable treatment or surgery

location. For example, patients may not expect a physician to treat them at home. Physicians also have the right to refuse service to new patients or existing patients with new problems unless they are on emergency room call, in which case they must continue to treat patients seen during this time. The subject of abandonment is discussed later. Doctors have the right to change their policies or availability as long as they give patients reasonable notice of the change. This can be done through a local newspaper advertisement and/or a letter to each patient. Box 2-1 lists the physician's responsibilities.

Patients' Bill of Rights

In 1998, the U.S. Advisory Commission on Consumer Protection and Quality in the Health Care Industry adopted the Consumer Bill of Rights and Responsibilities, also known as the Patients' Bill of Rights. The Patients' Bill of Rights has three major goals:

1. To help patients feel more confident in the U.S. health care system
2. To stress the importance of a strong relationship between patients and their health care providers
3. To stress the key role patients play in staying healthy by laying out rights and responsibilities for all patients and health care providers

The rights of the patient include the ability to choose a physician. This right may be limited to a list of participating providers under a patient's insurance plan. Patients have the right to determine whether to begin medical treatment and to set limits on that treatment. The patient also has the right to know in advance what the treatment will consist of, what effect it may have, and what dangers are to be expected. The concept of informed consent is discussed later in the chapter. Patients have the right to privacy. The Health Insurance Portability and Accountability Act of 1996 (HIPAA) outlines specific policies for protecting the privacy of electronic submissions of medical information. HIPAA is discussed at length in Chapter 8. Patients also have a right to emergency care. Box 2-2 outlines the Patients' Bill of Rights. It is important that you keep these rights in mind in all of your patient and physician encounters. Policies and procedures must incorporate these rights as well.

PATIENTS' BILL OF RIGHTS

The bill covers eight key areas:

1. Information
   You have the right to accurate and easily understood information about your health plan, health care professionals, and health care facilities. If you speak another language, have a physical or mental disability, or just don't understand something, help should be given so you can make informed health care decisions.
2. Choice of providers and plans
   You have the right to choose health care providers who can give you high-quality health care when you need it.
3. Access to emergency services
   If you have severe pain, an injury, or sudden illness that makes you believe that your health is in danger, you have the right to be screened and stabilized using emergency services. You should be able to use these services whenever and wherever you need them, without needing to wait for authorization and without any financial penalty.
4. Taking part in treatment decisions
   You have the right to know your treatment options and take part in decisions about your

(continued)

BOX 2-2 *(continued)*

care. Parents, guardians, family members, or others that you choose can speak for you if you cannot make your own decisions.

5. Respect and nondiscrimination
   You have a right to considerate, respectful care from your doctors, health plan representatives, and other health care providers that does not discriminate against you.

6. Confidentiality of private health information
   You have the right to talk privately with health care providers and to have your health care information protected. You also have the right to read and copy your own medical record. You have the right to ask that your doctor change your record if it is not correct, relevant, or complete.

7. Complaints and appeals
   In a health care system that protects consumer or patients' rights, patients should expect to take on some responsibilities to get well and/or stay well (for instance, exercising and not using tobacco). Patients are expected to do things like treat health care workers and other patients with respect, pay their medical bills, and follow the rules and benefits of their health plan coverage. You have the right to a fair, fast, and objective review of any complaint you have against your health plan, doctors, hospitals or other health care personnel. This includes complaints about waiting times, operating hours, the actions of health care personnel, and the adequacy of health care facilities.

8. Consumer responsibilities
   Having patients involved in their care increases the chance of the best possible outcomes and helps support a high-quality, cost-conscious health care system.

This Bill of Rights also applies to the insurance plans offered to federal employees. Many other health insurance plans and facilities have also adopted these values. Even Medicare and Medicaid stand by many of them.

Available at http://www.hcqualitycommission.gov/final.

Contracts

A **contract** is an agreement between two or more parties with certain factors agreed on among all parties. The physician–patient relationship is reinforced by the formation of a contract. All contractual agreements have three components:

1. Offer (contract initiation)
2. Acceptance (both parties agree to the terms)
3. Consideration (the exchange of fees for service)

A contract is not valid unless all three elements are present. A contract offer is made when a patient calls the office to request an appointment. The offer is accepted when you make an appointment for the patient. You have formed a contract that implies that for a fee, the physician will do all in his or her power to address the health concerns of the patient.

Certain individuals, such as children and those who are mentally incompetent or temporarily incapacitated, are not legally able to enter contracts. Patients in this category do not have the capacity to enter into a contract, and therefore, decisions about health care should be made by a competent party acting as a health care decision maker for the minor or incompetent person.

The two types of contracts between physicians and patients are implied and express.

Implied Contracts

Implied contracts, the most common kind of contract between physicians and patients, are not written but are assumed by the actions of the parties. For example, a patient calls the office and requests to see Dr. Smith for an earache. The patient arrives for the appointment, is seen by the physician, and receives a prescription. It is *implied* that, because the patient came on his own and requested care, that he wants this physician to care for him. The physician's action of accepting the patient for care *implies* that he acknowledges responsibility for his part of the contract. The patient *implies* by accepting the services that he will render payment even if the price was not discussed.

Express Contracts

Express contracts, either written or oral, consist of specified details. A mutual sharing of responsibilities is always stated in an express contract. The agreement you have with your creditors is an express contract. These kinds of contracts are not used as often in the medical setting as implied contracts.

 CHECKPOINT QUESTION

2. What action should be taken when a physician makes a change in his services?

Termination or Withdrawal of the Contract

A contract is ideally resolved when the patient is satisfactorily cured of the illness and the physician has been paid for the services. The patient may end the contract at any time, but the physician must follow legal **protocol** to dissolve the contract if the patient still seeks treatment, and the physician wishes to end the relationship.

Patient-Initiated Termination

A patient who chooses to terminate the relationship should notify the physician and give the reasons. You must keep this letter in the medical record. After the receipt of this letter, the physician should then send a letter to the patient stating the following:

- The physician accepts the termination.
- Medical records are available on written request.
- Medical referrals are available if needed.

If the patient verbally asks to end this relationship, the physician should send a letter to the patient documenting the conversation and, again, offering referrals and access to the medical records. Clear documentation is essential.

Physician-Initiated Termination

The physician may find it necessary to end the relationship. A physician may terminate the contract if the patient is noncompliant or does not keep appointments or for personal reasons. The physician must send a letter of withdrawal that includes:

- A statement of intent to terminate the relationship
- The reasons for this action
- The termination date at least 30 days from the date of receipt of the letter
- A statement that the medical records will be transferred to another physician at the patient's request
- A strong recommendation that the patient seek additional medical care as warranted

The letter must be sent by certified mail with a return receipt requested. A copy of the termination letter and the return receipt are placed in the patient's record. Figure 2-1 shows a sample letter of intent to terminate a physician–patient relationship.

Abandonment

If a contract is not properly terminated, the physician can be sued for **abandonment**. Abandonment may be charged if the physician withdraws from the contractual relationship without proper notification while the patient still needs treatment. Physicians must always arrange coverage when absent from the office for vacations, conferences, and so on. Patients may sue for abandonment in any instance that a suitable substitute is not available for care. Coverage may be provided by a **locum tenens**, a substitute physician.

Other examples of abandonment include:

- The physician abruptly and without reasonable notice stops treating a patient whose condition requires additional or continued care.
- The physician fails to see a patient as often as the condition requires or incorrectly advises the patient that further treatment is not needed.

Amy Fine, MD
Charlotte Family Practice
220 NW 3rd Avenue
Charlotte, NC 25673

October 11, 2012

Regina Dodson
Jones Hill Road
Charlotte, NC 25673

Dear Ms. Dodson,

Due to the fact that you have persistently failed to follow my medical advice and treatment of your diabetes, I will no longer be able to provide medical care to you. Since your condition requires ongoing medical care, you must find another physician within the next 30 days. I will be available to you until your appointment date with a new physician.

To ensure continuity of your care, I will make your records available to your new physician. As soon as you make an appointment with a new physician, please come by our office to sign an authorization form enabling us to send your records.

Sincerely,

Amy Fine, MD

Figure 2-1 Letter of intent to terminate physician–patient relationship.

 CHECKPOINT QUESTION

3. What five elements must be included in a physician's termination intent letter?

Consent

The law requires that patients must **consent** or agree to being touched, examined, or treated by the physician or agents of the physician involved in the contractual agreement. No treatment may be made without a consent given orally, nonverbally by behavior, or clearly in writing. Patients have the right to appoint a health care surrogate or health care power of attorney who may make health care decisions when the patient is unable to make them. A health care surrogate may be a spouse, a friend, a pastor, or an attorney. A **durable power of attorney** for health care gives the patient's representative the ability to make health care decisions as the health care surrogate. A patient's physician should be aware of the power of attorney agreement, and a copy of the legal documentation should be kept in the office medical record.

Implied Consent

In the typical visit to the physician's office, the patient's actions represent an informal agreement for care to be given. A patient who raises a sleeve to receive an injection implies agreement to the treatment. **Implied consent** also occurs in an emergency. If a patient is in a life-threatening situation and is unable to give verbal permission for treatment, it is implied that the patient would consent to treatment if possible. As soon as possible, informed consent should be signed by either the patient or a family member in this type of situation. When there is no emergency, implied consent should be used only if the procedure poses no significant risk to the patient.

Informed or Express Consent

The physician is responsible for obtaining the patient's **informed consent** whenever the treatment involves an invasive procedure such as surgery, use of experimental drugs, potentially dangerous procedures such as stress tests, or any treatment that poses a significant risk to the patient. A federal law discussed later requires that health care providers who administer certain vaccines give the patient a current vaccine information statement (VIS). A VIS provides a standardized way to give objective information about vaccine benefits and adverse events (side effects) to patients. The VIS is available online through the Centers for Disease Control and Prevention (CDC) in 26 languages. The Internet address can be found at the end of the chapter.

Informed consent is also referred to as **express consent**. Informed consent is based on the patient's right to know every possible benefit, risk, or alternative to the suggested treatment and the possible outcome if no treatment is initiated. The patient must voluntarily give permission and must understand the implications of consenting to the treatment. This requires that the physician and patient communicate in a manner understandable to the patient. Patients can be more active in personal health care decisions when they are educated about and understand their treatment and care.

A consent form must include the following information:

1. Name of the procedure to be performed
2. Name of the physician who will perform the procedure
3. Name of the person administering the anesthesia (if applicable)
4. Any potential risks from the procedure
5. Anticipated result or benefit from the procedure
6. Alternatives to the procedure and their risks
7. Probable effect on the patient's condition if the procedure is not performed
8. Any exclusions that the patient requests
9. Statement indicating that all of the patient's questions or concerns regarding the procedure have been answered
10. Patient's and witnesses' signatures and the date

As the medical assistant, you will frequently be required to witness consent signatures. A sample consent form is seen in Figure 2-2.

Figure 2-2 Sample consent form.

The informed consent form supplied for the patient's signature must be in the language that the patient speaks. Most physicians who treat multicultural patients have consent forms available in a variety of languages. Never ask a patient to sign a consent form if he or she:

- Does not understand the procedure
- Has unanswered questions regarding the procedure
- Is unable to read the consent form

Never coerce (force or compel against his or her wishes) a patient into signing a consent form. Figure 2-3 shows a certified medical assistant (CMA) obtaining consent from a hearing-impaired patient. The signing interpreter is assisting. Every patient has the right to be informed, and the medical assistant must be sure he or she understands.

Who May Sign a Consent Form

An adult (usually someone over age 18) who is mentally competent and not under the influence of medication or other substances may sign a consent form. Depending on state law a minor may sign a consent form if he or she is:

- In the armed services
- Requesting treatment for communicable diseases (including sexually transmitted diseases)
- Pregnant

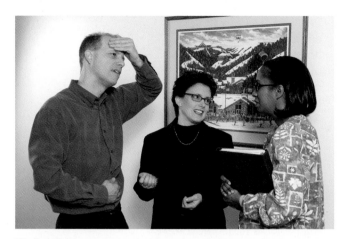

Figure 2-3 Using an interpreter, the CMA helps this patient understand the procedure.

- Requesting information regarding birth control, abortion, or drug or alcohol abuse counseling
- Emancipated

An **emancipated minor** is under the age of majority but is either married or self-supporting and is responsible for his or her debts. The age of majority varies from state to state and ranges from 18 to 21 years. Minors may give consent if any one of the above-listed criteria is present.

Legal guardians may also sign consent forms. A legal guardian is appointed by a judge when the court has ruled an individual to be mentally incompetent. Health care surrogates may also sign consent forms. Health care surrogates are discussed later in the chapter.

 CHECKPOINT QUESTION

4. Under what circumstances should a patient never be asked to sign a consent form?

Refusal of Consent

Patients may refuse treatment for any reason. Sometimes, patients make treatment choices based on religious or personal beliefs and preferences. For instance, a Jehovah's Witness may refuse a blood transfusion on religious grounds, or an elderly person may not want to undergo serious surgery because the potential complications may limit future lifestyle options. In this situation, the patient must sign a refusal of consent form indicating that the patient was instructed regarding the potential risks and benefits of the procedure as well as the risks if the procedure is not allowed. If the patient is a minor, the courts may become involved at the request of the physician or hospital and may award consent for the child. In this situation, the physician should follow legal counsel and document the incident carefully. In any instance that the patient refuses treatment, documentation must be made to protect the physician. The physician has a legal right to refuse to perform elective surgery on a patient who refuses to receive blood if needed.

Releasing Medical Information

The medical record is a legal document. Although the medical record itself belongs to the physician, the information belongs to the patient. Patients have the right to their medical information, and they have the right to deny the sharing of this information.

Requests for medical records are common. Other health care facilities, insurance companies, and patients themselves may need information from the medical chart. Staying within the law when releasing medical information is covered in Chapter 8.

Legally Required Disclosures

Even though patients have the right to limit access to their medical records, health care facilities have a responsibility to report certain events to governmental agencies without the patient's consent, which are referred to as **legally required disclosures**. You and other health care providers must report to the department of public health the situations described in the following sections.

 PATIENT EDUCATION

LEGALLY REQUIRED DISCLOSURES

Inform patients who have conditions that require legal disclosure about the applicable law. Assure them that you will protect their confidentiality. Educate them about why the disclosure is necessary, who receives the information, what particular forms will be completed, and any anticipated follow-up from the organization. For example, you are required to give the local health department the name, address, and condition of a patient with a sexually transmitted disease. The health department then contacts the patient to acquire the names of the patient's sexual contacts. These contacts are notified and counseled by the health department official. Patients who are educated about these legally required disclosures will better understand and accept the need to file official reports.

Vital Statistics

All states maintain records of births, deaths, marriages, and divorces. These records include the following:

- Birth certificates.
- Stillbirth reports. Some states have separate stillbirth forms; other states use a regular death certificate.
- Death certificates. These must be signed by a physician. The cause and time of death must be included.

You may assist the physician in completing a death certificate and filing the finished report in the patient's chart.

Medical Examiner's Reports

Each state has laws pertaining to which deaths must be reported to the medical examiner's office. Generally, these include the following:

- Death from an unknown cause
- Death from a suspected criminal or violent act
- Death of a person not attended by a physician at the time of death or for a reasonable period preceding the death
- Death within 24 hours of hospital admission

Infectious or Communicable Diseases

These reports are made to the local health department. The information is used for statistical purposes and for preventing or tracking the spread of these diseases. Although state guidelines vary, there are usually three categories of reports:

- Telephone reports are required for diphtheria, cholera, meningococcal meningitis, and plague, usually within 24 hours of the diagnosis. Telephone reports must always be followed by written reports.
- Written reports are required for hepatitis, leprosy, malaria, rubeola, polio, rheumatic fever, tetanus, and tuberculosis. Sexually transmitted diseases must also be reported. Notification is usually required within 7 days of the date of discovery.
- Trend reports are made when your office notes an unusually high occurrence of influenza, streptococcal infections, or any other infectious diseases. Box 2-3 is a sample of reportable diseases and their timeframes.

---

amebiasis—7 days
anthrax—24 hours
blastomycosis—7 days
botulism—24 hours
brucellosis—7 days
Campylobacter infection—24 hours
chancroid—24 hours
chlamydial infection (laboratory confirmed)—7 days
cholera—24 hours
dengue—7 days
diphtheria—24 hours
Escherichia coli infection—24 hours
encephalitis—7 days
food-borne disease, including but not limited to *Clostridium perfringens*, Staphylococcal, and *Bacillus cereus*—24 hours
gonorrhea—24 hours
granuloma inguinale—24 hours
Haemophilus influenzae, invasive disease—24 hours
hepatitis A—24 hours
hepatitis B carriage—7 days
hepatitis non-A, non-B—7 days
HIV infection confirmed—7 days
legionellosis—7 days
leprosy—7 days
leptospirosis—7 days
Lyme disease—7 days

The CDC keeps a watchful eye on the public health. When necessary, the CDC establishes directives for the protection of the public. For example, when the public appeared to be at risk for contracting anthrax in 2001, the CDC mandated that documented anthrax cases be reported immediately. Fax machines and e-mail help facilitate such urgent public health communication.

National Childhood Vaccine Injury Act of 1986

Health care providers who administer certain vaccines and toxoids must report to the U.S. Department of Health and Human Services (DHHS) the occurrence of any side effects listed in the manufacturer's package insert. In addition, health care providers must record in the patient's record the following information:

1. Date the vaccine was administered
2. Lot number and manufacturer of vaccine
3. Any adverse reactions to the vaccine
4. Name, title, and address of the person who administered the vaccine

---

BOX 2-3

REPORTABLE CONDITIONS

Chapter 19—Health: Epidemiology
Subchapter 19a—Communicable Disease Control
Section .0100—Reporting of Communicable Diseases
.0101 Reportable Diseases and Conditions
(a) The following named diseases and conditions are declared to be dangerous to the public health and are hereby made reportable within the time period specified after the disease or condition is reasonably suspected to exist:

acquired immune deficiency syndrome (AIDS)—7 days

BOX 2-4

VACCINATIONS REQUIRING VACCINE INFORMATION STATEMENTS

Anthrax
Chickenpox
Diphtheria, tetanus, and pertussis
Haemophilus influenzae type b (Hib)
Hepatitis A
Hepatitis B
Influenza
Lyme disease
Measles, mumps, and rubella
Meningococcal
Pneumococcal polysaccharide
Pneumococcal conjugate
Polio
Lymphogranuloma venereum—7 days
Malaria—7 days
Measles (rubeola)—24 hours
Meningitis, pneumococcal—7 days
Meningitis, viral (aseptic)—7 days
Meningococcal disease—24 hours
Mucocutaneous lymph node syndrome (Kawasaki syndrome)—7 days
Mumps—7 days

Excerpt from the North Carolina Administrative Code Regarding Reporting of Communicable Diseases.

Box 2-4 lists the vaccines and toxoids covered by the National Childhood Vaccine Injury Act.

Abuse, Neglect, or Maltreatment

Abuse, neglect, or maltreatment of any person who is incapable of self-protection usually falls under this category and may include the elderly or the mentally incompetent. Each state has its own regulations regarding what must be reported. Patient confidentiality rights are waived when the law requires you to report certain conditions.

Abuse is thought to be the second most common cause of death in children under age 5. The Federal Child Abuse Prevention and Treatment Act mandates that threats to a child's physical and mental welfare be reported. Health care workers, teachers, and social workers who report suspected abuse are not identified to the parents and are protected against liability. State laws vary regarding the procedure for reporting abuse. Local regulations should be outlined in the policies and procedures manuals at any outpatient facility. If you suspect a child is being abused, relay your suspicions to the physician. The physician will make the formal report. When authorities receive a report from a health care provider, they follow up by investigating the situation. For assistance in reporting suspected child abuse, you may call the national 24-hour hotline at 800-4 A CHILD (800-422-4453).

Spousal abuse is a significant problem in this country. Many women and children are trapped in a cycle of abuse. Mothers who are financially dependent on their abusers may see no way out. You should record any information gathered in the patient interview or anything observed in the course of dealing with the patient that may indicate abuse. Report these observations to the physician. Most communities have anonymous safe places for victims of domestic abuse, and you should be familiar with these services. With proper referrals, you may be able to help break the cycle of domestic abuse.

This country is also undergoing a rise in elderly parents being cared for by their adult children who also have the responsibility of raising young children. This phenomenon can cause great stress among caregivers. Abuse of the elderly can be in the form of mistreatment or neglect (not providing appropriate care). You should pay attention to observations and information provided by your elderly patients. If mistreatment is suspected, alert the physician. Support groups for those caring for the elderly are useful in dealing with the challenges of caring for others.

Violent Injuries

Health care providers have the legal duty to report suspected criminal acts. Injuries resulting from weapons, assault, attempted suicide, and rape must be reported to local authorities.

Other Reports

A diagnosis of cancer must be reported to assist in tracking malignancies and identifying environmental carcinogens. Just as the CDC keeps track of all communicable diseases reported, a database of treated tumors is kept in hospitals through a tumor registry. Some states also require that epilepsy (a seizure condition) be reported to local motor vehicle departments. The testing of newborns for phenylketonuria (PKU), which can cause mental retardation, is required in all states. Some states require positive PKU results to be reported to the health department so that close observation and follow-up care are ensured to prevent serious complications for the infant. Infantile hypothyroidism is also a reportable condition in some states.

 CHECKPOINT QUESTION

5. List six situations and conditions you are legally required to report.

COG Specific Laws and Statutes that Apply to Health Professionals

Medical Practice Acts

Although each state has its own medical practice act, the following elements are usually included:

- Definition of the practice of medicine.
- Requirements that the physician must have graduated from an accredited medical school and residency program and have passed the state medical examination.
- Description of the procedure for **licensure**.
- Description of the conditions for which a license can be suspended or revoked.
- Description of the renewal process for licensure. Most states require the physician to have attended a certain number of continuing education hours.
- Personal requirements necessary to become a licensed physician. Generally, a licensed physician must be a state resident, of good moral character, a U.S. citizen, and 21 years of age or older.

A physician may have his or her license revoked or suspended by the board of medical examiners in most states for a variety of reasons, including certain criminal offenses, unprofessional conduct, fraud, or professional or personal incompetence. Criminal offenses include but are not limited to murder, manslaughter, robbery, and rape. Examples of unprofessional conduct may include invasion of a patient's privacy, excessive use of alcohol or use of illegal drugs, and **fee splitting** (sharing fees for the referral of patients to certain colleagues). Fraud is a common reason for revoking a license. Fraud may include filing false Medicare or Medicaid claims, falsifying medical records, or professional misrepresentation. Examples of misrepresentation or fraud include advertising a medical cure that does not exist, guaranteeing 100% success of a treatment, or falsifying medical credentials. Incompetence is often a hard charge to prove. The three most common examples are insanity, senility, and other documented mental incompetence.

As a medical assistant, it is your responsibility to report illegal or unethical behavior or signs of incompetence in the medical office.

Licensure, Certification, and Registration

As discussed in Chapter 1, medical professionals can be licensed, certified, or **registered**. Licensure is regulated by laws, such as medical practice acts and nursing practice acts. If a particular profession is a licensed one, it is mandatory that one maintain a license in each state where he or she works. Each state determines the qualifications and requirements for licensure of a particular profession. A state agency will be responsible for issuing and renewing licenses. Most professionals are licensed to practice their profession according to certain guidelines and are limited to specific duties. For example, nurses are licensed. As mentioned earlier, in North Carolina, the Nursing Practice Act specifically prohibits a nurse from delegating professional authority to unlicensed personnel.

The term registered indicates that a professional has met basic requirements, usually for education, has passed standard testing, and has been approved by a governing body to perform given tasks within a state. X-ray technologists are registered as registered radiologic technologists. A national registry is available to verify a potential employee's status.

Certification is a voluntary process regulated through a professional organization. Standards for certification are set by the organization issuing the certificate. The CMA and registered medical assistant (RMA) credentials are nationally recognized and do not require any action when moving from one state to another. Remember, you must adhere to the laws regarding the CMA or RMA in the state where you work.

Remember, as a medical assistant, you are not licensed and therefore limited to certain duties. The physician-employer has the sole responsibility of setting any limits on the duties of a medical assistant. Take a look back at Figure 1-4 in Chapter 1. A medical assistant's scope of practice is determined by his or her training and his or her provider's discretion. Although most states do not require certification for employment, employers seek the CMA or RMA because certification indicates the achievement of certain standards of competence. A few states require that you take a test or short course before performing certain clinical duties.

Controlled Substances Act

The Controlled Substances Act of 1970 is a federal law enforced by the DEA. The act regulates the manufacture, distribution, and dispensing of narcotics and nonnarcotic drugs considered to have a high potential for abuse. This act was designed to decrease the illegal use of controlled substances and to prevent substance abuse by medical professionals. The law requires that any physician who dispenses, administers, or prescribes narcotics or other controlled substances be registered with the DEA.

Physicians who maintain a stock of controlled substances in the office for dispensing or administration must use a special triplicate order form available through the DEA. A record of each transaction must be kept and retained for 2 to 3 years. The record must be available for inspection by the DEA at any time. The act requires that all controlled substances be kept in a locked cabinet out of the patients' view and that the keys be kept secure.

Theft should be reported immediately to the local police and the nearest DEA office. Prescription pads used for prescribing controlled substances must remain in a safe place at all times. The Legal Tip box lists steps you can take to keep these prescription pads safe.

This act also requires a physician to return all registration certificates and any unused order forms to the DEA if the practice is closed or sold. Violation of this act is a criminal offense. Penalties range from fines to imprisonment.

 AFF LEGAL TIP

PRESCRIPTION PAD SAFETY TIPS

- Keep only one prescription pad in a locked cabinet in the examining room. All other pads should be locked away elsewhere. Do not leave prescription pads unattended.
- Keep a limited supply of pads. It is better to reorder on a regular basis than to overstock.
- Keep track of the number of pads in the office. If a burglary occurs, you will be able to advise the police regarding the number of missing pads.
- Report any prescription pad theft to the police and alert local pharmacies of the theft. If the theft involves the loss of narcotic pads, the Drug Enforcement Agency must be notified.

Good Samaritan Act

As the number of lawsuits against physicians began to rise, physicians feared that giving emergency care to strangers outside the office could lead to malpractice suits. To combat that fear, all states now have Good Samaritan acts. Good Samaritan acts ensure that caregivers are immune from liability suits as long as they give care in good faith and in a manner that a reasonable and prudent person would in a similar situation. Each state has specific guidelines. Some even set standards for various professional levels, such as one set of standards for a physician and another set of standards for emergency medical technicians. Your state's Good Samaritan Act will not protect you if you are grossly negligent or willfully perform negligent acts.

You are not covered by the Good Samaritan Act while you are working as a medical assistant, nor does it cover physicians in the performance of their duties. Liability and malpractice insurance policies are available to protect you in those situations. If you render emergency care and accept compensation for that care, the act does not apply.

The provisions only cover acts outside of the formal practice of the profession.

COG Basis of Medical Law

Tort Law

A tort is a wrongful act that results in harm for which restitution must be made. The two forms of torts are intentional and unintentional. An allegation of an unintentional tort means that the accuser (the **plaintiff**) believes a mistake has been made; however, the plaintiff believes the caregiver or accused party (the **defendant**) was operating in good faith and did not intend the mistake to occur. Consider the following scenario as an example of an unintentional tort: A medical assistant giving a patient a heat treatment for muscle aches inadvertently burns the arm of the patient because the equipment is faulty. This act was not intentional or malicious, but it caused damage to the patient. About 90% of suits against physicians fall into this category.

Negligence and Malpractice (Unintentional Torts)

Most unintentional torts involve negligence. These are the most common forms of medical malpractice suits.

Negligence is performing an act that a reasonable health care worker or provider would not have done or the omission of an act that a reasonable professional or provider would have done. Failure to take reasonable precautions to prevent harm to a patient is termed **negligence**. If a physician is involved, the term usually used is malpractice. Malpractice is said to have occurred when the patient is harmed by the professional's actions. There are three types of malpractice:

- Malfeasance—incorrect treatment
- Misfeasance—treatment performed incorrectly
- Nonfeasance—treatment delayed or not attempted

In a legal situation, the standard of care determines what a reasonable professional would have done. Standards of care are written by various professional agencies to clarify what the reasonable and prudent physician or health care worker would do in a given situation. For example, a patient comes to an orthopedist's office after falling from a horse and complains of arm pain. The standard of care for orthopedists would require an x-ray of the injured extremity after trauma. Standards of care vary with the level of the professional. A registered nurse is not held to the same standards of care as a physician, and a medical assistant is not expected to perform by the same standards as the registered nurse. Each must practice within the scope of their training. The representing attorney may seek an **expert witness** to state under oath the standards of care for a specific situation. Expert witnesses may be physicians, nurses, physical therapists, or other specialized practitioners who have excellent reputations in their field.

Expert witnesses are always used in malpractice cases, except when the doctrine of **res ipsa loquitur** is tried. This doctrine means "the thing speaks for itself." In other words, it is obvious that the physician's actions or negligence caused the injury. A judge must preapprove the use of this theory in pretrial hearings. An example of a case tried under this doctrine might be a fracture that occurred when the patient fell from an examining table.

For negligence to be proved, the plaintiff's attorney must prove that the following four elements were present: duty, dereliction of duty, direct cause, and damage. The courts place the burden of proof on the plaintiff; the physician is assumed to have given proper care until proven otherwise.

Duty

Duty is present when the patient and the physician have formed a contract. This is usually straightforward and the easiest of the elements to prove. If the patient presented to the physician's office and the physician sees the patient, there is duty.

Dereliction of Duty

The patient must prove that the physician did not meet the standard of care guidelines, either by performing an act inappropriately or by omitting an act.

Direct Cause

The plaintiff must prove that the derelict act directly caused the patient's injury. This can be difficult to prove if the patient has an extensive medical history that may have contributed to the injury.

Damage

The plaintiff must prove that an injury or **damages** occurred. Documentation must be available to prove a diagnosis of an injury or illness.

Jury Awards

There are three types of awards for damages:

1. *Nominal.* Minimal injuries or damages occurred, and compensation is small.
2. *Actual (compensatory).* Money is awarded for the injury, disability, mental suffering, loss of income, or the anticipated future earning loss. This payment is moderate to significant.
3. *Punitive.* Money is awarded to punish the practitioner for reckless or malicious wrongdoing. Punitive damages are the most costly. (Note: A physician may have committed a medical error, but if the patient suffered no injuries or damages, he or she cannot win the suit. Also, if the outcome was not as expected but the physician cannot be shown to be at fault, the patient will not be compensated.)

 CHECKPOINT QUESTION

6. What four elements must be proved in a negligence suit?

Intentional Torts

An **intentional tort** is an act that takes place with malice and with the intent of causing harm. Intentional torts are the deliberate violation of another person's legal rights. Examples of intentional torts are assault and battery, use of duress, invasion of privacy, defamation of character, fraud, tort of outrage, and undue influence. These are described next.

Assault and Battery

Assault is the unauthorized attempt or threat to touch another person without consent. **Battery** is the actual physical touching of a patient without consent; this includes beating and physical abuse. By law, a conscious adult has the right to refuse medical care. Care given without the patient's consent constitutes assault. An example of battery might be suturing a laceration against the patient's wishes.

Duress

If a patient is coerced into an act, the patient can possibly sue for the tort of **duress**. Following is an example in which a patient may be able to sue successfully for assault, battery, and duress. A 22-year-old woman arrives at a pregnancy center. She is receiving public assistance and has five children. Her pregnancy test is positive. The staff persuades her to have an abortion. She signs the consent form, and the abortion is performed. Later she sues, stating that she was verbally coerced into signing the consent form (duress) and that the abortion was performed against her wishes (assault and battery).

Invasion of Privacy

Patients have the right to privacy. Remember, HIPAA regulates the sharing of information. Most offices have patients sign an authorization to release information to their insurance company on their first visit. This covers each return visit unless the insurance carrier changes. Written permission must be obtained from the patient to:

- Release medical records or personal data
- Publish case histories in medical journals
- Make photographs of the patient (exception: suspected cases of abuse or maltreatment)
- Allow observers in examination rooms

For example, a 57-year-old woman is seen in your office for a skin biopsy. Her insurance company calls asking for information regarding the bill and asks for the biopsy report. You give the requested information and then find that the patient never signed a release form. She has a valid case for invasion of privacy.

Defamation of Character

Making malicious or false statements about a person's character or reputation is **defamation of character. Libel** refers to written statements, and **slander** refers to oral statements. For example, a patient asks for a referral to another physician. She states that she has heard, "Dr. Rogers is a good surgeon." You have heard that he has a history of alcoholism. You tell the patient that he is probably not a good choice because of his drinking. That is defamation of his character, and you could be sued for saying it.

Fraud

Fraud is any deceitful act with the intention to conceal the truth, such as:

- Intentionally raising false expectations regarding recovery
- Not properly instructing the patient regarding possible side effects of a procedure
- Filing false insurance claims

Tort of Outrage

Tort of outrage is the intentional infliction of emotional distress. For this tort to be proved, the plaintiff's attorney must show that the physician:

- Intended to inflict emotional distress
- Acted in a manner that is not morally or ethically acceptable
- Caused severe emotional distress

Undue Influence

Improperly persuading another to act in a way contrary to that person's free will is termed undue influence. For instance, preying on the elderly or the mentally incompetent is a common type of undue influence. Unethical practitioners who gain the trust of these persons and persuade them to submit to expensive and unnecessary medical procedures are practicing undue influence.

 CHECKPOINT QUESTION

7. What is the difference between assault and battery?

The Litigation Process

The litigation process begins when a patient consults an attorney because he or she believes a health care provider has done wrong or becomes aware of a possible prior injury. The patient's attorney obtains the medical records, which are reviewed by medicolegal consultants. (Such consultants may be nurses or physicians who are considered experts in their field.) Then the plaintiff's attorney files a complaint, a written statement that lists the claim against the physician and the remedy desired, usually monetary compensation.

The defendant and his or her attorney answer the complaint. The discovery phase begins with interrogatories and **depositions**. During this phase, attorneys for both parties gather relevant information.

Next, the trial phase begins. A jury is selected unless the parties agree to a **bench trial**. In a bench trial, the judge hears the case without a jury and renders a verdict (decision or judgment). Opening statements are given, first by the plaintiff's attorney, then by the defendant's attorney. The plaintiff's attorney presents the case. Expert witnesses are called, and the evidence is shown. Examination of the witnesses begins. Direct examination involves questioning by one's own attorney; cross-examination is questioning by the opposing attorney. When the plaintiff's attorney is finished, the defense presents the opposing arguments and evidence. The plaintiff's attorney may cross-examine the defendant's witnesses. Closing arguments are heard. Finally, a verdict is made.

If the defendant is found guilty, damages are awarded. If the defendant is found not guilty, the charges are dismissed. The decision may be appealed to a higher court. An **appeal** is a process by which the higher court reviews the decision of the lower court.

Defenses to Professional Liability Suits

The objective of all court proceedings is to uncover the truth. Many defenses are available to a health care worker who is being sued. These include the medical record, statute of limitations, assumption of risk, res judicata, contributory negligence, and comparative negligence, discussed next.

Medical Records

The best and most solid defense the caregiver has is the medical record. Every item in the record is considered to be a part of a legal document. Juries may believe a medical record regardless of testimony. Juries tend to believe these records because they are tangible items from the actual time the injury occurred. There is a common saying in the medicolegal world: "If it's not in the chart, it did not happen." This means that even negative findings should be listed. For example, instead of saying that the patient's neurologic history is negative, the documentation might say the patient reports no headaches, seizures, one-sided weakness, and so on. Entries in the medical record refresh the memory of the defendant and provide documentation of care. As a medical assistant, you must make sure that all of your documentation is timely, accurate, and legible. (See Chapter 8 for specific information regarding charting practices.)

Statute of Limitations

Each state has a statute that defines the length of time during which a patient may file a suit against a caregiver. When the **statute of limitations** expires, the patient loses the right to file a claim. Generally, the limits vary from 1 to 3 years following the alleged occurrence. Some states use a combination rule. Some states allow 1 to 3 years following the patient's discovery of the occurrence. States vary greatly when an alleged injury involves a minor. The statute may not take effect until the minor reaches the age of majority and then may extend 2 to 3 years past this time. Some states have longer claim periods in wrongful death suits.

Assumption of Risk

In the assumption of risk defense, the physician will claim that the patient was aware of the risks involved before the procedure and fully accepted the potential for damages. For example, a patient is instructed regarding the adverse effects of chemotherapy. The patient fully understands these risks, receives the chemotherapy, and wants to sue for alopecia (hair loss). Alopecia is a given risk with certain forms of chemotherapy. A signed consent form indicating that the patient was informed of all of the risks of a procedure proves this point.

Res Judicata

The doctrine of **res judicata** means "the thing has been decided." Once the suit has been brought against the physician or patient and a settlement has been reached, the losing party may not countersue. If, for instance, the physician sues a patient for not paying bills and the court orders the patient to pay, the patient cannot sue the physician for malpractice. The opposite may occur as well. If the physician is sued for malpractice and loses, he cannot countersue for defamation of character.

Contributory Negligence

With the **contributory negligence** defense, the physician usually admits that negligence has occurred; he or she will claim, however, that the patient aggravated the injury or assisted in making the injury worse. For example, the patient's laceration is stitched with only three sutures when 10 were needed. The physician instructs the patient to limit movement of the arm. The patient plays baseball; the laceration reopens, causing infection; and subsequently, extensive scar tissue forms. Both the patient and the physician contributed to the postoperative damages. Most states do not grant damage awards for contributory negligence. If an award is granted, the courts assess **comparative negligence**.

Comparative Negligence

In comparative negligence, the award of damages is based on a percentage of the contribution to the negligence. If the patient contributed 30% to the damage, the damage award is 30% less than what was granted. In the example in the previous paragraph, the courts may decide that the negligence is shared at 50%. Therefore, if the court assessed damages of $20,000, the physician would be responsible for $10,000.

In the past, contributory negligence, such as a patient not returning for appointments, was seen as absolute defense for the physician. This has changed over the years, however, and many defendants use the defense of comparative negligence, with the responsibility shared between the physician and the patient.

COG Defense for the Medical Assistant

Respondeat Superior or Law of Agency

The doctrine of **respondeat superior** literally means "let the master answer." This may also be called law of agency. This doctrine implies that physicians are liable for the actions of their employees, as discussed earlier. The physician is responsible for your actions as a medical assistant as long as your actions are within your scope of practice. If your actions exceed your abilities or training, the physician is not generally responsible for any error that you make. You must understand that you can be sued in this instance and that respondeat superior does not guarantee immunity for your actions.

For example, Mrs. Smith is a chronic complainer, calling your office frequently with minor concerns. Today, she calls complaining of tingling in her arms. The physician has left for the day, so you tell Mrs. Smith, "Don't worry about this; take your medication, and call us tomorrow." During the night, a blood vessel in Mrs. Smith's brain bursts. She has a cerebral hemorrhage (bleeding inside the brain) and dies. The family sues. The physician claims that you were instructed not to give advice over the telephone. You are not covered by respondeat superior because you acted outside of your scope of practice.

To protect yourself from situations such as this, have your job description in written form and always practice within its guidelines. Do not perform tasks that you have not been trained to do. Never hesitate to seek clarification from a physician. If you are not sure about something, such as a medication order, ask!

Malpractice insurance is available to allied health care professionals for further protection. Malpractice premiums are inexpensive and afford protection against losing any personal assets if sued. The insurance company would pay damages as assessed by a jury. Of course, as with any insurance policy, there will be conditions of coverage and maximum amounts the company will pay. The Legal Tip provides some additional advice for preventing lawsuits.

AFF LEGAL TIP
YOU CAN AVOID LITIGATION

- Keep medical records neat and organized. Always document and sign legibly.
- Stay abreast of new laws and medical technology.
- Become a certified or registered medical assistant (CMA or RMA, respectively).
- Keep both your cardiopulmonary resuscitation (CPR) and first-aid certification current.
- Never give any information over the telephone unless you are sure of the caller's identity and you have patient consent.
- Keep the office neat and clean. Make sure that children's toys are clean and in good condition to avoid injuries. Perform safety checks frequently.
- Limit waiting time for patients. If an emergency arises, causing a long wait, explain the situation to waiting patients in a timely and professional manner.
- Practice good public relations. Always be polite, smile, and show genuine concern for your patients and their families.

CHECKPOINT QUESTION

8. What is the law of agency, and how does it apply to the medical assistant?

COG Employment and Safety Laws

Civil Rights Act of 1964, Title VII

Title VII of the Civil Rights Act of 1964 protects employees from discrimination in the workplace. The Equal Employment Opportunity Commission (EEOC) enforces the provisions of the act and investigates any possible infractions. Employers may not refuse to hire, limit, segregate or classify, fire, compensate, or provide working conditions and privileges on the basis of race, color, sex, religion, or national origin. This act determines the questions that may be asked in a job interview. For example, a potential employee cannot be asked questions that would reveal age, marital status, religious affiliation, height, weight, or arrest record. It is acceptable, however, to ask if an applicant has ever been convicted of a crime. In the health care setting, employers can require a criminal records check and even drug screening to ensure the safety of the patients. The American Association of Medical Assistants (AAMA) has made recent changes to prohibit convicted felons from taking the CMA examination.

Sexual Harassment

In recent years, Title VII has been expanded to include sexual harassment. Sexual harassment is defined by the EEOC as unwelcome sexual advances or requests for sexual favors in the workplace. The definition includes other verbal or physical conduct of a sexual nature when such conduct is made a condition of an individual's employment, is used as a basis for hiring or promotion, or has the purpose or effect of unreasonably interfering with an individual's work performance. If such behavior creates an intimidating, hostile, or offensive working environment, it is considered sexual harassment. In the past two decades, court decisions have confirmed that this form of harassment is a cause for both criminal prosecution and civil litigation.

In the medical office setting, the office manager must be alert for signs of harassment and should have in place a policy for handling complaints.

Americans with Disabilities Act

Title VII also includes the Americans with Disabilities Act (ADA), which prohibits discrimination against people with substantial disabilities in all employment practices, including job application procedures, hiring, firing, advancement, compensation, training, benefits, and all other privileges of employment. The ADA applies to all employers with 15 or more employees. The law covers those with impairments that limit their major life activities. The statute also protects those with AIDS or HIV-positive status and individuals with a history of mental illness or cancer. ADA also requires that employers provide basic accommodations for disabled employees. Those basic accommodations include extra-wide parking spaces close to the door, ramps or elevators, electric or easily opened doors, bathroom facilities designed for the disabled, an accessible break room, and a work area with counters low enough for a person in a wheelchair.

The ADA also takes safety into consideration. Employers are permitted to establish qualification standards that will exclude individuals who pose a direct threat to others if that risk cannot be lowered to an acceptable level by reasonable accommodations. In the medical field, technical standards are established that outline physical requirements of a certain job. For example, if a particular job requires adequate vision to see the dials on a piece of laboratory equipment, it is unreasonable to expect an employer to hire a person who is sight impaired. The law is designed to protect employees, not to require unreasonable accommodations.

The ADA also requires that all public buildings be accessible to physically challenged people. Following is a partial list of ways the medical office can comply with this act:

- Entrance ramps
- Widened rest rooms to be wheelchair accessible

BOX 2-7   *(continued)*

and use the talents of other health professionals when indicated.

VI. A physician shall, in the provision of appropriate patient care, except in emergencies, be free to choose whom to serve, with whom to associate, and the environment in which to provide medical care.

VII. A physician shall recognize a responsibility to participate in activities contributing to the improvement of the community and the betterment of public health.

VIII. A physician shall, while caring for a patient, regard responsibility to the patient as paramount.

IX. A physician shall support access to medical care for all people.

Violations of these AMA principles may result in censure, suspension, or expulsion by the state medical board. Censure, the least punitive action, is a verbal or written reprimand from the association indicating negative findings regarding a specific incident. Suspension is the temporary removal of privileges and association with the organization. Expulsion is a formal discharge from the professional organization and is the maximum punishment. Many of these issues, however, deal with laws and the patient's rights as established by law. When violations of laws are involved, physicians may lose their license to practice, may be fined, or may be imprisoned. Serious consequences can arise from a breach of this code of ethics.

Medical Assistant's Role in Ethics

As an agent of the physician in the medical office, you are also governed by ethical standards and are responsible for:

* Protecting patient confidentiality
* Following all state and federal laws
* Being honest in all your actions

As a medical assistant, you must apply ethical standards as you perform your duties. You must realize that your personal feelings of right and wrong should be kept separate if they differ from the ethics of your profession. For example, a medical assistant who has a strong opinion against abortion would not be happy working in a medical facility that performs abortions. The care you give patients must be objective, and personal opinions about options must not be shared.

AFF **ETHICAL TIP**

An Ethical Dilemma

How would you handle the following hypothetical ethical dilemma?

You are the office manager for a well-respected family physician in a small town. He is 70 years old and is starting to show signs of senile dementia. He is forgetful and has even been disoriented and confused a few times. No one else seems to have noticed. Should you report your concerns? If so, to whom?

The AMA Principles of Medical Ethics require that physicians, and medical assistants through the law of agency, report unethical behavior among colleagues. The medical profession is also governed by the patient's right to safety and quality care. It is your ethical responsibility to report the doctor's condition to the administration of the hospital where the physician has privileges or to the state board of medicine. The physician's family should be involved in the situation.

Patient Advocacy

Your primary responsibility as a medical assistant is to be a patient advocate at all times. Advocacy requires that you consider the best interests of the patient above all other concerns. This often means setting aside your own personal beliefs, values, and biases and looking at a given situation in an objective manner. You should never, however, be asked or forced to compromise your own value system.

Patient Confidentiality

Confidentiality of patient information is one of the most important ethical principles to be observed by the medical assistant. As discussed earlier, information obtained in the care of the patient may not be revealed without the permission of the patient unless required by law. Whatever you say to, hear from, or do for a patient is confidential. Patients will reveal some of their innermost thoughts, feelings, and fears. This information is not for public knowledge. Family members, friends, pastors, or others may call the physician's office to inquire about a patient's condition. Many of these calls are made with good intentions; *no information*, however, should be released to anyone—friends, family, media, or insurance companies—without prior written approval from the patient (see Chapter 8).

WHAT IF?

A well-meaning family member asks for information about her mother's condition. What should you say?

Tell the family member that HIPAA's Privacy Rule does not allow you to discuss the patient without his or her permission. No information can be released to anyone—friends, family, media, or insurance companies—without prior written approval from the patient (see Chapter 8).

HIPAA also requires that each patient complete a form that establishes his or her wishes about giving information to family members and friends. If there is a particular family member who brings the patient to the office, the patient may sign a release form giving that person the right to receive information. Many physicians provide the patient with a short progress report including the patient's test results, diagnosis, treatment, and next appointment. A form could be designed for this purpose. This gives the patient the opportunity to share complete and accurate information if he or she chooses.

Honesty

One of the most important character traits for medical assistants is honesty. We all make mistakes at times; how we handle our mistakes is the indication of our ethical standards. If you make a mistake (e.g., giving the wrong medication), you must immediately report the error to your supervisor and the attending physician. The mark of a true professional is the ability to admit mistakes and take full responsibility for all actions. When speaking to patients concerning medical issues, be honest; give the facts in a straightforward manner. Never offer false expectations or hope. Never minimize or exaggerate the risks or benefits of a procedure. If you do not know the answer to a question, say, "I don't know, but I will find out for you," or refer the question to the physician. Treating the patient with dignity, respect, and honesty in all interactions will build trust in you and your professional abilities.

CHECKPOINT QUESTION

10. What are the three ethical standards a CMA, as an agent of the physician, should follow?

American Association of Medical Assistants Code of Ethics

Principles

The AAMA has published a set of five principles of ethical and moral conduct that all medical assistants must follow in the practice of the profession. They state that the medical assistant must always strive to:

1. Render services with respect for human dignity
2. Respect patient confidentiality, except when information is required by the law
3. Uphold the honor and high principles set forth by the AAMA
4. Continually improve knowledge and skills for the benefit of patients and the health care team
5. Participate in community services that promote good health and welfare to the general public

These principles are outlined in the AAMA creed seen in the Medical Assistants' Creed (see Box 2-8).

According to the *AAMA's Disciplinary Standards & Procedures for CMAs*, CMAs who violate the disciplinary standards may face possible sanctions including denial of eligibility for the certification examination, probation, reprimand, temporary revocation of the CMA credentials, and permanent revocation of the CMA credential. For more information, see the AAMA Web site.

COG Bioethics

Bioethics deals specifically with the moral issues and problems that affect human life. As a result of advances in medicine and research, many situations require moral decisions for which there are no clear answers. Abortion and genetic engineering are examples. The goal is to make the right decision in each specific instance as it applies to an individual's specific circumstances. What may be right for one patient may be wrong for another; that is the foundation of bioethics.

American Medical Association Council on Ethical and Judicial Affairs

Because of the broad scope of medical ethics and bioethical issues, the AMA formed a subcommittee to review AMA principles and to interpret them as they apply to everyday clinical situations. This subcommittee is called the Council on Ethical and Judicial Affairs. The council has formulated a series of opinions on various medical and bioethical issues that are intended to provide the physician with guidelines for professional conduct and responsibilities. These opinions, most recently revised in 1992, are divided into four general categories:

• Social policy issues
• Relations with colleagues and hospitals
• Administrative office procedures
• Professional rights and responsibilities

The following discussion provides a summary of these opinions along with questions designed to promote your ability to use reasoning to examine difficult ethical issues. These issues are not within the scope of decisions for medical assistants, but you will be faced with their consequences at some time in your career.

Social Policy Issues

The social policy section deals with various issues of societal importance and provides guidelines to aid the physician in making ethical choices. Five common societal topics and the opinion statements from the AMA Council on Ethical and Judicial Affairs follow.

Allocation of Resources

The term *allocate* means to set aside or designate for a purpose. Allocation of resources in the medical profession may refer to many health needs:

• *Organs for transplantation.* Who gets the heart, the college professor or the young recovering addict whose heart was damaged by his lifestyle? Should lifestyle or perceived worth be considered in the decision?
• *Funds for research.* Which disease should receive more funding for research, cancer or AIDS?
• *Funds for health care.* For what should the money be spent, for keeping alive extremely premature infants or making preventive health care available for a greater number of poor children?
• *Hospital beds and professional care.* With hospital care at a premium, who will pay for the indigent? How is it decided which patient is entitled to the last bed in the intensive care unit?

BOX 2-9

AMA COUNCIL ON ETHICAL AND JUDICIAL AFFAIRS VIEWPOINT

• When resources are limited, decisions for allocating health care materials should be based on fair and socially acceptable criteria. Economic or social position should not be a factor in the decision.
• Priority care is given to the person or persons who are more likely to receive the greatest long-term benefit from the treatment. Patients with other disease processes or who are not good candidates for treatment for whatever reason will be less likely to receive treatment than otherwise healthy patients. For instance, a patient with cancer in other sites would not be considered for a liver transplant, whereas a patient whose liver was damaged by trauma but who has no other involvement would probably be a good candidate.
• An individual's societal worth must not be a deciding factor during the decision process. A socially or politically prominent patient should not be considered a better recipient of treatment options than a young mother on welfare.
• Age must not be considered in the decision process. If the age of the patient is not a contraindication for the treatment, all ages should be considered on an even basis for most medical resources.

Box 2-9 outlines the judicial council's viewpoints on allocation of limited resources.

Clinical Investigations and Research

Physicians are frequently involved in studying the effectiveness of new procedures and medications, often called clinical investigations or research. New drugs and treatments are tested on animals first and then considered safe for human testing. The council's viewpoint on research investigation of new drugs and procedures states:

• *A physician may participate in clinical research as long as the project is part of a systematic program with controls for patient evaluation during all phases of the research. At all stages of the testing and at the completion of the study, a protocol must be in place to evaluate the immediate and the long-term effects of the study.*
• *The goal of the research must be to obtain scientifically valid data. The objectives of the study must be available to the physician and the patient, results must be provided to all participants on request, and the testing must serve a medically sound purpose to provide better patient care.*

- *Utmost care and respect must be given to patients involved in clinical research. They are entitled to be treated just as any other patient receiving health care.*
- *Physicians must obtain the patient's permission or consent before enrolling the patient in a research project.*
- *The patient's decision to participate in the program must be completely voluntary.*
- *The patient must be advised of any potential risks, side effects, and benefits of participating in the project.*
- *The patient must be advised that this procedure or drug is experimental. Patients must be made aware that research is not complete, that this is the purpose of the trials, and that the risks and benefits are not fully known at this time.*
- *The physician and the institution must have a check and balance system in place to ensure that quality care is always given and ethical standards are followed. Documentation of patient education and instruction for following testing guidelines and patient response to the treatment must be ongoing and thorough.*

Obstetric Dilemmas

Advances in technology have created legal and ethical situations that have polarized opinions and are difficult to bring to consensus. Issues such as the beginning of life, genetic testing and engineering, sex determination, the rights of the fetus, ownership of the fertilized egg, and so forth will not be easily answered. The council formulated an opinion regarding obstetric issues as fairly as possible that states the following:

ABORTION. As the law now stands, a physician may perform an abortion as long as state and federal laws are followed regarding the trimester in which it is performed. A physician who does not want to perform abortions cannot be forced to perform the procedure; that physician, however, should refer the patient to other health care professionals who can assist the patient.

GENETIC TESTING. If amniocentesis is performed on a mother and a genetic defect is found, both parents must be told. The parents may request or refuse to have the pregnancy terminated. (Amniocentesis is a procedure in which a needle is inserted in a pregnant woman's abdomen to remove and test amniotic fluid. Many abnormalities and disorders can be diagnosed early in pregnancy by this procedure.)

ARTIFICIAL INSEMINATION. Artificial insemination involves the insertion of sperm into a woman's vagina for the purpose of conception. The donor may be the husband (artificial insemination by husband [AIH]) or an anonymous donor (artificial insemination by donor [AID]). The council states that both the husband and wife must consent to this procedure. If a donor is used, the sperm must be tested for infectious and genetic disorders. Complete confidentiality for the donor and recipient must be maintained.

 CHECKPOINT QUESTION

11. What is the opinion of the AMA's Council on Ethical and Judicial Affairs regarding abortion?

Stem Cell Research

As we continue to find new technologies, ethical dilemmas continue to emerge. Stem cell research is an ethical issue resulting from our ability to program the immature and undifferentiated cells of a fetus to be muscle, liver, or cardiac cells. The implications of this ability have become a political issue in the last several years. Researchers have found that stem cells taken from the umbilical cord of a newborn are also useful. It is even possible for parents to have the umbilical cord of their infant frozen and stored for use in later years to cure any diseases encountered. Some people believe that the potential to cure such diseases as Parkinson's disease and cystic fibrosis is worth using embryonic stem cells. Others believe that using fetal cells and tissue is immoral. The political debate about government funding of stem cell research continues. As discussed in Chapter 1, today's research has made it possible to use a patient's own stems cells to regenerate cells, tissue, and even organs. This makes the use of stem cells for treatment a less sensitive issue.

Organ Transplantation

Organ transplantation became a medical option in the mid 1950s, although at that time, there were many problems with rejection of the organs by the recipient's immune system. When this postoperative complication was corrected by antirejection drugs, the practice became more common. Organs are viable (able to support life) for varying lengths of time, but most can be used successfully if transplanted within 24 to 48 hours. An organization in Richmond, Virginia, the United Network of Organ Sharing, coordinates local organ procurement teams that will fly to areas where organs are to be harvested to assist with the surgery if needed and to ensure the integrity of the organ. There are far fewer organs available than are needed, and every year, thousands of patients die who could have lived if an organ had been available.

The use of organs from a baby born without a brain (anencephaly) raises serious ethical issues. The council states that everything must be done for the infant until the determination of death can be made. For infant organs to be transplanted, both parents must consent.

The council's views on transplantation state:

- *The rights of the donor and organ recipient must be treated equally. The imminent death of the donor does not release the medical personnel from observing all rights that every patient is due.*
- *Organ donors must be given every medical opportunity for life. Life support is not removed until the*

patient is determined to have no brain activity and could not live without artificial support.

- *Death of the donor must be determined by a physician who is not on the transplant team to avoid a charge of conflict of interest.*
- *Consent (permission) must be received from both the donor, if possible, and recipient before the transplant. Family members may give consent if the donor is unable to do so.*
- *Transplants can be performed only by surgeons who are qualified to perform this complex surgery and who are affiliated with institutions that have adequate facilities for the surgery and postoperative care.*

Box 2-10 highlights the Uniform Anatomical Gift Act.

Withholding or Withdrawing Treatment

Physicians have a professional and ethical obligation to promote quality of life, which means sustaining life and relieving suffering. Sometimes, these obligations conflict with a patient's wishes. Patients have the right to refuse medical treatment and to request that life support or life-sustaining treatments be withheld or withdrawn. Withholding treatment means that certain medical treatments may not be initiated. Withdrawing treatment is terminating a treatment that has already begun. In 1991, congress passed the Self-Determination Act, which gave all hospitalized patients the right to make health care decisions on admission to the hospital. These decisions may be referred to as advance directives. Today, everyone is encouraged to participate in his or her own end-of-life decisions. You can go online and complete an advance directive. An **advance directive** is a statement of a person's wishes for medical decisions prior to a critical event. Advance directives may include specific wishes, such as whether a ventilator can be used, whether CPR should be initiated, and whether a feeding tube should be inserted. Just completing an advance directive does not ensure that the patient's wishes will be carried out. It is important to make family members aware of these wishes. The patient's next of kin should keep a copy of the advance directive, and one should be placed in the medical office chart with special notation. Figure 2-4 is a sample of an advance directive.

 CHECKPOINT QUESTION

12. What is an advance directive? How can a patient be sure his or her wishes will be followed?

BOX 2-10

UNIFORM ANATOMICAL GIFT ACT

Many organs can be transplanted, including the liver, kidney, cornea, heart, lung, and skin. To meet the growing need for organs and to allay the concern over donor standards, the National Conference of Commissioners for Uniform State Laws passed legislation known as the Uniform Anatomical Gift Act.

All acts include the following clauses:

- Any mentally competent person over age 18 may donate all or part of his or her body for transplantation or research.
- The donor's wishes supersede any other wishes except when state laws require an autopsy.
- Physicians accepting donor organs in good faith are immune from lawsuits against harvesting organs.
- Death of the donor must be determined by a physician not involved with the transplant team.
- Financial compensation may not be given to the donor or survivors.
- Persons wishing to donate organs can revoke permission or change their minds at any time.

In most states, the Department of Motor Vehicles asks applicants for a driver's license about organ donation and indicates their wishes on their license. In addition, an individual may declare the wish to donate all or parts of the body in a will or any legal document, including a Uniform Donor Card. Organ donors should make their families aware of their wishes to ensure they will be carried out.

Professional and Ethical Conduct and Behavior

The council states that all health care professionals are responsible for reporting unethical practices to the appropriate agencies. No health care professional should engage in any act that he or she feels is ethically or morally wrong.

Additionally, the council states:

- A physician must never assist or allow an unlicensed person to practice medicine.
- Hospitals and physicians must work together for the best care for patients. Hospitals should allow physicians staff privileges based on the ability of the physician, educational background, and the needs of the community. (Staff privileges allow physicians to admit their patients to a given hospital.) Issues of a personal nature must never be considered when accepting or declining a physician's application for privileges.
- It is unethical for physicians to admit patients to the hospital or to order excessive treatments for the sole purpose of financial rewards.

 CHECKPOINT QUESTION

13. What steps should be taken when a physician closes his or her practice?

ADVANCE DIRECTIVE

UNIFORM ADVANCE DIRECTIVE OF [list name of declarant]

To my family, physician, attorney, and anyone else who may become responsible for my health, welfare, or affairs, I make this declaration while I am of sound mind.

If I should ever become in a terminal state and there is no reasonable expectation of my recovery, I direct that I be allowed to die a natural death and that my life not be prolonged by extraordinary measures. I do, however, ask that medication be mercifully administered to me to alleviate suffering, even though this may shorten my remaining life.

This statement is made after full reflection and is in accordance with my full desires. I want the above provisions carried out to the extent permitted by law. Insofar as they are not legally enforceable, I wish that those to whom this will is addressed will regard themselves as morally bound by this instrument.

If permissible in the jurisdiction in which I may be hospitalized I direct that in the event of a terminal diagnosis, the physicians supervising my care discontinue feeding should the continuation of feeding be judged to result in unduly prolonging a natural death.

If permissible in the jurisdiction in which I may be hospitalized I direct that in the event of a terminal diagnosis, the physicians supervising my care discontinue hydration (water) should the continuation of hydration be judged to result in unduly prolonging a natural death.

I herewith authorize my spouse, if any, or any relative who is related to me within the third degree to effectuate my transfer from any hospital or other health care facility in which I may be receiving care should that facility decline or refuse to effectuate the instructions given herein.

I herewith release any and all hospitals, physicians, and others for myself and for my estate from any liability for complying with this instrument.

Signed:

_____
[list name of declarant]

City of residence: _____
                              [city of residence]

County of residence: _____
                                  [county of residence]

State of residence: _____
                              [state of residence]

Social Security Number: _____
                                      [social security number]

Date: _____

_____
Witness

_____
Witness

STATE OF _____

COUNTY OF _____

This day personally appeared before me, the undersigned authority, a Notary Public in and for _____County, _____ State,

_____   _____
                                                                              (Witnesses)

who, being first duly sworn, say that they are the subscribing witnesses to the declaration of [list name of declarant], the declarant, signed, sealed, and published and declared the same as and for his declaration, in the presence of both these affiants; and that these affiants, at the request of said declarant, in the presence of each other, and in the presence of said declarant, all present at the same time, signed their names as attesting witnesses to said declaration.

Affiants further say that this affidavit is made at the request of [list name of declarant], declarant, and in his presence, and that [list name of declarant] at the time the declaration was executed, in the opinion of the affiants, of sound mind and memory, and over the age of eighteen years.

Taken, subscribed and sworn to before me by _____(witness) and

_____ (witness) this _____ day of_____, 20_____.

My commission expires: _____

_____ Notary Public

Figure 2-4 Sample advance directive.

español SPANISH TERMINOLOGY

¿Usted entiende la información que acaba de recibir?

Do you understand the information I have given?

¿Usted nos autoriza a llevar a cabo este procedimiento médico?

Do you give us permission to perform this procedure?

¿Firme aquí, por favor.

Please sign here.

 MEDIA MENU

- **Student Resources on thePoint**
  - **CMA/RMA Certification Exam Review**
- **Internet Resources**

  Web sites to keep abreast of changes in the medical field:
  Go to your state's home page and click on the link to the state legislature to view pending state legislation.
  Go to The Library of Congress to view federal legislation to be considered in the coming week.
  http://Thomas.loc.gov

  Equal Employment Opportunity Commission
  http://www.eeoc.gov

  U.S. Department of Labor, Bureau of Labor Statistics
  http://stats.bls.gov

  To complete an advance directive
  http://www.legalzoom.com

  To download and print a Vaccination Information Statement
  http://www.cdc.gov/vaccines/pubs/vis/default.htm

  American Hospital Assocation
  http://www.aha.org

  AHA's Patient Care Partnership
  http://www.aha.org/aha/issues/Communicating-With-Patients/pt-care-partnership.html

  Patients' Bill of Rights
  http://www.hcqualitycommission.gov/final

PSY PROCEDURE 2-1: **Monitoring Federal and State Regulations, Changes, and Updates**

Purpose: To ensure compliance with regulations by keeping abreast of changes and actions affecting medical assisting issues and health care legislation

Equipment: Computer, Internet connection, search engine or Web site list

Steps	Reasons
1. Using a search engine, input the keywords for your state legislature, OR go to the homepage for your state government. Example: http://www.nc.gov	The best source for legislative changes is a state's legislative Web site.
2. Follow links to the legislative branch of your state.	The homepage will give you the appropriate links.
3. Search for such issues as health care finances, allied health professionals, outpatient medical care, Medicare, etc.	These general search words will lead you to information about current or pending legislation.
4. Read and share information from the Centers for Disease Control and Prevention (CDC), Occupational Safety and Health Administration (OSHA), your state medical society, and the American Medical Association (AMA).	Information you receive from outside sources will keep you abreast of changes and trends. For example, OSHA informed providers about changes in the regulations for needle disposal.
5. Create and enforce a policy for timely dissemination of information received by fax or e-mail from outside agencies.	OSHA and the CDC alert providers of vital information via fax or e-mail.
6. Circulate information gathered to all appropriate employees with an avenue for sharing information.	Any information obtained should be shared.
7. Post changes in a designated area of the office.	A break room or time clock area is a good place to display important information.
8. **AFF** Explain what you would say to a fellow employee who responds to a change in a current law with: "I will just keep doing it the old way. Who is going to care?"	Health care professionals must stay current and abreast of any changes in the law. As the saying goes, "ignorance is no excuse" when it comes to changes in statutes and laws. You are legally obligated to obey the new law after the effective date.

- The fields of medicine and law are linked in common concern for the patient's health and rights. Increasingly, health care professionals are the object of malpractice lawsuits.
- You can help prevent medical malpractice by acting professionally, maintaining clinical competency, and properly documenting in the medical record. Promoting good public relations between the patient and the health care team can avoid frivolous or unfounded suits and direct attention and energy toward optimum health care.
- Medical ethics and bioethics involve complex issues and controversial topics. There will be no easy or clear-cut answers to questions raised by these issues.

As a medical assistant, your first priority must be to act as your patients' advocate, with their best interests and concerns foremost in your actions and interactions. You must always maintain ethical standards and report the unethical behaviors of others.

- Many acts and regulations affect health care organizations and their operations. A medical office must keep current on all legal updates.
- Most states publish a monthly bulletin that reports on new legislation. Every state has a Web site that will link you to legislative action. Read these on a regular basis.
- Each office should have legal counsel who can assist in interpreting legal issues.

Warm Ups for Critical Thinking

1. An acquaintance who knows you work in the medical field asks you to diagnose her rash. What do you say?
2. A patient owes a big bill at your office. She requests copies of her records. What do you do?
3. You suspect that a new employee in the office is misusing narcotics. What do you do?
4. Mrs. Rodriguez has bone cancer. Her doctor has estimated that she has 6 months to live. Mrs. Rodriguez wants the physician to withhold all medical treatments. She does not want chemotherapy or any life-sustaining measures. Her family disagrees. Should her family have any input into her health care decisions?
5. You are on your lunch hour from your job at a Planned Parenthood clinic. You run into the mother of a friend who happened to be seen earlier that day in your clinic. You say, "Hi, I just saw Heather this morning." Heather's mother says, "Oh, yes? And where did you see her?" What now? Discuss the need to think before you speak where confidentiality is concerned.

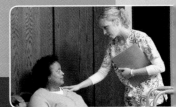

Learning Outcomes

Cognitive Domain

Note: AAMA/CAAHEP 2008 Standards are italicized.

1. Spell and define the key terms
2. List two major forms of communication
3. *Identify styles and types of verbal communication*
4. *Identify nonverbal communication*
5. *Recognize communication barriers*
6. *Identify techniques for overcoming communication barriers*
7. *Recognize the elements of oral communication using a sender-receiver process*
8. *Identify resources and adaptations that are required based on individual needs, i.e., culture and environment, developmental life stage, language, and physical threats to communication*
9. *Discuss the role of cultural, social and ethnic diversity in ethical performance of medical assisting practice*
10. *Discuss the role of assertiveness in effective professional communication*
11. Explain how various components of communication can affect the meaning of verbal messages
12. Define active listening
13. List and describe the six interviewing techniques
14. Give an example of how cultural differences may affect communication
15. Discuss how to handle communication problems caused by language barriers
16. List two methods that you can use to promote communication among hearing-, sight-, and speech-impaired patients

17. Discuss how to handle an angry or distressed patient
18. List five actions that you can take to improve communication with a child
19. Discuss your role in communicating with a grieving patient or family member
20. List the five stages of grief as outlined by Elisabeth Kübler-Ross
21. Discuss the key elements of interdisciplinary communication
22. *Explore issue of confidentiality as it applies to the medical assistant*

Psychomotor Domain

Note: AAMA/CAAHEP 2008 Standards are italicized.

1. *Respond to nonverbal communication*
2. *Use reflection, restatement and clarification techniques to obtain a patient history*

Affective Domain

Note: AAMA/CAAHEP 2008 Standards are italicized.

1. *Apply active listening skills*
2. *Use appropriate body language and other nonverbal skills in communicating with patients, family, and staff*
3. *Demonstrate awareness of the territorial boundaries of the person with whom one is communicating*
4. *Demonstrate sensitivity appropriate to the message being delivered*
5. *Demonstrate awareness of how an individual's personal appearance affects anticipated responses*
6. *Demonstrate recognition of the patient's level of understanding in communications*

7. *Analyze communication in providing appropriate responses/feedback*
8. *Recognize and protect personal boundaries in communicating with others*
9. *Demonstrate respect for individual diversity, incorporating awareness of one's own biases in areas including gender, race, religion, and economic standing*
10. *Demonstrate empathy in communicating with patients, family, and staff*
11. *Demonstrate sensitivity in communicating with both providers and patients*
12. *Respond to issues of confidentiality*

ABHES Competencies

1. Identify and respond appropriately when working/caring for patients with special needs
2. Use empathy when treating terminally ill patients
3. Identify common stages that terminally ill patients go through and list organizations/ support groups that can assist patients and family members of patients struggling with terminal illness
4. Advocate on behalf of family/patients, having ability to deal and communicate with family
5. Analyze the effect of hereditary, cultural, and environmental influences
6. Locate resources and information for patients and employers
7. Be attentive, listen, and learn
8. Be impartial and show empathy when dealing with patients
9. Communicate on the recipient's level of comprehension
10. Serve as liaison between physician and others
11. Recognize and respond to verbal and nonverbal communication

Key Terms

anacusis	discrimination	messages	presbycusis
bias	dysphasia	mourning	reflecting
clarification	dysphonia	nonlanguage	stereotyping
cultures	feedback	paralanguage	summarizing
demeanor	grief	paraphrasing	therapeutic

Communication is sending and receiving **messages** (information), verbally or otherwise. Until the message is received accurately, communication has not taken place. The ability to communicate effectively is a crucial skill for medical assistants. In your role, you must accurately and appropriately share information with physicians, other professional staff members, and patients. When communicating with patients, you must be able to receive messages correctly, interpret them, and respond to the sender appropriately. Proper grammar is important! Although you may speak in an informal way with family and friends, you must speak in a professional manner while at work. The medical assistant is usually the first person the patient meets in the medical office. Thus, your positive attitude, pleasant presentation, and use of good communication skills will set the tone for future interactions.

COG Basic Communication Flow

Communication requires the following elements:

- A message to be sent
- A person to send the message
- A person to receive the message

During the act of communicating, two or more people will alternate roles as sender and receiver as they seek **feedback** (responses) and **clarification** (understanding) regarding the message. The process of message exchange is like a swing moving back and forth between two people. Figure 3-1 illustrates the flow of communication and its common components.

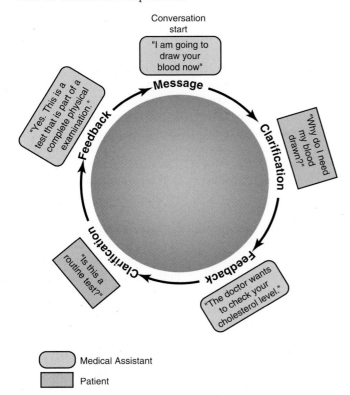

Figure 3-1 Flow of communication.

As a medical assistant, you will primarily be communicating in a therapeutic manner. This means that your communication will focus on conversations regarding pertinent topics relating to office procedures, policies, and patient care. Your other responsibilities for ensuring good communication include the following:

- Clarifying confusing messages
- Validating (confirming) the patient's perceptions
- Adapting messages to the patient's level of understanding
- Asking for feedback to ensure that the messages you sent were received by the patient or other persons as intended

CHECKPOINT QUESTION

1. What three elements must be present for communication to occur?

COG Forms of Communication

Verbal Communication

Verbal communication involves an exchange of messages using words or language; it is the most commonly used form and is usually the initial form of communication. You need good verbal communication skills when performing such tasks as making appointments, providing patient education, making referrals, and sharing information with the physician.

Oral communication is sending or receiving messages using spoken language. As a professional, you should use a pleasant and polite manner of speaking. Use proper English and grammar at all times; lapsing into slang and colloquialisms projects an unprofessional image.

Gear your conversation to the patient's educational level. A well-educated patient may resent your using other than the correct terms, yet a less educated patient may be confused and intimidated by the same phrases. Avoid using elaborate medical terminology if you think it might confuse or frighten a patient. Will this patient understand "myocardial infarction," or should you say heart attack? Do not talk down to the patient, but do phrase your communication appropriately.

Be aware, too, that the meaning of spoken messages may be affected by other components of oral communication, including paralanguage and nonlanguage sounds. The cliché that it's not what you say but how you say it is true. Research shows that the primary message is transmitted more by the way it is said than by the words that are used. This refers to paralanguage. **Paralanguage** includes voice tone, quality, volume, pitch, and range. **Nonlanguage** sounds include laughing, sobbing, sighing, grunting, and so on. Other nonlanguage clues to understanding can be found in a speaker's grammatical structure, pronunciation, and general articulation, which can indicate regional or cultural background and level of education. Knowing this information can help you adapt responses and explanations to the patient's level of understanding.

Written communication uses written language to exchange messages. The ability to write clearly, concisely, and accurately is important in the health care profession (see Chapter 7). Typically, patients receive oral instructions first, as you or the physician explain key points of concern. These verbal instructions are then reinforced with written instructions (Box 3-1).

If the instructions, oral or written, are not clear, the patient may misinterpret them. This misunderstanding can hinder treatment and recovery and possibly even require the patient to be admitted to the hospital. Here is an example of an unclear instruction: "Return to the office if you don't feel better." This provides the patient with no details. Clearer instructions would state, "If your fever and sore throat are not better in 24 hours, call the office to schedule a revisit." Even the most clearly outlined instructions can be misunderstood, particularly by those with deficient hearing or reading abilities. As a medical assistant, you are responsible for asking questions to verify that the patient has correctly understood the information. To verify that the patient understood these instructions, a good question to ask would be, "When should you call the office if you don't feel better?"

 CHECKPOINT QUESTION

2. List five examples of paralanguage.

Nonverbal Communication

Nonverbal communication—exchanging messages without using words—is sometimes called body language. Body language includes several types of behaviors, such as kinesics, proxemics, and the use of touch. Kinesics refers to body movements, including facial expressions, gestures, and eye movements. A patient's face can sometimes reveal inner feelings, such as sadness, happiness, fear, or anger, that may not be mentioned explicitly during a conversation. Gestures also carry various meanings. For instance, shrugging the shoulders can mean simple lack of interest or hopeless resignation. Eyes can often hint at what a person may be thinking or feeling. For example, a patient whose eyes wander away from you while you are talking may be impatient, lack interest, or not understand what you are saying.

Nonverbal communication may more accurately reflect a person's true feelings and attitude than verbal communication. In other words, people may say one thing but show a completely different response with their body language. For example, if the patient says, "The pain in my foot is not too bad," but the patient's face shows pain with each step, the nonverbal clues demonstrate an inconsistent message. Many patients mask their feelings, so you must learn to read their actions and nonverbal clues in addition to what they tell you. Be aware that patients are also acutely attuned to your facial and nonverbal reactions. Responding with an expression of disgust or shaking your head in a negative way can jeopardize communication and rapport between you and the patient.

How and where individuals physically place themselves in relation to others can affect communication as well. Proxemics refers to spatial relationships or physical proximity tolerated by humans. Generally, the area within a 3-foot radius around a person is considered personal space and is not to be invaded by strangers, although this area varies among individuals and people of various **cultures** (societies). To deliver care to a patient, physicians and medical assistants must enter a patient's personal space. After a patient task is completed, it is appropriate to take a few steps back and allow for more space between you and the patient.

BOX 3-1

EXAMPLE OF WRITTEN DISCHARGE INSTRUCTIONS

Main Street Pediatric Group
343 Main Street, Suite 609
King, NC 27021

Instructions for Otitis Media

Your child has an ear infection. It is easily treated with antibiotics. Get the prescription filled immediately. The first dose should be given as soon as you arrive home. Read the attached information on the antibiotic.

Here are some other important things to remember:

- Ear infections are not contagious.
- Symptoms usually resolve within 24 hours of beginning antibiotics. It is very important to make sure your child takes all of the prescription.
- If the pain persists for more than 48 hours, call the office.
- If you see any blood in the ear canal, call the office.

Make an appointment for a follow-up visit in 2 weeks.

_____   _____
Patient's signature   Physician's signature

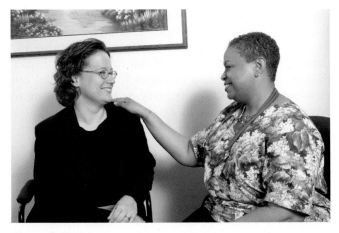

Figure 3-2 Therapeutic touch conveys caring and concern.

Ask another student to speak continuously for 1 to 2 minutes while you listen. (The student should discuss a topic with which you are unfamiliar.) When he or she finishes, wait silently for the same amount of time. Then try to repeat the message. If you have trouble doing this exercise, you need to practice listening.

AFF ETHICAL TIP

Don't Let Your Mouth Get You in Trouble

All patient communication is confidential. Patient information is sometimes discussed unintentionally, however. To avoid breaching confidentiality, follow these guidelines:

- Do not discuss patients' problems in public places, such as elevators or parking lots. A patient's friends or family members might overhear your conversation and misinterpret what is said.
- Keep the glass window between the waiting room and the reception desk closed.
- Watch the volume of your voice.
- When calling coworkers over the office intercom, do not use a patient's name or reveal other information. Avoid saying something like, "Bob Smith is on the phone and wants to know if his strep throat culture came back." Instead, say "There's a patient on line 1."
- Before going home, destroy any slips of paper in your uniform pockets that contain patient information (e.g., reminder notes from verbal reports).

Because some individuals become uncomfortable when their space is invaded, it is essential to approach the patient in a professional manner and explain what you plan to do. Explanations help ease patient anxiety about what will happen.

Related to proxemics is the use of touch, which can be **therapeutic** (beneficial) for some patients. It can indicate emotional support and convey concern and feeling. For some patients, however, being touched by a stranger is an uncomfortable or even negative experience. Many patients perceive touch in a medical setting as a prelude to something unpleasant, such as an injection. To change this negative perception, try offering a comforting touch when nothing invasive or painful is imminent. Before comforting a patient by touching, assess the patient's **demeanor** (expressions and behavior) for clues indicating that touch would be acceptable. In Figure 3-2, the certified medical assistant's (CMA's) touch is comforting to the patient.

COG Active Listening

Active listening is important to ensure that messages are correctly received and interpreted. Failure to do so can result in poor patient care. To listen actively, you must give your full attention to the patient with whom you are speaking. Interruptions should be kept to a minimum. You need to focus not only on what is being said, but also on what is being conveyed through paralanguage, body language, and other aspects of communication. Occasionally, a patient's verbal messages may seem to conflict with the nonverbal messages. For example, a patient who is wringing his hands while telling you that everything is fine is sending conflicting signals that require further exploration. If a patient's verbal response does not correspond to your observations, convey your concern to the physician.

Active listening is a skill that develops with practice. To test your listening ability, try the following exercise.

COG Interview Techniques

As a medical assistant, you are typically responsible for gathering initial information and updating existing information about the patients. This task is accomplished by interviewing the patient. The interview will consist of you asking certain questions and then interpreting the patient's responses. The initial interview includes many areas. The key areas are the patient's medical and family history, a brief review of the body systems, and a social history. The main goal is to obtain accurate and pertinent information. The interview for an established patient, however, is much different. First, you should review the chart to look at the patient's health problems. Make a list of questions regarding the pertinent medical problems. Reconfirm medication usage and any specific treatments the patient is supposed to be doing.

To conduct either type of interview, you must use effective techniques: listen actively, ask the appropriate

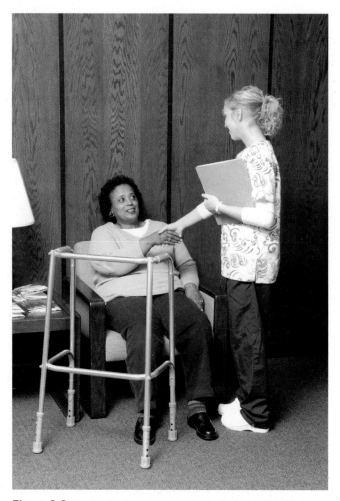

Figure 3-3 Begin the interview by introducing yourself.

questions, and record the answers. During the interview, you must demonstrate professionalism. Begin by introducing yourself (Fig. 3-3). Always conduct the interview in a private area. Know what questions you need to ask and in what order to ask them before you begin the interview. Be organized. It is also helpful to have an extra pen. And most important, do not answer phone calls or attend to other distractions until you have finished the interview. Last, when you leave the room, let patients know who will be in to see them and the approximate time, for example, "Dr. Sanchez will be in to see you in about 10 minutes."

The six interviewing techniques are reflecting, paraphrasing, clarification, asking open-ended questions, summarizing, and allowing silences.

Reflecting

Reflecting is repeating what you have heard the patient say, using open-ended statements. With this technique, you do not complete a sentence but leave it up to the patient to do so. For example, you might

say, "Mrs. Rivera, you were saying that when your back hurts you ...." Reflection encourages the patient to make further comments. It also can help bring the patient back to the subject if the conversation begins to drift. (Reflecting is a useful tool, but be careful not to overuse it, because some patients find it annoying to have their words constantly parroted back.)

Paraphrasing or Restatement

Paraphrasing or restatement means repeating what you have heard, using your own words or phrases. Paraphrasing can help verify that you have accurately understood what was said. It also allows patients the opportunity to clarify their thoughts or statements. Typically, a paraphrased statement begins with "You are saying that ...," or "It sounds as if ...," followed by the rephrased content.

Asking for Examples or Clarification

If you are confused about some of the information you have received, ask the patient to give an example of the situation being described. For instance, "Can you describe one of these dizzy spells?" The patient's example should help you better understand what the patient is saying. It also may give you an insight into how the patient perceives the situation.

Asking Open-Ended Questions

The best way to obtain specific information is to ask open-ended questions that require the patient to formulate an answer and elaborate on the response. Open-ended questions usually begin with what, when, or how. For example, "What medications did you take this morning?" "When did you stop taking your medication?" "How did you get that large bruise on your arm?" Be careful about asking "why" questions, because they can often sound judgmental or accusing. For example, asking "Why did you do that?" or "Why didn't you follow the directions?" may imply to patients that you have already made a negative value judgment about their behavior, and they could become defensive and uncooperative. Instead, you might ask, "What part of the instructions did you not understand?" or "How can we help you follow these instructions?"

Avoid closed-ended questions that allow the patient to answer with one word, such as yes or no. For example, suppose you ask the patient, "Are you taking your medications?" The patient can easily say yes but may not be taking all of them. However, suppose you ask, "What medications do you take every day?" The patient's answer will give you a clearer understanding of whether the patient is taking the correct medications.

Summarizing

Briefly reviewing the information you have obtained, or **summarizing**, gives the patient another chance to clarify statements or correct misinformation. This technique can also help you organize complex information or events in sequential order. For example, if the patient has been feeling dizzy and stumbling a lot, you might summarize by saying, "You told me that you have been feeling dizzy for the past 3 days and that you frequently stumble as you are walking."

Allowing Silences

Periods of silence sometimes occur during the interview. These can be beneficial. Some people are uncomfortable with prolonged silences and feel a need to break the silence with words in an effort to jump-start a stalled conversation. Silences are natural parts of conversations and can give patients time to formulate their thoughts, reconstruct events, evaluate their feelings, or assess what has already been said. During moments of silence, gather your thoughts and formulate any additional questions that you may have.

 CHECKPOINT QUESTION

3. What are the six interviewing techniques?

COG Factors Affecting Communication

Sometimes, despite your best efforts, others may not receive your message accurately. A common occurrence that causes messages to be misinterpreted is the use of a cliché. For example, suppose you are teaching a patient to use crutches and she is having difficulty managing them. A cliché comment may be, "Don't worry. Rome wasn't built in a day. This takes time." The cliché is innocent and not meant to be demeaning, but the patient may misinterpret it to mean that she is slow, ancient. A more positive message would be, "I can see that you are making progress. Let's try walking down the hallway."

Here are some reasons for miscommunication:

1. The message may have been unclear or inappropriate to the situation. For example, "I have scheduled you for a PET scan in radiology tomorrow at 8 a.m." Keep in mind that most of your patients do not understand medical abbreviations and terms. Because positron emission tomography (PET) is a newer technology, they may confuse it with computed tomography (CT). Also, where is radiology? A better message would be, "The doctor wants you to have a test done tomorrow. It is called a PET scan; here is a brochure that explains it. Go to the second floor of the outpatient center on Main Street. Do you know how to get there?"

2. The person receiving the message may have been distracted, anxious, or confused. A common cause of distraction is pain. For example, teaching a patient how to use crutches cannot be done if the patient's ankle or knee still hurts. The concentration will be on the pain, not on what you are saying. Patients who have just received positive news can also be anxious to contact loved ones. This is commonly seen with patients who have just been told that they are pregnant. The patient's focus is on calling family members and not on your conversation.

3. Environmental elements, such as noise or interruptions, may also distort messages. Environmental noises from staff lounges or break rooms can easily be overheard. Keep the doors to these areas closed. Cleaning staff should not be vacuuming or emptying trash while patients are present.

In addition to these three items, other factors may affect communication. They are discussed next.

Cultural Differences

The way a person perceives situations and other people is greatly influenced by cultural, social, and religious beliefs or firmly held convictions. Personal values (principles or ideals) are commonly developed from these same beliefs. As a medical assistant, you will interact with people from varied ethnic backgrounds and cultural origins who bring with them beliefs and values that may differ from your own. Understanding those differences can aid communication and thereby improve patient care (Table 3-1). It is very important that you not form preconceived ideas about a given culture. Remember that each of your patients is unique and that their health care needs differ.

Some cultures may be offended by the types of intensely personal questions necessary for a medical history and may perceive them as an inexcusable invasion of privacy. If this occurs, your physician may be required to intervene to allay the patient's concerns.

Looking someone else directly in the eyes, or eye contact, is also perceived differently by people of various backgrounds. Eye contact occurs more often among friends and family members than among acquaintances or strangers. In the United States, someone who maintains good eye contact is usually perceived as being honest, believable, and concerned. In contrast, in some Asian and Mideastern cultures, direct eye contact is perceived as sexually suggestive or disrespectful. In other cultures, lack of eye contact or casting the eyes downward is a sign of respect.

In addition to cultural differences in values, many differences occur among individuals. Some people are just more reserved or shy than others and may feel less comfortable in medical settings. To help avoid

TABLE 3-1   Cultural Factors That Affect Patient Care[a]

Cultural Group	Family	Folk and Traditional Health Care	Common Health Problems
White	Nuclear family is highly valued Elderly family members may live in a nursing home when they can no longer care for themselves	Self-diagnosis of illnesses Use of over-the-counter drugs, especially vitamins and analgesics Dieting, especially fad diets Extensive use of exercise and exercise facilities	Cardiovascular disease Gastrointestinal disease Some forms of cancer Motor vehicle accidents Suicide Mental illness Substance abuse
African American	Close and supportive extended-family relationships Strong kinship ties with nonblood relatives from church or organizational and social groups Family unity, loyalty, and cooperation are important Frequently matriarchal	Varies extensively and may include spiritualists, herb doctors, root doctors, conjurers, skilled elder family members, voodoo, faith healing	Hypertension Sickle cell anemia Skin disorders; inflammation of hair follicles, various types of dermatitis and excessive growth of scar tissue (keloids) Lactose enzyme deficiency resulting in poor toleration of milk products High rate of tuberculosis Diabetes mellitus Higher infant mortality rate than in the white population
Asian	Welfare of the family is valued above the individual person Extended families are common A person's lineage (ancestors) is respected Sharing among family members is expected	Theoretical basis in Taoism, which seeks balance in all things Good health is achieved through proper balance between yin (feminine, negative, dark, cold) and yang (masculine, positive, light, warm) An imbalance in energy is caused by an improper diet or strong emotions Diseases and food are classified as hot or cold, and a proper balance between them will promote wellness (e.g., treat a cold disease with hot foods) Many Asian health care systems use herbs, diet, and application of hot or cold therapy Many Asians believe some points on the body are on the meridians, or energy pathways; if the energy flow is out of balance, treatment of the pathways may be necessary to restore the energy equilibrium *Acumassage:* Manipulation of points along the energy pathways *Acupressure:* Technique for compressing the energy pathway points *Acupuncture:* Insertion of fine needles into the body at energy pathway points	Tuberculosis Communicable diseases Malnutrition Suicide Various forms of mental illness Lactose enzyme deficiency

TABLE 3-1	Cultural Factors That Affect Patient Care[a] *(continued)*		
Cultural Group	**Family**	**Folk and Traditional Health Care**	**Common Health Problems**
Hispanic, Mexican American	Familial role is important *Compadrazgo:* Special bond between a child's parents and grandparents Family is the primary unit of society	*Curanderas(os):* Folk healers who base treatments on humoral pathology: basic functions of the body are controlled by four body fluids, or humors—blood, hot and wet; yellow bile, hot and dry; black bile, cold and dry; and phlegm, cold and wet The secret of good health is to balance hot and cold within the body; therefore, most foods, beverages, herbs, and medications are classified as hot (caliente) or cold (fresco, frio); a cold disease will be cured with a hot treatment	Diabetes mellitus and its complications Problems of poverty, such as poor nutrition, inadequate medical care, and poor prenatal care Lactose enzyme deficiency
Hispanic, Puerto Rican	*Compadrazgo:* similar to Mexican-American culture	Similar to that of other Spanish-speaking cultures	Parasitic diseases, such as dysentery, malaria, filariasis, hookworms Lactose enzyme deficiency
Native American	Families large and extended Grandparents are official and symbolic leaders and decision makers A child's namesake may assume equal parenting authority with biological parent	Medicine men (shamans) are frequently consulted Heavy use of herbs and psychological treatments, ceremonies, fasting, meditation, heat, and massage	Alcoholism Suicide Tuberculosis Malnutrition Communicable diseases Higher maternal and infant mortality rates than in most of the population Diabetes mellitus Hypertension Gallbladder disease

Reprinted with permission from Taylor C, Lillis C, LeMone P. Fundamentals of Nursing, 2nd ed. Philadelphia: Lippincott-Raven, 1996:122–125.
[a]The beliefs and practices vary within each group, and no assumptions should be based on a patient's cultural background alone. The factors in this table are merely a guide to some commonly observed and documented cultural factors.

miscommunication and offending patients, you must be sensitive to these differences in all of your patient interactions.

Stereotyping and Biased Opinions

Medical assisting deals with people of different ages, races, and sexual orientation. Sometimes, your values may be in stark contrast to those held by a patient, but you should not let your personal values or **biases** (opinions) affect your communication or treatment of a patient. All patients must be treated fairly, respectfully, and with dignity, regardless of their cultural, social, or personal values. To treat them in any other fashion is **discrimination**.

Stereotyping is holding an opinion of all members of a particular culture, race, religion, age group, or other group based on oversimplified or negative characterizations. It is a form of prejudice. Examples of negative stereotypes include "All old people are frail and senile" and "Those people are always dirty and never bathe."

If you need to call a hearing-impaired patient, keep in mind that patients can make and receive calls using a special telephone with a service called converse communication center, which uses a system called telecommunication device for the deaf (TDD) or a text telephone (TTY). If your office has either of these types of phones, you call the patient and type in your message. The patient reads your message and types a response. If your office does not have one of these phones, your local telephone company can communicate with TDD/TTY users and nonusers. Check your telephone directory for more information. Most hospitals have TDD/TTY phones available.

 CHECKPOINT QUESTION

4. How does the TDD system work?

 AFF WHAT IF?

A patient is hearing impaired, and you cannot communicate with him to explain the procedure you are about to perform. What should you do?

If the patient does not understand the procedure, he or she is not *informed*. Legally, you have not met your responsibilities to obtain informed consent if the patient does not understand the information you are trying to convey (see Legal Tip box; also see Chapter 2 for more information about informed consent).

Most community colleges offer courses in sign language. The Internet offers a site for the deaf community that will direct you to resources in your area. The American Sign Language alphabet chart is available online. It can be printed out for use with hearing-impaired patients. Handspeak is another Web site that provides a visual language dictionary. These Web sites are listed at the end of this chapter in the Media Menu. Medicine and technology promise to continue to improve communication for the deaf in the form of cochlear inplants, computer software, and digital capabilities that we can only imagine. We should be doing everything we can to give the same experience to every patient. Prepare yourself to face the communication challenges you might encounter.

Sight-Impaired Patients

Sight impairments range from complete blindness to blurred vision. The changes in vision tend to be slow and progressive. Some common medical conditions that can cause visual impairment include cataracts, glaucoma, macular degeneration, retinal detachment, hyperopia (farsightedness), myopia (nearsightedness), nyctalopia (night blindness), retinopathy, strabismus, and presbyopia. Patients who cannot see lose valuable information from nonverbal communication. To improve communication with a sight-impaired patient, try these suggestions.

1. Identify yourself by name each time the patient comes into the office.
2. Do not raise your voice; the patient is not hearing impaired.
3. Let the patient know exactly what you will be doing at all times, and alert him or her before touching.
4. Orient the patient spatially by having him or her touch the table, the chair, the counter, and so forth.
5. Assist the patient by offering your arm and escorting him or her to the interview room.
6. Tell the patient when you are leaving the room and knock before entering.
7. Explain the sounds of machines to be used in the examination (e.g., buzzing, whirring) and what each machine will do.

Speech Impairments

Speech impairments can come from a variety of medical conditions. The medical term for difficulty with speech is **dysphasia**. Dysphasia is usually the result of a neurologic problem. A common neurologic condition that can result in dysphasia is a stroke. **Dysphonia** is a voice impairment that is caused by a physical condition, such as oral surgery, cancer of the tongue or voice box, or cleft palate. Stuttering is another medical condition that can impair the patient's ability to communicate.

Here are some suggestions to help you communicate with a patient who has a speech impediment:

- Allow such patients time to gather their thoughts.
- Allow plenty of time for them to communicate.
- Do not rush conversations.
- Offer a note pad to write questions.
- Discuss with the physician the potential benefits for getting a speech therapist referral for the patient.

 CHECKPOINT QUESTION

5. What is the difference between dysphasia and dysphonia?

Mental Health Illnesses

Many mental illnesses and psychiatric disorders can impair a patient's ability to communicate. These illnesses produce a broad range of communication challenges. Some illnesses can cause the patient to have uncontrollable outbursts, whereas others can cause a mute condition in which the patient will not communicate at all. Some patients may hear voices that direct their communication to a given topic, whereas others may see objects that do not exist and will want confirmation from you that you see the objects. Communicating with patients with moderate to severe psychiatric disorders requires in-depth training. It is important to stress that not all patients with mental illnesses will be challenges. Most mental illnesses can be controlled and treated with medications and other therapies. Here are a few suggestions for communicating with patients who have mild mental illnesses.

- Tell the patient what to expect and when things will happen.
- Keep conversations focused and professional.
- Do not force or demand answers from patients who are withdrawn or mute.
- If you feel unsafe communicating with a given patient, speak to either your supervisor or the physician regarding your concerns.
- Do not confirm hearing voices or seeing nonexistent objects.
- Orient the patient to reality as appropriate.

Patients with a history of substance abuse, alcoholism, and other addictions can also present a communication challenge. Patients may have euphoria and communicate with a flight of ideas. Or they may demonstrate aggression and agitation while they are withdrawing from the addiction. Your responsibility in communicating with patients who have any of these conditions is to identify the reasons for today's visit and follow your regular assessment duties. It is not the role of the medical assistant to recommend treatments or counseling for these patients. Your communication should be professional, nonjudgmental, and encouraging when appropriate.

Angry or Distressed Patients

Patients' emotions can run the spectrum from polite and cordial to angry and upset. There are numerous reasons for the latter. Prolonged waiting times, financial issues, and illness can spark untoward emotions. At some time in our lives, we all have had a cold, felt terrible, and snapped angrily at an innocent bystander. The key to communicating with upset patients is to prevent an escalation of the problem. Keep your patients informed about waiting times, billing and insurance changes, and other office policies that might trigger untoward emotions (Box 3-2).

It is understandable that patients will become upset on hearing sad or unfortunate news about their health. Most patients take sad news in a calm manner. It is important to offer assistance as needed. Provide written instructions and information for the patient to read later. This material should consist of information on the diagnosis, causes of the illness, treatment options, and phone numbers that the patient may call for additional information.

AFF **BOX 3-2**

CASE SCENARIO: COMMUNICATING WITH A PATIENT WHO IS UPSET

Mr. Hunt, an elderly, long-time patient, calls the office and asks to speak to the doctor. When you inquire about the nature of his call, he begins to get louder and more upset.

Note: When patients ask to speak directly to the doctor, it is usually because they don't understand the workings of the office. Let the patient know that it is your job to screen the doctor's calls.

Mr. Hunt: "I just got this bill in the mail, and it says that I owe Dr. Smith $152.00. He is crazy if he thinks I'm paying this."

Note: Patients will say things they regret later. You may want to just let this one go.

Medical Assistant (MA): "I would be glad to help you with this, Mr. Hunt. Please hold while I look at your account."

Note: Putting the patient on hold may calm him down.

Mr. Hunt: "I'm not holding on very long."

Note: You can assure him that you will be right back.

MA: "I see that your balance is $152.00, Mr. Hunt, but you may make arrangements to pay this over several months."

Note: Giving the patient options may calm him down.

Mr. Hunt: "I'm not paying it at all because Dr. Smith didn't help me. I'm no better."

Note: A statement like this is upsetting, but you must remain professional.

MA: "I'm so sorry you are not feeling better, but Dr. Smith performed a service that you agreed to pay for. I will be happy to make you another appointment to come in and talk with him about a different course of treatment."

Note: Be firm but kind. Hopefully being firm will let the patient know who is in charge, but kindness will help defuse the anger.

Mr. Hunt: "I'll make an appointment, but I am not paying until I talk to the doctor."

Note: Again, you must not show your own feelings.

MA: "I will make a note of that on your account, and we can see you tomorrow at 9:30. Is that all right?"

Note: Documenting the patient's call will alert anyone working with the account. You would not want to add fuel to the flame by sending him another bill right away or making a collection call.

(continued)

BOX 3-2 *(continued)*

Mr. Hunt: "I'll be there, but you can tell that doctor that I'll have a thing or two to say to him."

Note: Document the conversation in the chart and be sure that the physician knows what to expect during the visit.

MA: "I hope we can resolve this, Mr. Hunt. We will see you tomorrow."

Note: You must remain calm and in control of the conversation.

Here are some suggestions that will help you communicate with an angry or distressed patient.

- Be supportive.
- Be open and honest in all communication.
- Do not provide false reassurances.
- Do not belittle the problem or concern.
- Ensure your own safety if the angry patient becomes aggressive or threatening.

Children

Levels of comprehension vary greatly during childhood, and therefore, communication needs must be tailored to the specific child's needs. The following suggestions will help facilitate communication:

1. Children are responsive to eye-level contact. Either raise them to your height or lower yourself to theirs (Fig. 3-5).
2. Keep your voice low-pitched and gentle.
3. Make your movements slow and keep them visible. Tell children when you need to touch them.
4. Rephrase your questions until you are sure that the child understands.

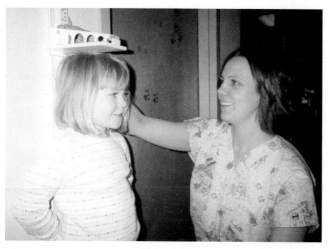

Figure 3-5 The medical assistant communicates at the child's eye level.

5. Be prepared for the child to return to a lower developmental level for comfort during an illness. For example, a child may revert to thumb sucking during a stressful event.
6. Use play to phrase your questions and to gain the child's cooperation. (For example, if the child appears shy and does not want to talk, start by asking the child how a stuffed animal feels today. "How does teddy feel today?" Follow up on the child's answer with "And how do you feel?" Offering to take the teddy's temperature first may lessen any fear of thermometers.)
7. Allow the child to express fear, to cry, and so on.
8. Many adolescents resent authority. During the interview, some teenagers may not want a parent in the room. Assess the situation before including the parent.
9. Never show shock or judgment when dealing with adolescents; this will immediately close communication.

COG Communicating with a Grieving Patient or Family Member

Occasionally, you will need to support patients who are in **grief** or great sadness caused by a loss. Grieving starts when a person experiences a significant loss, such as the loss of a loved one through death or the end of a relationship, a body part, or personal health. Grief includes such emotional responses as anger, sadness, and depression, and each emotion may trigger certain behaviors. For example, anger may result in outbursts, sadness may cause crying, and depression may lead to unusual quietness or isolation.

Dr. Elisabeth Kübler-Ross identified five distinct stages in the human grieving process. In her book *On Death and Dying*, she lists these stages that follow the realization that a person has a terminal illness: denial, anger, bargaining, depression, and acceptance. Dr. Kübler-Ross believed that these stages are also found in those experiencing change. Box 3-3 outlines these stages with examples. These stages may spread over months or years. It is possible to go through stages more than once. Sometimes, the collective signs of grief are referred to as **mourning**.

In medical settings, expect to see grief displayed in many ways. Know, too, that several factors can influence how a patient demonstrates grief and that different cultures and individuals demonstrate their grief in a variety of ways, ranging from stoic, impassive responses to loud, prolonged wailing and fainting. Other responses may reflect religious beliefs about the meaning of death. Grieving is a unique and personal process. There is no set time period for grieving, and there is no "right" way to grieve. It is very important to remember that everyone grieves in their way at their own pace.

BOX 3-3

THE FIVE STAGES OF GRIEVING AS IDENTIFIED BY ELISABETH KÜBLER-ROSS

Mechanism	Quote
Denial	"The doctor must have read the test wrong." "I don't have cancer; I feel fine."
Anger	"I hate the doctor." "This is a terrible place."
Bargaining	"God, I will be the best person I can be if you take away this disease."
Depression	"I don't care if I live anymore."
Acceptance	"I understand that I have terminal disease and am going to die."

Grieving patients may want to talk about their feelings and review events. Terminally ill patients may want to discuss their fears of dying and concerns for surviving loved ones. Many times, it is too difficult to discuss dying with family members. Dying patients may want to spare their family's feelings. To support grieving patients, allow time for them to express themselves and actively listen to what they say. When appropriate, consider using touch to convey your understanding. If patients' concerns stem from a lack of understanding about their condition, provide pertinent education for them and for their caregivers (if appropriate). You should also become familiar with available community resources, such as grief or other counseling services and hospice care, so you can assist the patient and physician when these services are necessary.

It is normal for you to feel sad when a patient dies. It is important that your communication focuses on empathy, not sympathy. Many psychologists describe sympathy as feeling *for* someone and empathy as feeling *with* someone. In the health care setting, empathy means trying to understand what patients are feeling so you can help them. Empathy can help you recognize a patient's fear and discomfort so you can do everything possible to provide support and reassurance.

Sympathy, or pitying your patient, may compromise your professional distance and cause you to become personally involved. Box 3-4 offers suggestions for helping grieving patients.

CHECKPOINT QUESTION

6. What are the five stages of grieving?

BOX 3-4

COMMUNICATING WITH A GRIEVING FAMILY MEMBER OR PATIENT

Patients and families faced with great loss can be helped through a variety of community resources. Hospice is a national program that offers support to patients and family members dealing with a loss. Hospice deals with all types of medical conditions and with people of all ages. The earlier the patient is introduced to a hospice program, the more beneficial. Hospice does have a palliative component. Hospice staff and volunteer grief counselors are trained to answer the questions, acknowledge the fears and anger, ease the transition, and offer respite for caregivers. A patient must never be forced to use hospice or other community resources. Grieving is an individual experience. Your local hospital may also have grief counselors or social workers who can help your patients. Other community resources may be available. The knowledgeable medical assistant will, with the physician's permission, direct the patient and the family to the proper organization.

COG Establishing Positive Patient Relationships

Your approach to patients conveys a message about who you are and how you feel about yourself and your profession. Medical assistants can be role models, earning the trust and admiration of patients. To establish and maintain positive relationships with patients, speak respectfully and exhibit an appropriate demeanor during all interactions. See Box 3-5 for guidance in communicating with patients on an individual basis.

Proper Form of Address

The way you address patients provides clues about your attitude and how you will likely provide care. When greeting patients, use a proper form of address, for example, "Good morning, Mr. Jones!" or "How are you feeling, Mrs. Smith?" This type of address shows respect and sets a professional tone. In contrast, calling patients by pet names, such as sweetie, granny, gramps, or honey, can offend the person. These terms denigrate the individual's dignity and put the interaction on a personal, not professional, level. Always call patients by their last name unless and until they instruct you otherwise. Some people are bothered or offended by being addressed by their first names; others prefer it. When patients indicate

AFF **BOX 3-5**

CHECK YOUR BEHAVIOR WHEN RESPONDING TO NONVERBAL COMMUNICATIONS

Consider this scenario:

You are interviewing a patient having a complete physical. You can sense that the 75-year-old man is nervous about his exam. He is obviously a shy man. He makes no eye contact. He keeps his arms folded on his chest. He asks that his 82-year-old wife remain with him. She provides the answers to your questions, and he seems to be more nervous as you progress through the patient history. His wife reports a previous head injury 5 years ago, and you realize that he is limited in his mental abilities.

How will you communicate with this patient now that you know more about his individual situation?

1. Watch for nonverbal cues before touching him. He needs to be calmed, but his shyness may make the touch uncomfortable.
2. Because he depends on his wife for understanding, speak to both of them.
3. Speak slowly and calmly.
4. Use simple language.
5. Try to calm his nerves by explaining what he can expect.
6. Give written instructions and materials with contact information if they have questions later.

a preference or ask you specifically to use their first name, document this in the chart so others will know.

Other inappropriate forms of address include referring to the patient as a medical condition, such as "the gallbladder in room 2" or "the broken arm in the waiting room." Patients often come to the medical office feeling anxious, so they may be particularly sensitive to everything they see and hear (or overhear). Referring to the patient as a medical condition sends the message that the staff values the patient as nothing more than an illness, which can lead to heightened anxiety.

Professional Distance

As discussed in Chapter 1, you must stay within certain boundaries when dealing with patients. How people interact with each other is influenced by the level of emotional involvement between them. For instance, communication between a husband and wife is more intimate than the personal level of communication between friends or the social level of communication between acquaintances. In the health care setting, you must establish an appropriate level of communication to be effective. You should not become too personally involved with patients because doing so may jeopardize your ability to be objective. It is easy to become overattached, especially to elderly patients who are lonely. For example, do not offer to drive patients to appointments, pick up prescriptions, or do their grocery shopping. Keeping a professional distance allows you to deal objectively with patients while creating a therapeutic environment. To keep this distance, avoid revealing intimate information about yourself (e.g., marital woes, financial troubles, family conflict) that might shift the dynamics of the relationship to a more personal level. Small talk may put a patient at ease, and you may need to distract a patient who is going through an unpleasant treatment or procedure, but be careful to choose general topics and keep the conversation light. Often, in an attempt to comfort a patient, we might say, "My grandmother was diagnosed with cancer too, but she is fine; it's not a big deal. You will be okay too." Every situation is different. The patient may misinterpret this to mean that you don't think that his or her diagnosis of cancer is a big deal. But at that moment, it is a very big deal to the patient!

Teaching Patients

One of the fundamental communication skills you will need is the ability to teach patients about their medical conditions (see Chapter 4). Teaching patients might involve something as relatively simple as explaining how often they should take a medication or instructing a newly diagnosed diabetic patient about self-injection. The guidelines listed below incorporate such key communication skills as interviewing and active listening. Follow these to provide effective patient education.

1. Be knowledgeable about current medical issues, discoveries, and trends.
2. Be aware of special services available in your area.
3. Have pertinent handouts or information sheets available.
4. Allow enough teaching time so that you are not interrupted or rushed.
5. Find a quiet room away from the main office flow if at all possible.
6. Give information in a clear, concise, sequential manner; provide written instructions as a follow-up.
7. Allow the patient time to process this new information.
8. Encourage the patient to ask questions.
9. Ask open-ended questions in a way that will allow you to know whether the patient understands the material.
10. Invite the patient to call the office with additional questions that may arise.

COG Professional Communication

Assertiveness in Professional Communication

The line between being assertive and being aggressive is very thin. The key to effective communication in a professional setting is learning the difference between the two and ensuring that you never cross the line.

An assertive person:

- Sets clear boundaries for himself or herself and others
- Knows how to set limits
- Clearly and politely communicates his or her wants and needs
- Can say "no" without offending another person
- Understands the appropriate time for assertiveness versus passive compliance
- Refuses to be inappropriately dominated or "handled"
- Considers the feelings and roles of others
- Voices differences of opinion without being rude or overbearing
- Stands up for what he or she believes when appropriate
- Holds himself or herself with confidence and maintains eye contact
- Looks for compromise, not conflict
- Speaks firmly but pleasantly
- Respects others
- Understands when he or she is about to "step over a line" and pulls back
- Is honest and fair

An aggressive person, however, is hostile, threatening, demanding, loud, annoying, sarcastic, angry, and, often, mean. Aggressive employees want everything *their* way and, although they may listen to other people, they don't *hear* other people.

For instance, say your boss has asked you to work the last two weekends to process a backlog of claims and is now asking you to work next weekend as well. You do not want to work yet another weekend. A meek, unassertive person would swallow her anger and work the weekend, all the while building up resentment. An aggressive person would announce in front of his or her coworkers, "No, I'm not working one more weekend; it's not in my job description." An assertive person, however, would meet with his or her boss privately, explain his or her desire to return to normal business hours, and help find another solution to the claims backlog.

Which type of person are you?

Communicating with Peers

Communication among your peers must remain professional and appropriate throughout the workday. Discussions of non-work-related topics should be kept to a minimum and occur only during designated break times. It is not appropriate to discuss last night's TV shows, family issues, shopping lists, and so on in front of patients. Excessive laughing, high-pitched voice tones, and whispering can produce an unprofessional atmosphere.

During your career, you may come across a situation that requires communication with your supervisor about another peer's actions. Your communication must always be honest and accurate when reporting facts to a supervisor. Embellishing or hiding information can result in termination of your employment.

An excellent way to promote communication among your peers is to become active in your local professional organization. Your involvement at the local level can spread to national exposure. Involvement in local community organizations and support groups is also beneficial to promoting you and your profession.

Communicating with Physicians

Physicians and other health care practitioners will rely on you to communicate pertinent information to patients in a timely manner to provide quality care. Your communication must always be professional. The physician should always be addressed as doctor unless he specifies otherwise. The use of inappropriate terms is never acceptable. When possible, the correct medical terminology should be used. If you are unsure of the correct medical term, however, explain the condition rather than use a term that you do not understand. For example, if a patient comes into the office with a chief complaint of difficulty urinating, simply say, "Mr. Bowen is complaining of trouble urinating." Never use a slang expression, such as "He is having trouble peeing."

Do not feel intimidated when speaking to a physician. Speak slowly and confidently and you will develop a professional rapport. Be honest. It is better to say, "I am not sure what to do with this specimen" than to assume and make a mistake.

Remember, there is a time and place for everything. The physician may be the biggest jokester or sports fan in the office, but it is not appropriate to draw on these topics in front of patients or family members.

Communicating with Other Facilities

The medical administrative staff often makes referrals to other facilities or physicians. When contacting other facilities, follow these key points:

- Maintain patient confidentiality. Make sure you have appropriate patient consent.
- Observe all legal requirements for dispensing patient data.

- Use caution with fax machines, e-mail, and other electronic devices. Make sure the intended receiver is the one who gets the communication.
- Provide only the facts. Do not relay suspicions or assumptions.
- Always be nonjudgmental.
- Confirm that the message was received and that the referral will be handled.

español SPANISH TERMINOLOGY

Hable despacio, por favor.
　　Please speak slowly.

Sí, hablo un poco de español.
　　Yes, I speak Spanish a little.

No, no entiendo.
　　No, I don't understand.

¿Entiende?
　　Do you understand?

¿Cuándo?
　　When?

¿De qué tipo?
　　What kind?

¿Porqué?
　　Why?

¿Cuántos?
　　How many?

¿Cuánto?
　　How much?

¿Qué?
　　What?

¿En qué puedo ayudarlo?
　　What can I help you with?

¿Dígame, porque está aquí?
　　Tell me, why are you here?

¿Cómo?
　　How?

MEDIA MENU

- **Student Resources on thePoint**
  - **CMA/RMA Certification Exam Review**
- **Internet Resources**

　National Institute of Deafness and Other Communication Disorders
　http://www.nidcd.nih.gov
　National Association for the Deaf
　http://www.nad.org
　American Speech-Language-Hearing Association
　http://www.asha.org
　Hearing, Speech and Deafness Center
　http://www.hsdc.org
　National Hospice and Palliative Care Organization
　http://www.nhpco.org
　Handspeak: American Sign Language Online Dictionary
　http://www.handspeak.com

- Communication is a complex and dynamic process involving the sending and receiving of messages. It includes verbal and nonverbal forms of expression and is influenced by personal and societal values, individual beliefs, and cultural orientation.
- In the medical practice, important aspects of patient communication are interviewing and active listening.
- You will need to overcome many communication challenges to communicate with all patients. These challenges include patients with hearing, sight, and speech impairments.
- Children, angry or distressed patients, and patients with mental illnesses can also present a challenge to communication.
- To communicate effectively, you must understand the various factors that can affect the exchange of messages and use the communication techniques that are most appropriate for each individual situation.

Warm Ups for Critical Thinking

1. Dr. Hedrick has just told a patient that she has breast cancer. The words "breast cancer" can spark many emotions and fears. Write three sample questions that you could ask the patient to promote open communication about her feelings.

2. Dr. Yevin has just discharged a patient with specific instructions for crutch walking. How would you determine the patient's understanding of these instructions? Can nonverbal clues help you determine whether the patient is confused?

3. A mother brings in her 3-year-old child for a checkup. The child refuses to open her mouth so the doctor can examine her throat. How would you go about communicating the importance of this? What if the child was 6 years old?

4. A patient arrives in your office demanding to see the physician immediately. He is yelling and obviously very angry. The doctor is with another patient. Write three statements that you could say that might help the situation. Write three statements that would escalate the situation.

5. List five local resources that can assist a grieving patient or family member. Include the name of the agency, type of help that it offers, any special information, and its phone number.

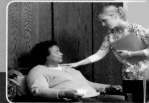

Patient Education

Outline

The Patient Education Process
Assessment
Planning
Implementation
Evaluation
Documentation
Conditions Needed for Patient Education
Maslow's Hierarchy of Needs
Environment
Equipment
Knowledge

Resources
Factors that Can Hinder Education
Existing Illnesses
Communication Barriers
Age
Educational Background
Physical Impairments
Other Factors
Teaching Specific Health Care Topics
Preventive Medicine

Lifestyle Changes
Medications
Alternative Medicine
Stress Management
Patient Teaching Plans
Developing a Plan
Selecting and Adapting Teaching Material
Developing Your Own Material
Locating Community Resources and Disseminating Information

Learning Outcomes

Cognitive Domain

Note: AAMA/CAAHEP Standards are italicized.

1. Spell and define the key terms
2. Explain the medical assistant's role in patient education
3. Define the five steps in the patient education process
4. Identify five conditions that are needed for patient education to occur
5. Explain Maslow's hierarchy of human needs
6. List five factors that may hinder patient education and at least two methods to compensate for each of these factors
7. Discuss five preventive medicine guidelines that you should teach your patients
8. Explain the kinds of information that should be included in patient teaching about medication therapy
9. Explain your role in teaching patients about alternative medicine therapies
10. List and explain relaxation techniques that you and patients can learn to help with stress management

11. Describe how to prepare a teaching plan
12. List potential sources of patient education materials
13. Locate community resources and list ways of organizing and disseminating information
14. *Recognize communication barriers*
15. *Identify techniques for overcoming communication barriers*
16. *Identify resources and adaptations that are required based on individual needs, i.e., culture and environment, developmental life stage, language, and physical threats to communication*

Psychomotor Domain

Note: AAMA/CAAHEP 2008 Standards are italicized.

1. *Document patient education (Procedure 4-1)*
2. *Develop and maintain a current list of community resources related to the patient's health care needs (Procedure 4-2)*

Affective Domain

Note: AAMA/CAAHEP 2008 Standards are italicized.

1. *Use language/verbal skills that enable patients' understanding*
2. *Demonstrate respect for diversity in approaching patients and families*
3. *Demonstrate empathy in communicating with patients, family, and staff*
4. *Demonstrate sensitivity appropriate to the message being delivered*
5. *Demonstrate recognition of the patient's level of understanding in communications*
6. *Demonstrate sensitivity to patient rights*

ABHES Competencies

1. Identify and respond appropriately when working/caring for patients with special needs
2. Adapt to individualized needs
3. Communicate on the recipient's level of comprehension
4. Be impartial and show empathy when dealing with patients

Key Terms

alternative medicine	documentation	learning objectives	planning
assessment	evaluation	noncompliance	psychomotor
disseminates	implementation	placebo	stress

In the current health care climate of short hospital stays, patients seen in the medical office typically have acute conditions requiring intensive and extensive education from their health care provider. This will be one of your most challenging and rewarding roles as a medical assistant. Of course, you will not be responsible for teaching patients everything they need to know about health care. Patient education is performed under the direction of the physician. The amount and types of education that you will be expected to do will vary greatly from office to office. This chapter will give you the foundation needed for providing patient education.

COG The Patient Education Process

Patient education involves more than telling patients which medications they need to take or which lifestyle behaviors they need to change and expecting them to follow these instructions blindly. To educate patients effectively, you need to help them accept their illness, involve them in the process of gaining knowledge, and provide positive reinforcement. Ultimately, that knowledge should lead to a change in behavior or attitudes.

The process of patient education involves five major steps:

- Assessment
- Planning
- Implementation
- Evaluation
- Documentation

These five steps collectively produce the teaching plan. The plan may be formally written as the process is occurring or may be documented after the event. You must follow all these steps to achieve effective patient education.

Assessment

Before you begin to teach, you must assess your feelings and attitudes about the patient and the topic to be taught. Sometimes in your career as a medical assistant, you may encounter situations or patients that make you feel uncomfortable. Your role as an educator, however, requires that you set aside your own personal feelings and life experiences to instruct the patient objectively and to the best of your ability. Always consider how your responses and actions will affect the patient, and be sure to treat each patient impartially.

Assessment requires gathering information about the patient's present health care needs and abilities.

In addition to knowing the present health care needs, you must also look at these other areas:

- Past medical and surgical conditions
- Current understanding and acceptance of health problems

- Needs for additional information
- Feelings about their health care status
- Factors that may hinder learning (covered in detail later in the chapter)

You may obtain this information from a number of sources. The most comprehensive source will be the medical record. The patient's medical record consists of all information regarding current diagnoses, treatments, medications, past medical history, and a variety of other documentation. Some medical records have a problem list on the inside cover. This will provide you with a snapshot of the patient and save you time from reading the entire document. Other sources of information will be the physician, family members, significant others, and other members of the health care team. When you have collected all of the assessment data, you are ready to start the next step of the education process: planning.

 CHECKPOINT QUESTION

1. What is the purpose of the assessment step during patient education?

Planning

Planning involves using the information you have gathered during the assessment phase to determine how you will approach the patient's learning needs. If possible, involve the patient in this part of the process. Learning goals and objectives that are established with input from the patient are most meaningful. A patient's learning goal is what the patient and educator want to be the outcome of the program. The patient's **learning objectives** include procedures or tasks that will be discussed or performed at various points in the program to help achieve the goal. Make certain the objectives you establish are specific for each individual patient and are measurable in some manner. If the objectives are measurable, you will be able to evaluate when or whether the patient successfully completed them.

For example, consider a patient who needs to limit his fluid intake. Which of the following objectives is more specific and would allow you to evaluate the patient's progress? (1) The patient understands why he should limit his fluid intake, or (2) the patient is able to prepare a schedule for daily fluid intake and explain why it is important that he limit his fluids. The second objective is more specific and not only evaluates the patient's understanding but also requires the patient to demonstrate understanding. Having patients prepare their own schedule gets them involved in their health care. It allows them to customize the schedule to fit their lifestyle, which is likely to increase compliance.

Implementation

After you establish the need for patient teaching and agree on the goals and objectives, you begin implementation. **Implementation is the process used to perform the actual teaching.** The teaching usually is carried out in several steps. Box 4-1 presents some commonly used teaching strategies. For example, you may start by telling the patient how to use crutches, followed by a demonstration, and finally, the patient may do a return demonstration. Patients also benefit from the use of teaching aids (drawings, charts, graphs, pamphlets) that they can take home and use as reference material. You can also use videos and audiocassettes to supplement the implementation process.

Miscommunication or misinterpretation can lead to serious complications or injury. For example, assume you are teaching a patient to use crutches. It is very important that you stress to the patient that the crutch must not press directly into the axillary area. (There should be a two-finger distance between the crutch and the armpit.) If the patient does not comprehend the

---

BOX 4-1

IMPLEMENTATION STRATEGIES

Implementing the learning process should be individualized to the patient's best method of comprehension and retention. These may include:

1. *Lecture and demonstration.* This method presents the information in the most basic form but requires no patient participation for reinforcement and retention.
2. *Role playing and demonstration.* The patient watches you perform a medical procedure, then performs it to ensure understanding. Information is more likely to be recalled if the patient actively participates in the process.
3. *Discussion.* This two-way exchange of information and ideas works well for lifestyle changes (e.g., making dietary changes to lower cholesterol) rather than for medical procedures.
4. *Audiovisual material.* Audiocassettes or videos can often be taken home and reviewed by the patient and family members as needed. This allows for reinforcement of teachings and provides both visual and auditory stimulation.
5. *Printed material and programmed instructions.* All information should be discussed with the patient to clarify points and to elicit questions before assuming that the instructions are understood.

dangers of nerve damage to the axillary area from pressing the crutch into the armpit, a serious complication to the patient could occur. Miscommunication about medications can have fatal consequences. The implementation stage may occur once or over a longer period. The disease process and the patient's ability to comprehend information will dictate the length of teaching. For example, teaching a patient about diabetes takes place over multiple sessions. The first session may focus on what diabetes is, while subsequent teachings may include topics such as diet, foot care, glucose monitoring, and insulin injection.

After implementation of a given skill or knowledge, you must determine whether your teaching was effective. This step is called evaluation.

Evaluation

Is the patient progressing? Did the teaching plan work? Does the plan need any changes? These are a few of the questions you may ask yourself when you begin to evaluate. **Evaluation is the process that indicates how well patients are adapting or applying new information to their lives.**

In the medical setting, where contact with patients is limited, part of the evaluation may have to be done by patients at home. For example, if office visits for direct observation are not scheduled, patients will be responsible for telephoning and reporting their status. In other words, can patients do the task they were taught, or are they having troubles? If they voice concern or appear unclear about their instructions, you should either redirect them on the phone or schedule them for an office appointment.

During the evaluation, you may discover **noncompliance**. Noncompliance is the patient's inability or refusal to follow a prescribed order. After determining that the given order is not being followed, your first step is to determine why the order is not being followed. It may be a misunderstanding. For example, a patient who is to take a certain medication twice a day may be taking it only twice a week because that is what he or she thought you said. If the noncompliance is because the patient refuses to follow these orders, however, you must notify the physician. Remember that the patient has the right to refuse medical treatment unless the patient is determined to be mentally incompetent. The physician will determine the next appropriate action in these cases. Evaluation is an ongoing process, so you should expect to update and modify your plan periodically.

 CHECKPOINT QUESTION

2. What is the purpose of evaluation during patient education?

 AFF WHAT IF?

You are instructing a 60-year-old gentleman in the use of a Holter monitor (an ambulatory heart monitor) when he tells you that he has not been taking his heart medication because it makes him feel tired. You have heard Dr. Jones tell other patients that this particular medication can cause fatigue at first, but that the patient should keep taking it, and after several weeks, he will have more energy. Should you give the patient this information?

As long as you are sure that your information is correct, you should share this with the patient. The patient then says that he still does not want to take the medication, but he asks that you not to tell the doctor because he may get angry. Since the patient needs this medication for a serious problem, the doctor must be notified. A physician cannot force a patient to take his medication, but he may be able to convince him to take the medication. Perhaps the patient could try another medication that may not have the same effect. Remember to document the details of the encounter in the patient's chart.

Documentation

Documentation includes the recording of all teachings that have occurred. It should consist of the following information:

- Date and time of teaching.
- What information was taught, e.g., "Diabetes foot care was discussed. It consisted of the proper method for toenail cutting and regular examination by a podiatrist."
- How the information was taught, e.g., "ADA [American Diabetes Association] foot care video shown to the patient."
- Evaluation of teaching. For example, "Patient verbalized the need to make an appointment with a podiatrist."
- Any additional teaching planned, e.g., "Patient will return on Monday to the office with his wife for glucose monitoring instructions."

 AFF LEGAL TIP

ALWAYS REMEMBER TO DOCUMENT YOUR ACTIONS

There is a common saying in health care: "If it is not in the chart, it did not happen." In a court of law, the medical record is a health care professional's best defense. Always take special care to

(continued)

succinctly and accurately record every interaction with a patient and to give patients their instructions in writing. When patients receive a new diagnosis, provide educational materials about their disorder and direct them to appropriate Web sites. Document any instructions, information, or written materials given to the patient.

Box 4-2 has a charting example for patient education. Your signature implies that you performed the teaching. If this is untrue or if another staff member assisted you in teaching, make sure that information is clearly noted. Also include the names of any interpreters who were used. You must also document all telephone conversations (e.g., "I spoke with this patient via the telephone today, and he said he is testing his blood sugar every morning without problems.").

Documentation is essential because, from a legal viewpoint, procedures are only considered to have been done if they are recorded. Documentation should become second nature to you as you interact with patients each day. A complete and accurate medical record indicates good care and attention to detail.

COG Conditions Needed for Patient Education

Learning is the process of acquiring knowledge, wisdom, or skills through study or instruction. This process does not occur without certain conditions. Learning cannot occur without motivation or a perceived need to learn. For example, suppose you want to teach a patient about the need to adopt a low-sodium diet because of hypertension. Patients who feel that hypertension is not a problem, however, will not be motivated to learn the diet because they have not accepted the need for the teaching. For such patients to be taught, the following steps must occur:

1. The patient must accept that the hypertension has to be managed.
2. The patient must accept that there is a correlation between high sodium intake and hypertension.
3. The patient must accept and be willing to make this dietary change.

Only if these steps have occurred can teaching begin. In addition to patient motivation, basic human needs must be met first.

Maslow's Hierarchy of Needs

Abraham Maslow, an American psychiatrist, recognized that people are motivated by needs and that certain basic needs must be met before people can progress to higher needs, such as taking personal responsibility for their health (self-actualization). Maslow arranged human needs in the form of a pyramid, with basic needs at the bottom and the higher needs at the top (Fig. 4-1). The patient progresses upward, fulfilling different levels of needs toward the highest level, which results in a state of health and well-being. In your responsibility as an educator, you need to be aware that patients must have the basic needs satisfied before they are willing or able to learn to take care of their own health. Not everyone will start at the bottom of the pyramid. Some patients will never reach the top, while others may be at the top and slide backward as a result of unfortunate circumstances.

Physiologic needs are air, water, food, rest, and comfort. If these basic needs are unmet, the patient cannot begin the process. Everyone has a different tolerance and expectation for these needs. For example, one person

---

BOX 4-2

CHARTING EXAMPLE

11/27/12

Patient arrived in the office for teaching on the glucose meter; brought meter from home. Following steps were demonstrated by me: calibration of meter strips, battery change, finger sticks, strip insertion into machine, use of the patient logbook. Normal BGM ranges were reviewed along with the treatment of low blood sugar. Pt returned demonstration without problem. Reviewed glucose meter instructions manual with pt. Pt instructed to bring logbook to each MD appointment.—Margaret Blackwell, CMA

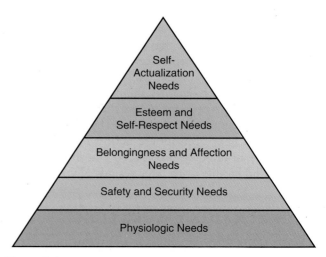

Figure 4-1 Maslow's hierarchy pyramid.

may expect that their food is served over three meals with full courses, while another person may accept that they will have one meal a day from a soup kitchen. If the patient perceives that these needs are met, we need to accept that and not judge the situation.

Safety and security needs include a safe environment and freedom from fear and anxiety. Patients are susceptible to fear and anxiety that accompany many medical conditions. For example, patients diagnosed with cancer may be so frightened that they are unable to think of anything but dying. Patients who have undergone some sort of trauma or disaster (hurricane, fire, motor vehicle accident) may place the need to feel safe above all other needs.

Affection needs, or the need for love and belonging, are essential for feeling connected and important to others. A sense of love or belonging can often be a powerful motivation for patients to try to regain good health.

Esteem needs involve our need to feel self-worth. Esteem can be self-generated, or it can come from those who admire us. If others value us or if we value ourselves, we are more likely to strive to maintain good health. Patients who lack self-esteem are less likely to want or accept education that targets improving their health. Thus, they will not see this as important information and will not be motivated to learn.

Self-actualization is the pinnacle of the pyramid, at which a person has satisfied all the other basic needs and feels personal responsibility and control over his or her own life. Self-actualized patients will strive to control their state of wellness by following all health directives and may even help others to achieve wellness. Not all patients will reach this level. Patients who have met this level will be ready to learn a multitude of health care skills and will strive to follow preventive health care maintenance guidelines.

After determining where on the pyramid the patient is, you can determine the appropriateness of education. For example, if the patient has not met the basic physiologic needs, you should help the patient meet these needs before beginning to teach. Patients who are in the middle levels may be able to focus and learn certain skills but may not be ready for complex teachings. If possible, you should involve family members or significant others in the teaching process.

 CHECKPOINT QUESTION

3. What are the basic physiologic needs outlined in Maslow's pyramid?

Environment

The environment where you teach must be conducive to learning. The room should be quiet and well lit and have limited distractions. It is not appropriate to teach patients a skill in a hallway, waiting room, or other high-traffic area. These areas produce distractions and prohibit confidentiality.

For patients to acquire knowledge, they must feel relaxed and comfortable. For example, it would be inappropriate to attempt to teach a patient who is sitting on an examination table with the stirrups in place. She will not feel comfortable. Reset the stirrups and direct the patient to dress and have a seat in a chair. If the patient had a procedure done in the room and bloody dressings or suture equipment is still present, clean the area and then return for teaching.

Equipment

A common type of education is teaching patients to perform a **psychomotor** skill. A psychomotor skill requires the participant to physically perform a task. Some examples include crutch walking, glucose monitoring, eye drop instillation, and dressing changes. The equipment for the skill must be present and functional. If possible, the equipment should be from the patient's home or be the exact replica of it.

The steps to teach a psychomotor skill are as follows:

1. Demonstrate the entire skill.
2. Demonstrate the skill step by step, explaining each step as you complete it.
3. Have the patient demonstrate the skill with your help.
4. Have the patient demonstrate the skill without your help.

Provide positive reinforcement throughout the steps. Always provide written step-by-step instructions. Always include instructions from the manufacturer for use and maintenance of any equipment.

Knowledge

The person teaching the skill must have a solid knowledge of the material. Imagine how difficult it would be to learn to ski from an instructor who did not know how to put skis on. The same is true in medical assisting. If you are not comfortable or do not feel knowledgeable about the topic, ask for help before starting to teach a patient. Be reassured that you do not have to be an expert on the topic, but you do need to feel comfortable with the information. If you start teaching a given topic and the patient asks you a question that you are not able to answer, state that you are not sure about that specific piece but you will get the answer. Then, either research the answer or ask for help from another health care professional. Never guess or imply that you know something that you do not know.

Resources

For patient education to be effective, it must consist of multiple techniques or approaches. The more techniques that are used, the more the patient will learn and retain. The three ways that we can learn are through hearing, seeing, and touch. If you can apply at least two of these senses in your teaching, your patient will be more stimulated to learn and will remember more information. For example, if you were teaching a patient about the dangers of smoking, which of the following would be more effective: (1) giving the patient a pamphlet that explains the dangers of smoking along with statistical data, or (2) showing a patient a diagram of what a nonsmoker's lung looks like versus a smoker's and providing the patient with pamphlets about local smoking cessation programs? The teaching in the second approach would be more beneficial. The patient sees the dangers of smoking and receives a brochure that contains practical hands-on information.

Fortunately, there is a wealth of information available for patient education. Tools to help teach patients include audiocassettes, compact discs, food labels, Internet and Web sites, manikins, models (heart, lungs), plastic food settings, pamphlets, and videos.

In addition to the five conditions already discussed, these factors will be necessary for the patient to learn:

- Family or significant others should be present if the information is complex or if it will require their assistance. Family members are essential if the patient is confused or unreliable.
- Patients should be wearing any sensory devices that they need (glasses, hearing aids).
- Qualified interpreters should be present if needed.
- Written instructions and materials should be prepared.

COG Factors That Can Hinder Education

Many factors or circumstances can hinder learning. It is important to recognize these factors and intervene as appropriate. In certain cases, teaching may have to be delayed, or your teaching plan may have to be revised.

Existing Illnesses

The type of illness that patients have will play a large role in their ability and willingness to learn. Generally, patients with acute short-term illnesses will be motivated to learn a skill that will accelerate healing. Examples of short-term illnesses are orthopedic injuries (uncomplicated fractures, sprains), colds, and viruses.

These are six examples of illnesses or conditions that will affect learning:

- *Any illness in which the patient has moderate to severe pain.* Examples of these illnesses include neuropathies, bone cancer, kidney stones, and recent surgical procedures. The patient's pain level must reach a tolerable stage before teaching can start and the patient can concentrate on learning.
- *Any illness or condition with a poor prognosis or limited rehabilitation potential.* Examples include progressive neurologic disorders, certain cancers, and large traumatic events. It is important that you assess such patients' readiness to learn and their level of acceptance of their illness before you proceed with your teaching.
- *Any illness or condition that results in weakness and general malaise as a primary symptom.* Examples include gastrointestinal disorders that cause vomiting and diarrhea, anemia, Lyme disease, and recent blood transfusion. For these patients, teaching should be limited to the essential information and expanded on as the patient regains strength.
- *Any illness or condition that impairs the patient's mental health or cognitive abilities.* Examples of these conditions include brain tumors, Alzheimer's disease, substance abuse, and psychiatric disorders. In these patients, education should be provided to patients at their ability level. Family members or significant others should be brought in to complement the learning process.
- *Any patient who has more than one chronic illness.* For example, patients with diabetes often have cardiac, renal, and integumentary complications. In patients with multiple system failures, it is important to prioritize the learning needs. Focus your education on the main problem and work from there.
- *Any illness or condition that results in respiratory distress or difficult breathing.* Examples of these conditions include chronic obstructive pulmonary disease, pneumonias, lung cancer, and asthma. The priority goal is first to establish optimal oxygenation for the patient. Once this is met, you can begin teaching. These patients tend to become exhausted easily during acute exacerbations of their illnesses. Keep the teaching time short and to the point and expand teachings as their activity tolerance allows.

✓ CHECKPOINT QUESTION

4. List six types of conditions or illnesses that may hinder your ability to educate patients effectively.

Communication Barriers

Effective communication skills are essential for patient education. Any barriers to communication must be resolved before you can start teaching the patient. If an interpreter is needed for language translation or for hearing-impaired patients, schedule a time convenient to all parties (see Chapter 3).

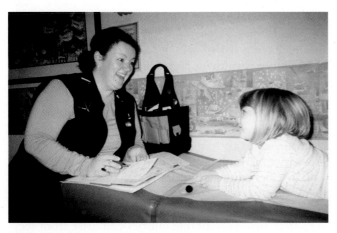

Figure 4-2 Establishing rapport with the child.

Age

The age of the patient plays a very important part in the amount and type of education that you can do. Small children need to be educated at an age-appropriate level (Fig. 4-2). For example, it would be inappropriate to teach a 2-year-old child how to assemble an asthma nebulizer. The parent or caregiver must be taught. It would be appropriate, however, to explain to the 2-year-old child that the nebulizer is not a toy and that it contains medication. Safety education is a prime teaching focus for small children and their parents. Box 4-3 presents some tips for communicating with and teaching children.

As children mature at different speeds, you should assess what information this child can handle and what information should not be shared with the child. Communication with the parents is essential. They know the

---

BOX 4-3

TIPS FOR TEACHING CHILDREN

Children require special communication skills and different teaching strategies. Here are a few tips to help you:

- Encourage the child to be part of the teaching process.
- Speak directly to the child.
- Avoid confusing medical terms.
- Avoid using baby language.
- Teach only age-appropriate information.
- Discuss with the parents the child's knowledge base about the illness and any feelings the parent may have regarding what they want the child to know. (This should not be done in front of the child.)
- Demonstrate skills on stuffed animals or dolls.

---

child's developmental stage. For example, a 7-year-old child who has just been diagnosed with diabetes needs to know the signs and symptoms of low blood sugar and how to treat it. The child may not be ready, however, to learn about the long-term complications (e.g., blindness, renal failure). It is important to teach the child that the disease must be well controlled to prevent future problems, but not to the extent that the child develops fear.

The challenge in teaching adults is that they often have multiple responsibilities to their children, spouses, or aging parents. Obligations at work, school, church, and other activities may also limit their free time. These obligations and responsibilities can interfere with willingness to learn and attentiveness. Your teaching may have to occur in short sessions over long periods. This age group may benefit from electronic resources that they can access on their own time schedule.

Elderly patients can be a challenge to teach for a variety of reasons. These reasons include confusion, lack of interest, and overall poor health. Some older patients, however, can be the most attentive and curious learners. It is fairly common for this age group to address items that they have heard on the news. For example, a patient may hear an advertisement for a new medication for arthritis and request clarification from you regarding its effectiveness.

 CHECKPOINT QUESTION

5. What is the primary teaching focus for small children and their parents?

Educational Background

Most initial health assessment forms ask patients what level of education they have obtained. This information may help you to determine the patient's ability to read. Caution is essential because graduation alone does not guarantee that the patient can read. You will need to use your tact and diplomacy to evaluate the situation.

Patients who have completed some college courses, however, are likely to be interested in preventive health care. Patients with an educational background in health care will still need the same attention and teaching from you. Do not assume that, since the patient is a nurse or a physician, you can skip teaching a skill. Their specialty may be in an unrelated area.

Physical Impairments

Numerous physical impairments may hinder learning. For example, patients with severe arthritis in their hands may have difficulty performing certain psychomotor skills, like giving themselves insulin. An occupational therapist is the best resource to assist you. Speak to the physician to obtain the proper referrals.

Other Factors

Other factors may hinder your ability to teach patients. The patient's culture may affect willingness to learn or the family's involvement in learning. Patients with financial troubles may not be ready to focus on learning new skills or knowledge. It is important that you assess the patient's readiness to learn and either try to remove or work around any obstacles that may be present.

COG Teaching Specific Health Care Topics

Your role in patient education will vary greatly. The topics that you will teach will depend on the patient, type of medical office, and physician's preferences. Staying well is a topic often discussed in the exam room. Medical assistants provide information and support about nutrition, exercise, and wellness. These topics are discussed in Chapter 16. Next are some other topics commonly taught by medical assistants.

Preventive Medicine

Preventing health problems is the key to living a long, healthy life. But the advantages to good preventive medicine extend much further. There are huge economic benefits to preventing illnesses. Millions of people are hospitalized each year. Caring for sick patients at home costs Medicare billions of dollars annually. These statistics affect everyone. They lead to higher taxes, higher health care insurance premiums, and limited programs for low-income families.

These are some commonly recommended preventive health care tips that you should teach all of your patients:

- Regular physical examinations for all age groups
- Annual flu and regular pneumonia vaccinations
- Adult immunizations for tetanus and hepatitis B
- Childhood immunizations
- Regular dental examinations
- Monthly breast self-examinations for women and regular physician examinations
- Cancer screening to include:
  - Mammograms
  - Colonoscopy
  - Annual Pap tests
  - Prostate-specific antigen blood tests for all men, along with need for regular digital rectal examinations

The frequency and age at which these procedures will be recommended to patients vary with the patient's medical history and genetics and the physician's preference. Some insurance will pay for these procedures, while others will not pay unless the procedure

is deemed diagnostic. Many hospitals and clinics offer free preventive screenings to patients. Your office should have a list of which free screenings are available. Public health departments may also have this information available for your patients. Most providers and insurance coverage base the frequency and type of testing on the guidelines set forth by the American Cancer Society.

Your role as a medical assistant is to promote preventive screenings. The physician you work with will instruct you in his or her recommendations for these tests.

Another large part of preventive medicine is teaching safety tips. Preventable injuries can arise from bicycle and car accidents, poisoning, fires, choking, falls, drownings, firearms, and lawn mowers. Toys can lead to injuries when they are broken or used by a child of an inappropriate age. The American Academy of Pediatrics (AAP) offers injury prevention tips for parents and health care providers. While working as a medical assistant, you will find valuable teaching tips to give to parents from their Web site. The AAP also provides numerous educational materials that can be mailed to physician offices and given to your patients.

According to the American Academy of Orthopaedic Surgeons (AAOS), falls cause 90% of the hip fractures that occur each year in the United States. By 2050, the AAOS estimates that the number of hip fractures per year will reach 650,000. Hip fractures require long hospitalizations and often rehabilitation in a nursing home. Most falls occur at home and are preventable. Fall prevention tips should be taught to all older patients or any patient who has a problem with maintaining balance or uses an ambulation device (cane, walker). Here are some tips that you can use to teach fall prevention:

- Encourage patients to remove all scatter rugs in their home. Remind patients to keep hallways clutter free.
- Instruct the patient to ensure adequate lighting in all rooms and hallways.
- Encourage the patient to avoid steps. Encourage one-floor living.
- Ensure that the patient has well-soled shoes or sneakers. Advise the patient to avoid wearing heels.
- Instruct the patient to place nonskid surfaces in bathtubs or purchase a shower chair.
- Instruct the patient to install handrails or grab bars in hallways and stairwells.
- Advise patients taking medications that lower their blood pressure to stand up slowly and get their balance, and then begin to walk.
- Advise patients to have regular eye examinations and have their glasses adjusted as needed.
- Encourage patients to have a plan for power outages and severe storms.

Lifestyle Changes

In addition to instructing patients, in many cases, you will be asking them to make changes in their lifestyle. Change is difficult for anyone. It is easier to continue doing what you have always done. Some patients view illness as strong motivation to follow the physician's orders. Others are resistant to eating less and moving more to lose extra pounds or beginning a walking program to help their arthritis. You can help with the difficult process of change. Encouragement and close follow-up are effective ways to keep a patient on the right track. When a patient sees results from his changes, he is encouraged and wants to continue. Eventually, the changes become habits, and the patient has been successful in making a lifestyle change that will probably add years to his life. Giving up foods you love, pushing yourself to work hard, and resisting addictions are difficult and continuous battles. Patients should be reminded to strive for small successes at first, monitor their progress weekly, and take one day at a time.

AFF ETHICAL TIP

Be Supportive, Not Judgmental

Even with your best efforts, some patients do not follow the doctor's orders. It is hard to understand a lung cancer patient who is still smoking or a patient with high cholesterol levels who continues to eat fried food. As a health care professional, you should never judge a patient or offer your personal opinions. Avoid showing negative feelings or distaste for patients or their actions. Provide patients with as much information, support, and encouragement as possible. People respond to positive reinforcement, and your interest and concern may be just what they need to help them make difficult lifestyle changes.

 CHECKPOINT QUESTION

6. To which patients should you teach fall prevention tips?

Medications

With the increasing number of medications available, the possibilities for teaching patients in this area are virtually endless. Pharmaceutical companies offer in-depth medication information for health care providers and patients concerning the chemical makeup of the drug, physiologic reactions in the body, prescribed dosage and route, and possible side effects. This information comes from the pharmaceutical companies either by mail or from the sales support team. In addition, some of this information will come in package inserts. If this information is not available, the patient may not understand the importance of the medication therapy, and this could lead to noncompliance, drug interactions, or other serious side effects. You may be responsible for gathering the information needed and preparing teaching materials for your patients to help prevent such complications.

When preparing a medication therapy teaching tool, you must consider such factors as the patient's financial abilities, social or cultural demands, physical disabilities, and age. Be sure to include the following information in any teaching:

- Medication name (generic or brand)
- Dosage
- Route
- What the medication is for
- Why the medication must be taken as prescribed
- Possible changes in bodily functions (e.g., colored urine)
- Possible side effects
- Other medications, such as over-the-counter drugs, herbal supplements, and so on, that might interfere with the action of the medication
- Foods or liquids to be avoided
- Activities to be avoided
- Telephone number to call for any questions or concerns

Figure 4-3 shows a medication therapy teaching tool that incorporates all of these elements.

Medication teaching should also include any over-the-counter medications or herbal supplements the patient is taking. This information should consist of the same items listed above. Many patients have the misconception that over-the-counter medications (e.g., aspirin, ibuprofen, cough syrup) are 100% safe and no dangers

Medication Therapy Teaching Tool

Trade name/Brand name: _____

Circle the one that applies:
Take by mouth   Apply to affected area   Drop into ear
Insert rectally   Place under tongue   Insert vaginally
Drop in eye   Other _____

The dosage of this medication is:
This medication was ordered for you because:
It may cause:
You should not take this medication if:
If you notice any of the following, you should call Dr. Smith's office at 555-1111.

The above information has been explained to me, and I understand the importance of following the prescribed treatment.

_____   _____
(patient's signature)   (date)

_____
(signature of person teaching patient)

Figure 4-3 Medication therapy teaching tool.

TABLE **4-1** Herbal Supplements[a]	
Supplement	**Reported Benefits**
Alfalfa	Relief from arthritis pain; strength
Anise	Relief of dry cough; treatment of flatulence
Black cohosh root	Relief of premenstrual symptoms; rheumatoid arthritis
Chamomile	Treatment of migraines, gastric cramps
Cholestin	Lowers cholesterol and triglycerides
Echinacea	Treatment of colds; stimulates immune system; attacks viruses
Garlic	Treatment of colds; diuretic; prevention of cardiac diseases
Ginkgo	Increased blood flow to brain; treatment of Alzheimer disease
Ginseng	Mood elevator, antihypertensive
Glucosamine	Treats arthritis symptoms; improves joint mobility
Kava	Treatment of anxiety, restlessness; tranquilizer
Licorice	Soothes coughs, treats chronic fatigue syndrome
St. John's wort	Treats depression, premenstrual symptoms; antiviral

[a]This box lists some commonly used herbal supplements and their reported benefits. Research is an ongoing process to document these findings. Some of these herbal supplements may have side effects or may interact with prescribed medications.

- Stress of treatments, procedures, and possible hospitalization
- Changes in role identity and self-image
- Loss of control and independence
- Changes in relationships with friends and family

Patients with chronic conditions may need more time to adjust than patients with acute illnesses. If patients are able to deal with stress factors, they are more likely to adapt and adjust to lifestyle changes.

Many other causes besides illness or injury can place patients under stress. The best way to cope with stress is by living a healthy lifestyle. When the body is healthy, it can handle stress more easily. Unfortunately, most of the reasons that hinder learning are the same factors that hinder patients' ability to comply with patient education. Patients who are not capable of coping with stress on their own or with the help of instruction provided by the medical office staff may need professional counseling.

Positive and Negative Stress

Two types of stress affect all of us daily: positive stress and negative stress. Positive stress motivates individuals to work efficiently and perform to the best of their abilities. Examples of positive stress include working on a challenging new job or assignment, getting married, and giving a speech or performance. In fact, many people work best under positive stress. Under positive stress, the brain releases chemicals that increase the heart rate and breathing capacity. The body also releases stored glucose that gives an energy boost. Once the job (or wedding) is over, though, time must be taken to relax and

prepare for the next project. If relaxation techniques are not incorporated into the daily routine, positive stress can become negative stress.

Negative stress is the inability to relax after a stressful encounter. Left unchecked, it can lead to such physiologic responses as:

- Headache
- Nausea, diarrhea
- Sweating palms
- Insomnia
- Malaise
- Rapid heart rate

Long-term physical effects of unrelieved stress include increases in blood pressure, glucose levels, metabolism, intraocular pressure, and finally exhaustion. There is also an increased risk of heart attack, stroke, diabetes, certain cancers, and immune system failure. If the stress is not relieved, patients will progress to higher anxiety levels and will require all of their energy and attention to focus solely on the problem at hand. Most mental and physical activity will be directed at relief of the stress to avoid the ultimate anxiety level known as panic—a sudden, overwhelming state of anxiety or terror.

It may be difficult to escape completely from stress-causing factors, but management of them is possible. For a patient suffering from the physiologic effects of negative stress, you can offer the following coping strategies:

- Encourage patients to attempt to reduce stressors, but emphasize that it is not possible to remove all stressors. Warn them to avoid attempting to make everything perfect; perfectionism adds its own stress.

- Encourage patients to organize and limit activities as needed.
- Try to lessen patients' fear of failure so they just do the best they can.
- When patients are feeling anxious, encourage them to talk to someone about their problems and let off steam.

Any one of these tips may help patients to regain control over stressors. In addition, a number of relaxation techniques described in the following sections may help.

Psychological Defense Mechanisms

Humans employ the use of defense mechanisms to cope with the painful and difficult problems life can bring. Freud's unconscious awareness theory says that we unconsciously avoid conflict and situations that cause us feelings of anxiety. Patients can use defense mechanisms to hide from or ignore their problems, especially those resulting from illness. We all use defense mechanisms from time to time, but psychologists say that the key to good mental health is to face our real conflicts and problems. You may encounter patients who are using such mechanisms to hide their true feelings. You must keep this possibility in mind as you attempt to understand and help patients. Table 4-2 outlines some common defense mechanisms.

Relaxation Techniques

Patients can use any of several types of relaxation techniques. To determine what works best for them, they must first consider how much time they have and what type of relaxation they need. Next are three examples of relaxation techniques.

TABLE 4-2	Common Defense Mechanisms	
Defense Mechanism	**Explanation**	**Example**
Denial	Refusing to acknowledge an unpleasant fact of life in order to delay facing it. Allowing yourself to believe that the problem does not exist.	A parent of a teen ignores or trivializes physical signs of drug abuse.
Displacement	Taking out your anger and frustration on someone other than the person responsible for the bad feelings.	A medical assistant is angry with her physician-employer. Later, she yells at her husband when he asks about dinner.
Intellectualization	Analyzing a difficult situation to try to make sense of it.	A daughter spends hours researching Alzheimer disease after her mother's diagnosis.
Projection	Blaming others for your unacceptable qualities.	A medical assisting graduate blames her teachers when she has trouble finding a job because of poor personal work history.
Rationalization	Using excuses for unacceptable behavior.	A patient says it is alright for him to smoke because he has a high-stress job.
Regression	Behaving in an immature way when faced with difficulty.	A patient pouts when she has to wait because the doctor has been called to the hospital.
Repression	Blocking out bad memories.	An abused wife remembers only "the good times" when she thinks about leaving her abuser.
Sublimation	Changing unwanted aggressive or sexual drives by finding an outlet through creative mental work.	A recovering abuser volunteers at a shelter and counsels abused spouses.
Withdrawal	Physically or emotionally pulling away from difficult situations.	A child sits alone on the playground because he is not as good at kickball as the others.

Breathing Techniques

Breathing exercises can be done anywhere. Most people are shallow breathers and need to be instructed on deep-breathing techniques. To perform these breathing exercises, the patient should sit up straight with hands placed on the stomach and take a deep breath in through the nose, feeling the hands being pushed away by the stomach. (This may feel awkward because most people do just the opposite.) The patient holds the breath for a few seconds and then exhales through pursed lips as the hands are felt being pulled in. This exercise allows for good control of the rate of exhalation. Sometimes, getting the oxygen flowing through the body at a faster rate is all that is needed to relieve boredom, tension, and stress.

Visualization

Visualization is a relaxation technique that involves allowing the mind to wander and the imagination to run free and focus on positive and relaxing situations. It is similar to daydreaming. It can "remove" the patient from a stressful situation and put him or her in a place where, if nothing else, the mind can relax. Instruct the patient to find a quiet place, close the eyes, and then visualize a soothing scene. Sometimes, background music helps. Remind the patient that it is important to choose appropriate times for this daydreaming technique. For example, it would be dangerous to use this technique when driving a car or operating heavy equipment.

Physical Exercise

There is no better tranquilizer than physical exercise. Walking at least 30 minutes 3 times a week is a great stress reliever. Most people who exercise regularly say that it helps them reduce tension, relax, and rest better at night.

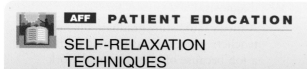

AFF PATIENT EDUCATION

SELF-RELAXATION TECHNIQUES

Here are two examples of self-relaxation techniques for you and your patients.

1. Sit with both feet on the floor, place your hands in your lap, and close your eyes. Visualize yourself standing at the top of a staircase with six steps. Now imagine that you are going down each step very slowly. With each step down, your body becomes more relaxed. When you feel completely relaxed for a minute or so, imagine going back up the steps. With each step up, you feel more alert and ready to take on the world. It takes practice, but after awhile, the process can be done in the time it takes to take a bathroom break. You will be refreshed and ready to sail through the rest of the day.

2. In a sitting position, concentrate on relaxing the muscles in your body. Beginning with the top of your head and moving down, concentrate on relaxing your shoulders, your arms, your hips, your legs, etc. Try this technique when you are having trouble getting to sleep or you're anxiously sitting in the dentist's chair.

COG Patient Teaching Plans

Developing a Plan

Because medical assistants are usually allotted only minimal time for patient teaching, you may often find yourself teaching without a written plan. To ensure that teaching is done logically, always use the education process to help you formulate a plan in your mind. Also remember to document in the patient's record whatever teaching you perform and the patient's response.

Many facilities use preprinted teaching plans for common problem areas, such as "Controlling Diabetes," "Living With Multiple Sclerosis," and "Coping With Hearing Loss." Although these save time, they are not individualized to the patient. If you use preprinted teaching plans, be sure to adapt them to your particular patient's learning needs and abilities.

If preprinted plans are not an option, consult teaching plan resource books, which contain the necessary information in outline form. You can take the plans from these sources and transfer them as needed to your facility-approved teaching plan format, adding your own comments to fit the patient's needs.

All teaching plans, no matter what the design, should contain the following elements:

- *Learning goal.* A description of what the patient should learn from implementation of the teaching plan.
- *Material to be covered.* All major topics to be discussed.
- *Learning objectives.* Steps or procedures the patient must understand or demonstrate to accomplish the learning goal.
- *Evaluation.* Appraisal of the patient's progress.
- *Comments.* Remarks concerning circumstances that may be preventing successful completion of the objectives.

Teaching plans must also include an area for documenting when the information was presented to the patient and when the patient successfully completed each objective. Figure 4-4 is an example of a teaching plan.

Selecting and Adapting Teaching Material

An enormous amount of teaching material is available. Although the physician or institution may select much

Teaching Plan: 32-year-old female with Iron Deficiency Anemia
Patient Learning Goal: Increase patient's knowledge of Iron Deficiency Anemia, its complications and treatments
Material to be Covered: Description of disorder, complications, diet, medications, procedures

Learning Objectives Comments	Teaching Methods/Tools	Procedure Explained/Demonstrated Date/Initial	PT Demonstrated/ Objectives Met Date/Initial
1. Patient describes what happens when body's demand for oxygen is not met. a. oxygen and hgb concentration decrease b. signs/symptoms of anemia c. anemia occurs only after body stores of iron are depleted	Instruction		
2. Patient describes complications caused by decrease of oxygen concentration a. chronic fatigue b. dyspnea c. inability to concentrate, think d. decrease in tissue repair e. increase of infection f. increase in heart rate	Instruction		
3. Patient discusses importance of diet in prevention of iron deficiency anemia a. including iron-rich foods in diet (beef, poultry, green vegetables) b. including foods that contain ascorbic acid to assist in absorbing iron in body (fruits) c. importance of limiting large meals if fatigued; stress importance of several small meals	Instruction/Video: "Your Diet: Why It Is Important"		
4. Patient describes prescribed medication, its purpose, dosage, route, and side effects	Instruction/Pamphlet: *Taking Your Iron Supplements*		
5. Patient aware of importance of follow-up appointments for evaluation of prescribed plan of treatment	Instruction/Appointment slip with next scheduled appointment		

Figure 4-4 Teaching plan.

of the material you will use, you may be responsible for selecting some teaching aids. Assess your patients' general level of understanding to choose materials appropriately. When using preprinted material, consider the format, headings, illustrations, vocabulary, and writing style for overall clarity and readability. Also, ensure that the information provided on commercial materials is truthful and in agreement with the policies and procedures of your facility. A good rule of thumb is to use commercial material only from nationally recognized organizations or government agencies.

Many patient education textbooks are available from your clinic library. If you do not have access to a library, you can order most texts from local bookstores or through the Internet. Many of these sources list addresses for other patient education materials available from companies or associations. These materials commonly include printed items as well as videos, audiocassettes, and compact discs. Use commercially prepared materials to start a patient teaching library in the physician's office so you will have information at your fingertips when needed.

Developing Your Own Material

Sometimes, you may need to create your own teaching materials. Review available resources and teaching aids, and adapt the information to benefit your patients. When developing teaching material, remember to do the following:

- Indicate the objective of the information.
- Personalize the information so the patient wants to learn.
- Make sure information is clear and well organized.
- Use lists and outlines, which are easier to read and remember than paragraphs.
- Avoid medical jargon as much as possible.
- Focus on the key points.
- Select appropriate printing type.
- Use diagrams that are simple, clear, and well labeled.
- Include the names and telephone numbers of people or organizations that patients can call with further questions or concerns.

After patients have been using the material for a while, periodically evaluate its effectiveness and modify your teaching plan as needed.

Not all of the patient teaching materials you create will have to be in print form. Patients must be motivated to read, but many will be more receptive to audiovisual instruction. Take advantage of any opportunity to develop teaching materials in other media.

 CHECKPOINT QUESTION

8. List the elements of a written teaching plan.

PSY Locating Community Resources and Disseminating Information

Patients have access to many services that sometimes they do not even realize are available. Many communities have a central agency that coordinates and **disseminates** or distributes information about many or all community resources. If this is not the case in your area, you will want to gather the information and create an information sheet for patients to take home. The patient and his family can then examine the resources, decide if they want to participate, and contact the appropriate community resource. Support groups not only provide assistance for patients and their families in coping with illness, but they also give the patient an opportunity to meet and exchange ideas with others who are experiencing the same issues such as Alzheimer disease, cancer, and diabetes.

Most local telephone directories include a section that outlines the agencies and resources available through the city and state. Information for patients who need financial assistance or assistance with transportation would be found in a telephone directory. The Internet is an excellent resource for local, state, and national agencies that provide information, support, and services to patients. Box 4-5 lists some of the agencies that might be available in your area. For information about local support, the Web sites of these agencies are listed as well.

---

español SPANISH TERMINOLOGY

Tres veces al día.
Three times a day

Antes/después de las comidas
Before/after meals

Al acostarse
At bedtime

Tómela con la comida.
Take this with food.

Dele la medicina cada cuatro horas.
Give him the medicine every 4 hours.

 MEDIA MENU

- **Student Resources on thePoint**
  - **CMA/RMA Certification Exam Review**
- **Internet Resources**

  American Academy of Pediatrics
  http://www.aap.org

  American Cancer Society
  http://www.cancer.org

  American Heart Association
  http://www.heart.org

  American Lung Association
  http://www.lungusa.org

  U.S. Food and Drug Administration
  http://www.fda.gov

  National Center for Complementary and Alternative Medicine
  http://www.nccam.nih.gov

  National Council on Patient Information and Education
  http://www.talkaboutrx.org

BOX 4-5

COMMUNITY RESOURCES

Council on Aging; http://www.ncoa.org
American Red Cross; http://www.redcross.org
Hospice; http://www.hospicefoundation.org
American Cancer Society; http://www.cancer.org
American Heart Association; http://www.heart.org
Civic organizations
Public health department
Social services
Home health agencies

Various support groups can be located in the telephone directory or local newspaper. Cancer centers would have information about the support they offer.

PSY PROCEDURE 4-1:   Document Patient Education

Purpose: To record teaching that has occurred.
Equipment: Patient's chart, pen, student partner

Steps	Reasons
1. Record the date and time of teaching.	To refresh the memory, make a legal and permanent note of your actions, and to facilitate the continuity of the patient's care.
2. Record the information taught, e.g., "Diabetes foot care was discussed. It consisted of the proper method for toenail cutting and regular examination by a podiatrist."	To refresh the memory, make a legal and permanent note of your actions, and to facilitate the continuity of the patient's care.
3. Record the manner in which the information was taught, e.g., "ADA [American Diabetes Association] foot care video shown to the patient."	To refresh the memory, make a legal and permanent note of your actions, and to facilitate the continuity of the patient's care.
4. Record your evaluation of your teaching. For example, "Patient verbalized the need to make an appointment with a podiatrist."	To refresh the memory, make a legal and permanent note of your actions, and to facilitate the continuity of the patient's care.
5. Record any additional teaching planned, e.g., "Patient will return on Monday to the office with his wife for glucose monitoring instructions."	To refresh the memory, make a legal and permanent note of your actions, and to facilitate the continuity of the patient's care.
6. **AFF** Explain what you would do if you forgot to document an action you took during the patient education process.	Go back to the original entry and make the addition on a new line with today's date. For example: Current date. Addendum to 8/1/12 note: Also demonstrated back strengthening exercises. Patient voiced understanding and performed satisfactorily. Dierdre Hall, RMA In an electronic record, you can edit the original entry with the above information.

PSY PROCEDURE 4-2: **Develop and Maintain a Current List of Community Resources Related to Patient's Health Care Needs**

Purpose: To assist patients to identify and obtain assistance from available community resources
Equipment: Computer with Internet access

Steps	Reasons

1. Assess the patient's needs. Does he or she need:
  a. Education
  b. Someone to talk to
  c. Financial information
  d. Support groups
  e. Home health needs
	You must know what resources the patient needs. If there are several, organize the information to avoid confusion.

2. Be prepared with materials already on hand. Create a resource for patients using Word or an Excel sheet, for example.	With each resource located, place the information in a manual so that you will have general information about the resources available to patients.
3. Check the local telephone book for local and state resources.	Most telephone directories include a section for local, county, and state resources. It is difficult for some patients to sort all of the information out.
4. Check for Web sites for the city and/or county in which the patient lives.	Many patients do not have access to a computer, but phone numbers can be obtained from Web sites.

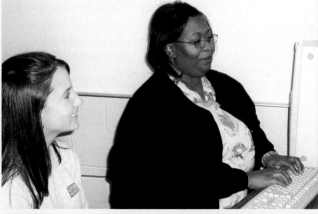

Step 4:   Check Web sites for information.

Steps	Reasons
5. Disseminate the information to patients at their level of understanding.	Remember that communication is not effective unless it is understood.
6. Give the patient the contact information in writing.	Instructions for patients should be in writing to avoid any confusion or memory loss.
7. Document your actions and the information you gave the patient.	If it's not in the chart, it did not happen.
8. Instruct the patient to contact the office if there is any difficulty.	Always make sure the patient knows how to contact you. This is good customer service.
9. **AFF** Explain what suggestions or assistance you would offer to a patient who would benefit from online patient education resources but does not own a computer.	The patient could go to a public library, Internet café, or copy shop for public computer use. You could offer to print information for the patient if feasible.

Chapter Summary

- Your role in teaching depends on the clinical setting in which you work. Never pass up an opportunity to teach.
- Encourage patients to ask questions.
- Periodically check to ensure that your teaching has been effective.

- Do not overstep your role as a medical assistant. The teaching you provide should clarify and complement information provided by the physician.
- A well-planned patient education program helps ensure that patients receive the high-quality health care they deserve.

Warm Ups for Critical Thinking

1. Look at the Maslow's hierarchy pyramid. What level are you on? What steps can you take to reach the self-actualization level? If you are at that level, what steps can you take to ensure that you remain there?

2. Review the list of information that you should teach patients about their medications. Choose two medications, herbal supplements, or vitamins that you have taken. (The medication can be over-the-counter or prescribed.) Using all available resources, write the information for these two medications or supplements.

3. Review the material on fall prevention and preventing childhood injuries. Make a checklist of at least 10 safety tips for both groups. Take your list and visit an elderly family member, friend, or neighbor's home. Review these tips with the person. Inspect the home for safety. What improvements or recommendations were you able to provide?

4. Make a list of preprinted educational materials that every office should have. What professional organizations (e.g., American Heart Association, American Cancer Society) could help provide these materials?

5. From information found at the American Cancer Society's Web site, develop a patient education information sheet for the current guidelines for breast cancer screening.

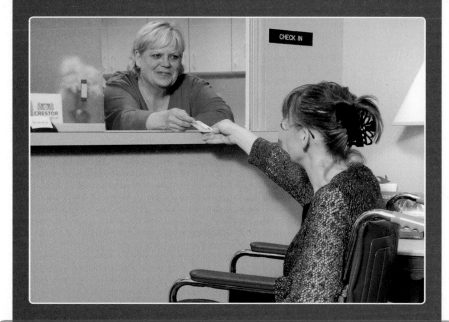

The
Administrative
Medical
Assistant

Fundamentals of Administrative Medical Assisting

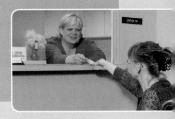

A well-run medical office requires that everyone works together as a team. Unit Two consists of six chapters that address administrative duties performed in the medical office. These duties include telephone and reception, appointment management, written communications, health information management, computer use, and medical office management. Some of these duties are shared with clinical personnel. This unit will help you to perform these duties whether you work in the front desk area or in the clinical area.

CHAPTER 5

The First Contact: Telephone and Reception

Outline

Professional Image
Importance of a Good Attitude
The Medical Assistant as a Role Model
Courtesy and Diplomacy in the Medical Office
First Impressions

Reception
The Role of a Receptionist

Duties and Responsibilities of the Receptionist
Ergonomic Concerns for the Receptionist
The Waiting Room Environment
The End of the Patient Visit

Telephone
Importance of the Telephone in the Medical Office

Basic Guidelines for Telephone Use
Routine Incoming Calls
Challenging Incoming Calls
Triaging Incoming Calls
Taking Messages
Outgoing Calls
Services and Special Features

Learning Outcomes

Cognitive Domain

Note: AAMA/CAAHEP 2008 Standards are italicized.

1. Spell and define the key terms
2. Explain the importance of displaying a professional image to all patients
3. List six duties of the medical office receptionist
4. List four sources from which messages can be retrieved

5. Discuss various steps that can be taken to promote good ergonomics
6. Describe the basic guidelines for waiting room environments
7. Describe the proper method for maintaining infection control standards in the waiting room
8. Discuss the five basic guidelines for telephone use
9. Describe the types of incoming telephone calls received by the medical office

10. Discuss how to identify and handle callers with medical emergencies
11. Describe how to triage incoming calls
12. List the information that should be given to an emergency medical service dispatcher
13. Describe the types of telephone services and special features
14. Discuss applications of electronic technology in effective communication

Psychomotor Domain

Note: AAMA/CAAHEP 2008 Standards are italicized.

1. Handle incoming calls (Procedure 5-1)
   * *Demonstrate telephone techniques*
2. Call Emergency Medical Services (Procedure 5-2)
   * *Demonstrate self awareness in responding to emergency situations*
   * *Recognize the effects of stress on all persons involved in emergency situations*
3. Explain general office policies (Procedure 5-3)
   * *Report relevant information to others succinctly and accurately*
4. Verify eligibility for managed care services

Affective Domain

Note: AAMA/CAAHEP 2008 Standards are italicized.

1. *Demonstrate empathy in communicating with patients, family, and staff*
2. *Implement time management principles to maintain effective office function*
3. *Communicate in language the patient can understand regarding managed care and insurance plans*
4. *Demonstrate awareness of the consequences of not working within the legal scope of practice*
5. *Demonstrate sensitivity in communicating with both providers and patients*
6. *Demonstrate sensitivity to patient rights*

ABHES Competencies

1. Use proper telephone technique
2. Receive, organize, prioritize, and transmit information expediently
3. Apply electronic technology

Key Terms

attitude	diplomacy	ergonomic	teletypewriter (TTY)
closed captioning	emergency medical service (EMS)	receptionist	triage
diction			

As a medical assistant, you are the patient's primary contact with the physician. In certain situations, the patient may spend more time with you than with the physician. Your interaction with the patient sets the tone for the visit and directly influences the patient's perception of the office and the quality of care the patient will receive. Therefore, it is vital that you project a caring and competent professional image at all times. You will have various responsibilities and duties when working as a receptionist. These duties will vary among physician offices. Proper telephone etiquette and use is an essential skill for all medical assistants. You must be able to handle incoming and outgoing calls correctly and efficiently.

The Health Insurance Portability and Accountability Act (HIPAA), which is discussed throughout this text, requires all health care settings to ensure privacy and security of patient information. HIPAA's Privacy Rule affects every area of the office. In waiting areas where conversations can be overheard or information can be seen by patients, you must take precautions to protect patient confidentiality.

COG Professional Image

Importance of a Good Attitude

An **attitude** is a state of mind or feeling regarding some matter. It can be either positive or negative. Attitudes can be formed by past or present experiences; they can be transmitted from one person to another. How you feel influences how you act; thus, your attitude shapes your behavior. You transmit your attitude to others through your behavior, thereby influencing their attitudes and behaviors.

The medical assistant must be able to transmit a positive attitude to the patient. This requires acceptance of the patient as a unique individual who has the right to be treated with dignity and compassion in a nonjudgmental manner. Ask yourself how you would feel in a similar situation and how you would want to be treated. By demonstrating empathy, interest, and concern, you tell the patient that he or she is important to you and that you care. This exerts a positive influence on the patient's own attitude, behavior, and response.

For example, let's assume that you are working as a receptionist in a busy family practice office. It is the peak of the flu and cold season. Which of the following interactions between the medical assistant and the patient transmits a positive attitude to the patient:

- "I know you feel terrible, Mr. Smith, but so does everyone else in the waiting room. It's the flu season. Just have a seat, and the doctor will see you shortly."
- "I'm sorry you don't feel well. Do you feel well enough to sit in the waiting room for about 10 minutes? The doctor will be ready to see you then."

The second interaction shows the patient that you care about how he feels and reassures him that he will be seen by the physician shortly. In the first interaction, the attitude that was transmitted made Mr. Smith feel like just another sick patient. Your positive attitude will influence the patient's attitude, behavior, and response.

The Medical Assistant as a Role Model

Another way in which you as a medical assistant influence the patient's perception of the medical office is your personal appearance. Good health and good grooming present a positive image to the patient. Taking care of yourself by eating well, exercising regularly, and getting enough rest is important not only for your appearance but also for your job performance. If you are tired or sluggish, you cannot give good patient care.

Pay particular attention to your personal hygiene to avoid offending your patients. A person who is ill is often acutely sensitive to odors, even those normally considered pleasant. A daily bath or shower is essential, followed by an unscented deodorant. Keep your hair clean and styled. Good oral hygiene is important, and during the day you should avoid foods that may give an offensive odor. Keep your fingernails clean and trimmed, with clear or neutral polish. Long nails polished with vivid colors are not appropriate for the medical office. Natural nail tips must be less than a quarter inch long, according to the Centers for Disease Control and Prevention (CDC). Artificial nails may increase

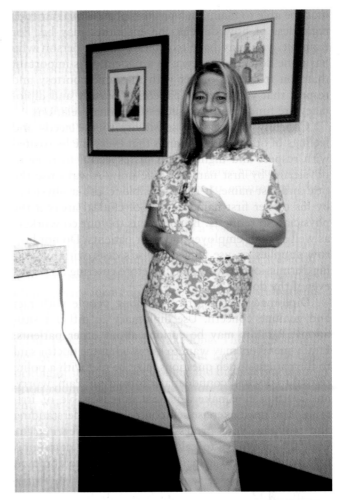

Figure 5-1 The properly dressed medical assistant presents a professional and positive image to patients.

the potential for infection transmission to you and your patients. The CDC recommendation is for health care providers not to wear artificial nails if high-risk patient care is required. If you wear makeup, keep it natural, and apply it lightly. Do not wear perfume, cologne, scented lotion, hair spray, or the like.

Most offices have a dress code. Whether you wear a uniform or street clothes, they should be clean, neat, pressed, and in good repair (Fig. 5-1). Wrinkles, missing buttons, split seams, torn hems, and stains project a negative image. Always wear clean, polished shoes. Stockings should be full length, of a neutral shade, and free from runs and holes. Jewelry such as dangling earrings, large rings, long chains, and ornate or multiple bracelets are not appropriate in the health care environment.

Courtesy and Diplomacy in the Medical Office

Being a medical assistant requires excellent human relations skills. In the course of a day, you will interact with a variety of personalities in a variety of situations, and you

the emergency messages to the physician, generally by beeper. Other messages are left for the office staff to obtain the following morning. Examples of messages that could be left here are:

- Patients calling the office for a sick appointment (not an emergency, such as an earache or flulike symptoms)
- Calls from hospitals or skilled nursing facilities about changes in patient status (new wounds or bed sores or patient falls without injury)

Voice Mail Systems

A voice mailbox is a type of answering machine in which the caller can leave a detailed message. You will need to know the security access code to obtain messages. After you obtain the messages, delete them from the recorder unless otherwise directed by office policy. Examples of messages that could be left here are:

- Patients wishing to change or cancel their appointments
- Patients requesting prescription refills
- Family members or patients calling to ask for additional information or clarification about their medical care or test results

Electronic Mail

The computer is a vital link for physicians to communicate with all health care professionals. E-mail messages are sent from other physicians, professional organizations, and hospital personnel. Some physician offices provide patients with their e-mail addresses. Examples of messages left here are:

- Memos from professional organizations
- Pharmaceutical representatives' updates or announcements

- Medical staff meeting minutes, announcements from hospital administration
- Upcoming continuing education courses for physicians
- Insurance representatives regarding billing issues

Facsimile Machines

All physician offices have a fax machine. The most common messages left here are:

- Patient referrals
- Consultation reports
- Laboratory and radiology reports

 CHECKPOINT QUESTION

2. What four locations should you retrieve messages from?

Prepare the Charts

Your next duty will be to gather charts. Gather the charts of all of the patients scheduled to be seen for the day and put them in order by appointment. Review each chart to ensure that it is complete and up to date. Check that adequate clinical data sheets are available for the doctor to record any notes. Test results received since the patient's last appointment and any other new information are placed in the front of the chart for the doctor's review. Make up a chart for each new patient and have the appropriate registration forms ready for the patient to complete. Once the charts are prepared, they are usually kept at the reception desk and given to the doctor or clinical assistant as the patient arrives, although some doctors prefer to have all charts on their desk at the start of the day (see Chapter 8).

Welcome Patients and Visitors

Make every attempt to greet patients personally and by name, e.g., "Good morning, Ms. Misko." A smile and cheerful greeting promote a positive image and make the patient feel welcome. Try to remember something personal about each patient, such as hobbies, pets, or special interests about which you can ask. Sometimes, you will not be at your desk when a patient arrives. Check the waiting room for new arrivals upon your return. Many offices install a bell or chime on the door and post a sign requesting patients to check in with the receptionist. Even if you cannot greet them immediately, acknowledge them with a smile and a nod until you can help them. You would not let someone walk into your home without greeting them immediately. If it is your responsibility to greet patients, you should make this a top priority.

Register and Orient Patients

Patients who are new to the office will have to complete a registration form, also called a patient information sheet. On this form, the patient provides name, address, and telephone number; the name, address, and telephone number of the insurance company or other party responsible for payment; employer names and addresses; marital status; spouse's name; social security number; and name of the person who referred the patient. Some information sheets include questions about medical history. In some cases, you may complete the form while interviewing the patient. Most offices have the patients fill in these forms and ask for your help if questions arise.

After registration, orient the patient to the office. Brochures that give the names of the doctor and staff, office hours, and telephone numbers are helpful. Explain any pertinent office policies or procedures, such as billing procedures, how to make or cancel appointments, and parking. Ask if the patient has any questions. Procedure 5-3 outlines the steps for explaining office policies to a new patient. Tell the patient where the water fountain and restrooms are, but caution the patient against using the restroom without checking with you to determine whether a urine specimen is needed. Urine specimens are generally needed for pregnant patients, patients with lower back or abdominal pain or back injuries, and patients being seen for drug or pre-employment health examinations. At the appropriate time, you may be responsible for taking patients to the examination room unless another health care worker escorts the patients.

Manage Waiting Time

Patients expect to be seen at the appointed time. They have allotted time in their schedule to see the doctor and do not want to be kept waiting. One of the major complaints of patients is the length of time they must wait to see the physician. Be sure to tell the patients if the doctor is behind schedule. If you expect the wait to be 30 minutes or more past the scheduled time, offer waiting patients some choices. Some choose to leave and come back in an hour, and some choose to reschedule the appointment for another time. Be honest with waiting patients. Tell them why there is a delay. If the provider has been called away for an emergency, patients will respect his dedication and appreciate the fact that if they need their doctor in an emergency, he will be there for them.

Ergonomic Concerns for the Receptionist

For most of the day you will be sitting at your desk performing these tasks. Occasional lifting of delivery boxes, paper supplies, and so on is required. The duties of the receptionist require you to twist from your primary desk to other areas to reach for files or to answer the telephone. These actions can lead to back injuries and other musculoskeletal disorders. Medical professionals are at

high risk for such injuries. Having a good **ergonomic** workstation and good body mechanics, however, can prevent most injuries.

An ergonomic workstation is designed specifically to prevent injuries and often results in increased employee satisfaction and work efficiency. The Occupational Safety and Health Administration (OSHA) has many recommendations for preventing such injuries. Here are some other suggestions to prevent injuries:

- Keep items that you must lift at waist level when possible. Keep the load close to the body. Bend at your hips.
- Instruct delivery people to place packages in locations that will not require movement.
- Carry only small loads of paper. Make additional trips as needed.
- Place items that you frequently use within easy reach. Moves from side to side are safer than twisting to a desk behind you. Avoiding storing charts above chest level to limit reaching over your head. Use a step stool to reach high shelves instead of stretching.
- Telephones with headsets will keep your head upright and allow your shoulders to relax. If you use a stationary phone, a long handset cord can reduce muscle strain. Do not rest the telephone on your shoulder while talking, since this causes neck and back injuries.

 CHECKPOINT QUESTION

3. What is the purpose of having an ergonomic workstation?

The Waiting Room Environment

General Guidelines for Waiting Rooms

The reception area should be designed for the comfort, safety, and enjoyment of all patients. It should be kept clean and uncluttered, with the furniture arranged to allow ample room for walking. A coat rack and umbrella stand should be present. Restrooms and a water fountain should be easily accessible.

Furniture should be aesthetically pleasing, comfortable, and durable. Chairs are preferable to sofas because most people find sharing a sofa with strangers uncomfortable. Chairs allow patients to maintain a degree of privacy and personal space. There should be a variety of soft chairs and firm chairs and chairs with and without arms. Some patients find it hard to stand up from a soft chair; others prefer the comfort. Some need chair arms to push themselves up, and others are more comfortable without chair arms.

A low-key color scheme is advisable. Muted pastels are preferable to bright primary colors, although the latter work well in pediatric offices (Fig. 5-2). Lighting should be bright but not harsh. The room should be well

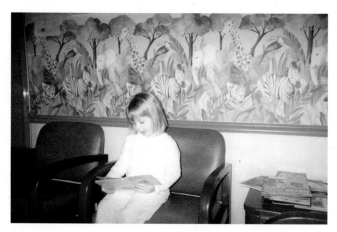

Figure 5-2 Children will respond to a doctor's visit more positively if the office is decorated for them.

ventilated and kept at a comfortable temperature. Many offices provide soothing background music.

Landscapes, waterscapes, and floral and animal pictures make better wall décor than abstract art. Lamps and plants can add interest to corners. Keep plants in good condition, and remove any dead leaves. An office with dead or dying plants does not project a comforting image.

A good selection of reading material should be available. Have a variety of current magazines that are appropriate for your patients. The doctor's professional journals should not be included. The reception area is a good place to set out patient education materials.

Some offices provide television for patients who prefer not to read. Most patients find television relaxing and entertaining, but other patients find it annoying. Television can serve as an education tool. Here are a few tips that you should follow regarding television:

- The volume should be set to allow a group of people to hear the television but not at a distracting volume for the whole waiting room.
- A simple sign placed on the television, "Please do not touch the controls; see the receptionist for channel changes" will prevent patients from selecting inappropriate programs.
- Only family-oriented programs should be shown. It is acceptable to select a news channel. No shows with violence, strong language, or sexual content should be on. Soap operas are not suitable for medical office waiting rooms.
- Some offices leave the television off unless a patient asks to have it on.
- Patients with hearing impairments must be offered the option of **closed captioning** if they choose to watch television. (Closed captioning is the translation of the spoken word into a written format. Most televisions have this capability under their options menu.)

You should check the waiting room several times during the day to make sure it is clean and tidy. Also check the entrance, hallways, and stairs. These areas too must be well lighted and maintained. Liability is a concern if patients slip on ice or snow coming into the office. Remember, the patient's privacy must be protected in the reception and waiting areas of the office as well (see Box 5-1).

 PATIENT EDUCATION

TELEVISION AS A TEACHING TOOL

A television in the reception area can entertain patients while they wait for an appointment, but it can also be a patient education tool. There are a variety of educational DVDs available. Here are some points to keep in mind:

- Be sure all material has been previewed by the physician.
- Select DVDs and videos that are geared toward the specialty of the practice (e.g., a video about heart attacks is appropriate for a cardiologist's office but not for a dermatologist's office).
- Carefully assess the graphic nature of certain videos. (A film of the birth of a child may interest you, but it might be too much for some patients.)
- Keep in mind the age of the patients and family members who will be in the waiting room. Caution must be used if small children are often in the area. For example, a video about preventing sexually transmitted diseases may provide information appropriate for a family practice office, but it would not be appropriate to show the video in the reception area.

 CHECKPOINT QUESTION

4. What option should you offer hearing-impaired patients if they wish to watch television?

Guidelines for Pediatric Waiting Rooms

Pediatric offices tend to be very busy practices with a multitude of reasons for patient visits. Generally, visits to the pediatrician can be divided into three types: well child checks, sick child visits, and follow-up visits. Because of the large volume of sick child visits, most pediatric waiting room areas are broken into two sections, one for well children and the other for sick children. Parents may have to be instructed by you as to which side of the waiting room they should sit in. According to the American Academy of Pediatrics (AAP), no studies document the effectiveness of segregated waiting room areas.

The recommendation of the AAP is to move children with a communicable disease into an examination room as quickly as possible. Your employer will provide you with instructions and guidelines for dealing with sick children.

A children's play area must be closely watched and monitored. Toys should be kept away from the general seating area. Here are some guidelines for toys:

- Toys should be simple and easy to clean, without sharp edges.
- A policy must be in place for routine cleaning of these toys.
- Toys should be checked daily to ensure that they are not broken. Toys that are broken must be thrown away. Toys should never be glued or taped together.
- Battery-powered toys that make loud noises are not permissible.
- Toys can be a choking hazard. According to the American Heart Association, small children should never to be given toys that can fit inside a standard toilet paper roll. Although older children would like to play with toys like Legos®, these toys should not be present. Older children should be expected to sit quietly while waiting for their appointment.

A good selection of books should be present for parents to read to their children. Books must be checked periodically to ensure that they are clean and no pages have been torn out. A small table and chairs will give children a place to read or color.

Americans with Disabilities Act Requirements

The U.S. Department of Justice is responsible for ensuring that all people are treated without discrimination of any kind. Under this department is the Americans with Disabilities Act (ADA). This act prohibits discrimination on the basis of a person's disability. The ADA Title III act requires that all public accommodations be accessible to everyone. This includes access into medical facilities. It is important that you be aware of the basic concept of the ADA rules. Table 5-2 lists some of the basic facility requirements. Additional information is available on the ADA Web site.

The existing structural dimensions are not something that you have control of, but you need to ensure that there is a clear path to the physician's office at all times. Here are some steps that you can take to ensure this:

- Check that deliveries are left in a safe place. They must not be left in the waiting area or block the door.
- Keep toys clear of entrance pathways.

TABLE 5-2	Summary of Americans with Disabilities Act Requirements for Public Buildings	
Area	**Specifics**
Access	Route must be stable, firm, and slip resistant.
	Route must be 36 inches wide.
Ramps	Ramps longer than 6 feet must have two railings.
	Railings must be 34–38 inches high.
	Ramp must be 36 inches wide.
	Ramps and elevators must be available to all public levels.
Entrance and door	Door must be 32 inches wide.
	Door handle must be no higher than 48 inches and must be operable with a closed fist.
	Interior doors must open without excessive force.
Miscellaneous	Carpeting must be no more than 0.5 inch high.
	Emergency egress system must have flashing lights and audible signals.
	Space for wheelchair seating must be available.
	Tables or counters must be 28–34 inches high.
Restrooms	Tactile signs must identify restrooms.
	Doorway must be at least 32 inches wide.
	All doors (including stall doors), soap dispensers, hand dryers, and faucets must be operable with a closed fist.
	Wheelchair stall is required and must be at least 5 feet by 5 feet.

- Check that chairs are not moved, creating obstacles that might limit wheelchair accessibility.
- Ensure that doors are not blocked or propped opened with objects.
- Limit the amount of stacked papers on counters that may limit the patient's access to you.
- Check the restroom regularly to make sure the entrance is open and not obstructed.

 CHECKPOINT QUESTION

5. What act prohibits discrimination of patients with disabilities?

Infection Control Issues

To prevent the spread of disease, aseptic technique must be used in every aspect of work in the medical office. During the clinical portion of your training, you will learn detailed information about infection control. As a receptionist, however, you need to be aware of a few key points:

- Always follow standard precautions. This means that you must treat all body fluids with precautionary measures.
- Handwashing is the most important practice for preventing the transmission of diseases. You must wash your hands following all direct patient contact (touching the patient) (Fig. 5-3). Since it is not always possible to leave the desk to wash your hands, the CDC has approved the use of alcohol-based antiseptic handwashing solutions for health care providers.
- Patients are often told to bring specimens to the office. Never touch a specimen container without proper gloves and personal protective equipment.
- Patients who arrive coughing and sneezing should be given tissues and instructed to cover their mouth and nose when coughing. Communicate with the clinical staff to have these patients taken directly into examination rooms. Patients who are vomiting, bleeding, or discharging other body fluids must not be left in the waiting room.

Biohazard Waste

All body fluids must be considered infectious and be managed appropriately. All body fluid spills and blood-stained papers must be disposed of in a biohazard container. The spills must be cleaned with an approved germicidal solution. If you have not been trained in handling such waste, do not touch it. Allow the clinical staff to handle the waste. If possible, contain the spill and prevent other patients from touching the area. Here are some examples of biohazard waste that you may encounter:

- Dressing supplies with bloodstains from cuts or wounds
- Tissues from patients with acute nosebleeds

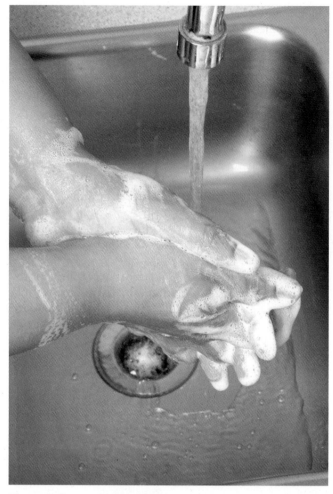

Figure 5-3 Good handwashing skills are essential to prevent disease transmission.

- Urine-saturated diapers left in the restroom
- Vomit
- Saturated tissues with sputum

Communicable Diseases

Depending on the type of office you work in, the amount of exposure to communicable diseases will vary. Family practice physicians and pediatricians, for example, treat acute communicable diseases regularly. If you work as a receptionist for a pediatrician, you will need to learn how to look at rashes and determine whether they are contagious.

Good communication between you and the clinical staff is essential to manage patients with communicable diseases. The clinical staff is often aware of patients with such diseases and will communicate it to you. Most infectious diseases cannot be transmitted with routine physical contact (handshaking, talking, touching, sharing pencils, using the telephone). Examples of infectious diseases that cannot be transmitted by routine physical contact include HIV, hepatitis, and the common cold. Some diseases can be easily transmitted, however, and

BOX 5-2

PATIENTS WHO SHOULD NOT BE LEFT IN THE WAITING ROOM

Patients with any of the following diseases or conditions should not be left in the waiting room. These patients should be taken to an examination room as soon as possible.

- Chickenpox
- Conjunctivitis
- Influenza
- Measles and rubella
- Meningitis (or suspected cases)
- Mumps
- Pertussis
- Pneumonia (if patient is coughing)
- Smallpox
- Tuberculosis
- Wounds (if open and draining)

patients with these diseases should not be left in the waiting room. Box 5-2 lists patients who should not be left in the waiting room.

Patients who have an impaired immune system or are taking medications that hinder their immune system (chemotherapy agents) may require immediate placement in an examination room to prevent exposure to otherwise benign organisms. The clinical staff will alert you to these patients.

CHECKPOINT QUESTION

6. What is the most antiseptic technique for preventing the transmission of diseases?

The End of the Patient Visit

After physicians have completed the examination or other procedures, they generally direct patients to get dressed and wait for their discharge information. In some offices, physicians provide all discharge instructions, while in other office settings, nurses or medical assistants may be assigned to discharge patients. Chapter 4 discusses the information you need to teach your patients. After the medical portion is completed, the patient is escorted to the front desk. It is generally at this time that any fees or copayments are collected by the receptionist. If the doctor has requested a follow-up visit, the appointment should be scheduled. An appointment reminder card is helpful for the patient. You or other administrative personnel may do these tasks. You should bid the patient goodbye in a warm and friendly

manner. As patients leave the office, they should feel they have been well cared for by a competent and courteous staff.

COG TELEPHONE

Importance of the Telephone in the Medical Office

The medical office is filled with expensive scientific equipment used in the diagnosis and treatment of disease, but one of the most important instruments is the telephone. It allows the patient rapid and easy access to medical care. A patient can schedule an appointment, seek medical advice, request prescription refills, obtain test results, question a bill, or report an emergency simply by picking up the telephone. The telephone also links the physician's office to the rest of the medical community, including hospitals, pharmacies, and other doctors.

You must be able to communicate a positive image of the physician and staff over the telephone without the aid of nonverbal cues such as appearance, facial expressions, body language, and gestures. You must be able to use the tone and quality of your voice and speech to project a competent and caring attitude over the telephone.

Basic Guidelines for Telephone Use

Telephone communication is not effective if either party does not fully understand what is being said. Misunderstandings can be embarrassing, frustrating, or even life threatening. To have effective telephone communication, you must be able to overcome various obstacles, such as a noisy environment, a poor telephone connection, a patient's emotional distress, or a patient's hearing or speech impairments

Diction

Diction refers to how words are spoken and enunciated. You should speak clearly and distinctly and use proper grammar. Talk clearly into the mouthpiece; do not prop the handset between your chin and shoulder. Never chew gum or eat while you speak on the telephone. Speak at a moderate pace to avoid slurring your words. Your grammar should be correct.

Pronunciation

Make sure you pronounce words correctly to avoid misunderstandings. Avoid using unfamiliar words, slang, and idiomatic expressions. Most patients do not understand medical terminology, so it is best to use lay terms whenever possible. For example, do not ask the patient, "Are you dyspneic?" Instead ask, "Are you having trouble breathing?"

Expression

Put a smile in your voice by sitting up straight and putting a smile on your lips. Speak with a modulated pitch and volume. Use proper inflection to avoid a droning, monotonous speaking style.

Listening

Be an attentive listener. Focus on the conversation and ignore outside distractions. Guide the conversation to obtain the information you need from the caller. Do not interrupt the speaker. You may have to ask the caller to repeat what was said. Verify your understanding by repeating the message. Some people tend to flood you with information. In order to keep the call concise and to the point, you will need to guide the conversation without being rude. For example, Mrs. Jones calls for an appointment. When you ask her why she needs to see the doctor, she begins a detailed history of her headaches. You have what you need. You could say, "Mrs. Jones, let me interrupt you because I don't want you to have to repeat this to several people. The certified medical assistant will record all of this when you see the doctor." Although listening carefully is important, you are handling several telephone lines at the same time.

Courtesy

Always speak politely and courteously. Address the caller by title and last name. Although many telephone calls interrupt your work, do not allow your voice to portray impatience or irritation (Fig. 5-4). Remember that you are there to help the patient.

Never answer the telephone and immediately put the caller on hold. If you need to answer another line or finish a task before you can engage in conversation, ask if the caller would mind holding. Courtesy demands that you wait for an answer before you place the call on hold. Also of great importance, you must determine whether the call is an emergency. If you are unable to take the call after 90 seconds, check back with the caller and ask whether he or she would like to continue holding. Again, wait for an answer before you place the call on hold. If the hold exceeds 3 minutes, you should apologize to the caller for the delay and offer to return the call as soon as you are available.

If you are already engaged in a telephone conversation and have to answer another line, ask the party with whom you are speaking if he or she would mind holding. Again, wait for a reply before answering the second call. Explain to the second caller that you are on the other line and need to complete that call. Do not handle the second call while the first party waits unless the second call is an emergency, a long distance call that cannot be referred to another worker, or a physician calling to speak with your physician.

Quite often you will find that you are juggling the telephones and patients who are in the office. Exercise

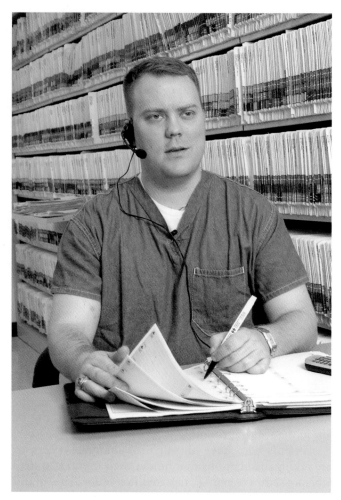

Figure 5-4 While speaking on the telephone, be courteous and professional.

your best judgment in balancing the tasks. If the call is going to take a long time, ask the caller to wait a moment, address the needs of the patient in the office, and then return to the call. Remember, all information about and conversations with patients are confidential. Use caution when talking on the telephone in front of patients.

 CHECKPOINT QUESTION

7. What are the five basic guidelines for telephone use?

Routine Incoming Calls

An incoming call should be given the same courtesy and attention as an arriving visitor. Just as you would not keep a patient waiting without acknowledging his or her presence, so too must you acknowledge an incoming call promptly. Answer the telephone by the second ring if at all possible. Identify both the office and yourself to assure the caller that the correct number has been reached, and offer your assistance. The following are examples of common calls that come into a medical office.

Appointments

New patients call to make appointments, and established patients call to schedule return visits (see Chapter 6). Always obtain a new patient's telephone number and verify an established patient's number in case you need to reach the patient before their appointment.

Billing Inquiries

In some offices, you may be responsible for handling routine inquiries concerning billing, fees, services, and insurance. You may be asked for specific information concerning the cost of services; do not quote exact prices, but tell the patient that costs depend on the type of examination and diagnostic tests performed. Sometimes, third-party callers request information about the patient; remember that no patient information can be given to anyone without a specific release from the patient.

Diagnostic Test Results

Many laboratory and radiology reports are called in to the physician's office before the written copy is sent. Record the information and post it on the front of the chart for the physician to review. If the results are needed at once, bring the information to the physician's attention immediately upon receiving the report. Having at hand a blank laboratory slip or specially designed forms listing the most frequently ordered reports for your office will save time and make it easier to accurately record the results as they are relayed from the laboratory or radiology department. Administrative personnel will place a written copy of test results in the patient's chart.

Routine and Satisfactory Progress Reports

At the end of an office visit, a patient may be told to call in a progress report within a few days. If the patient says he or she is feeling better or getting stronger or the symptoms have resolved, take down the information, record it in the patient's chart, and place it on the physician's desk for review. You may also handle routine progress reports from hospitals, home health agencies, and other allied health professionals. For example, a home care nurse may call and report that a patient's blood pressure is now within normal limits, or a physical therapist may call the office and say that a patient's range of motion is improving. Again, record the information and place it on the physician's desk for review.

Test Results

Patients often call for their test results, and many doctors allow the medical assistant to report favorable test

11/7/2012　Per Dr. Hedrich, called pt & told her that lab work was normal. She had no questions.

GRM, CMA

Figure 5-5 Charting example.

results to patients. Your office will have a specific policy for handling these calls. It is illegal to give information to anyone other than the patient without the patient's specific consent. This consent should be in the form of written permission in the chart, in accordance with HIPAA regulations. Always document the call, as in Figure 5-5.

Unsatisfactory Progress Reports and Test Results

The doctor must speak with patients whose progress or test results are unsatisfactory. The urgency of the patient's condition determines whether the call requires the physician's immediate attention. The physician will discuss serious unsatisfactory test results with the patient. In less serious cases, the physician may ask you to speak with the patient. Never discuss unsatisfactory test results with a patient unless the doctor directs you to do so.

Prescription Refills

As a medical assistant, you can handle requests for prescription refills if they are indicated on the chart. Most offices have an established protocol for refilling maintenance medications. If there is any doubt, tell the pharmacy or the patient that you will check with the doctor and call back.

Other Calls

Other calls you ordinarily handle include requests for referrals to other physicians, clarifying instructions for patients, and calls concerning routine administrative matters.

Ask the physician which calls he or she prefers to have transferred immediately and which calls can be returned later. Calls from other physicians should be directed to the physician immediately or according to office policy (Box 5-3). Physicians also receive personal calls. Your employer will tell you which calls should be put through immediately. Otherwise, take a message and tell the caller that the doctor will return the call.

BOX 5-3

AFF TELEPHONE ETIQUETTE

- When another physician calls, it is customary to give the call top priority. Many physicians instruct their receptionists to interrupt them. This shows the physician that you respect his time. Always ask the physician if you need to pull a patient chart before you get your doctor. If the call is about a patient, your doctor will need a chart. If it is a personal call or about something other than a patient, the calling doctor will say no. This way you do not have to ask the nature of the call.
- Never put a patient on hold without first asking if they can hold and then waiting for a response.
- Include office extensions in the patient informational brochure so that patients do not have to listen to a long list of options. They can dial an extension to be put through immediately.
- Be respectful of the caller's time.
- Ensure that automated answering systems give the patient instructions to immediately bypass the recorded greetings in case of an emergency. For example, the first thing the caller should hear is "If this is an emergency, please dial '0' now."
- Make an effort to add the human touch to automated systems.

Challenging Incoming Calls

Unidentified Callers

Sometimes, callers who ask to speak with the physician refuse to state their name or the nature of their business. In such instances, you should politely but firmly tell the caller that you cannot interrupt the physician and politely explain that you would be happy to take a message. If the caller persists, ask the caller to call back at a specific time when the physician will be available. Alert the physician that there will be a call for him or her at the specified time. Unidentified callers may be sales representatives.

Irate Patients

When a caller is angry, you must be careful to keep your own temper in check. Try to calm the patient and offer assurance that you want to help. Listen carefully and take notes. If you cannot resolve the situation, let the patient know you must consult with the physician and offer to call back. The physician will probably want to speak with the patient personally. Always tell the physician about complaints regarding fees or care.

 AFF WHAT IF?

An upset patient calls with questions about her bill and demands to speak with the employee who handles accounts receivable, who is at lunch. What should you say?

Patient: "Give me that woman who gets all of my money!"

Medical Assistant (MA): "Mrs. Smith in the Accounts Receivable Department is out of the office for lunch. May I transfer you to her voice mailbox?"

Patient: "Absolutely not! Someone else there must know something about the billing."

MA: "I'll be glad to try and help you, Mrs. McGuire."

If you cannot answer Mrs. McGuire's questions, tell her exactly when she can expect a call from Mrs. Smith. Make sure that happens. By cross-training all employees to understand the billing process, you can give patients better service. Making notes in a memo area of your office computer's system will give every employee an opportunity to look at the patient's account and help patients when they call.

Medical Emergencies

As a medical assistant, you must be able to differentiate between routine calls and emergencies. To do this, first try to calm the caller and ask specific questions concerning the patient's condition. Severe pain, profuse bleeding, respiratory distress, chest pain, loss of consciousness, severe vomiting or diarrhea, and a temperature above 102.0 °F are all emergencies, and you should immediately put the call through to the physician or an appropriate health care professional. In some offices, nurses will be assigned to handle these calls.

Determine the patient's name, location, and telephone number as quickly as possible in case you are disconnected or the patient is unable to continue the conversation. This will allow you to direct emergency personnel to the patient's aid. The office should have a policy for handling emergency calls when the doctor is not in the office. Most policies advise you to direct patients to go to the nearest emergency room or walk-in center.

Ask the physician to list instances that might constitute an emergency in his or her specialty and to describe how they should be handled. For example, if you work for a cardiologist, most of your emergency calls will be patients with chest pain and trouble breathing. The cardiologist may instruct you to ask the patient standard questions, have you instruct patients to take certain medications, and then instruct the patient to dial for an ambulance. If you are working for an obstetrician, your emergency calls will be related to patients who have labor concerns or sudden onset of bleeding. Most obstetricians have precise recommendations for when patients in labor should go to the hospital (e.g., contractions lasting more than 1 minute with a frequency of every 5 minutes). Once you have the list of the most common calls and what your response should be, put the list in a prominent place near the telephone.

Triaging Incoming Calls

Usually the office telephone has multiple lines, and frequently, several patients call at the same time. You must be able to **triage** (sort) them into a priority order. For example, any patient with a potentially life-threatening problem, such as chest pain, needs to be taken first. Follow your office policy for emergencies. Patients with serious but non–life-threatening problems should also be handled promptly according to office protocol. Callers who are upset or angry will become increasingly upset the longer they have to wait; handle these calls as quickly as possible. If you need to get back to the caller, do so in a timely manner. Do not leave messages unresolved.

 PSY **TRIAGE**

While answering the telephone, you must handle callers on four different lines:

A. Line 1 is a home care nurse calling the office with a patient status update.

B. Line 2 is a pharmacist questioning a prescription.

C. Line 3 is the mother of a 3-year-old child who has been vomiting for 24 hours.

D. Line 4 is a patient who is having trouble breathing.

How would prioritize these calls? Which one should be handled first? Last?

First, handle the patient on line 4. After gathering information about the patient's complaint and following office protocol, determine the best action. Instruct the patient to come in immediately or to report to the emergency department of a hospital. Next, handle Line 3 using office guidelines as mentioned earlier. Line 2 can be handled next. Even though the patient may be waiting at the pharmacy, the other two calls are more important since they involve the patients' conditions. Lastly, you may record the information on Line 1.

Taking Messages

Taking messages for the physician or other health care professionals will be a large part of your daily responsibilities. Taking messages is easier using notepads designed for this task. Office supply companies have an assortment of pads, or your physician may choose to design his or her own. Carbonless copies give you a record of the messages taken during the day and the action taken.

The minimum information needed for a telephone message includes the name of the caller, date and time of the call, telephone number where the caller can be reached, a short description of the caller's concern, and the person to whom the message is routed.

Before you end the call, tell the patient when to expect a return call. Callback times vary from office to office. Some physicians return calls only at the end of the day, while others return calls randomly. Learn the policy of the office in which you are working.

The patient's chart must document all calls. If you return the call to the patient, document your conversation in the medical record. Some message pads are designed to be added to the progress note on the patient's chart when the call is complete. See Figure 5-5 for a charting example for documenting a call.

 CHECKPOINT QUESTION

8. What is the minimum information needed for taking messages?

Outgoing Calls

General Guidelines for Outgoing Calls

You will make outgoing calls as well as receive incoming calls. You should prepare for your calls carefully; have all information gathered and know what you want to say before you dial the number. If you are calling a patient to reschedule an appointment, be able to explain why the change is necessary and be prepared to offer a new appointment time.

At times, you may have to make long distance calls. You may be required to document calls for the office records. Keep in mind the difference in time zones; if you do not know the time zone of the city you are calling, check the front of the telephone directory. Long distance calls should be dialed directly, without operator assistance. If you dial a wrong number or become disconnected during the call, notify the long distance operator immediately to avoid charges. Never make a long distance call unless you are authorized to do so.

Your employer may ask you to place a conference call, which connects three or more people. Notify all parties of the date and time the call will be made to ensure that everyone will be available to participate.

SPANISH TERMINOLOGY

español

¡Hola!
Hello!

¿Cómo se llama usted?
What is your name?

¿En qué puedo servirle?
May I help you?

¿Cuál es su dirección?
What is your address?

¿Cuál es el código postal?
What is the zip code?

¿Cuál es su número de teléfono?
What is your phone number?

¿Fecha de nacimiento?
What is your birth date?

¿Cuántos años tiene?
How old are you?

Por favor, sientese en la sala de espera.
Please have a seat in the waiting room.

Necesito hacerle unas preguntas.
I need to ask you some questions.

Por favor, llene estos papeles.
Please fill out these papers.

MEDIA MENU

- **Student Resources on thePoint**
  - **CMA/RMA Certification Exam Review**
- **Internet Resources**

  American Academy of Pediatrics
  http://www.aap.org

  American Heart Association
  http://www.heart.org

  Centers for Disease Control and Prevention
  http://www.cdc.gov

  Federal Communications Commission
  http://www.fcc.gov/cib/dro

  Institute for Disabilities Research and Training
  http://www.idrt.com

  Online Yellow Pages
  http://www.yellowpages.com

  Occupational Safety and Health Administration
  http://www.osha.gov

  Telecommunications for the Deaf
  http://www.amrad.org/

  U.S. Department of Justice/Americans with Disabilities Act
  http://www.ada.gov

PSY PROCEDURE 5-1: | **Handling Incoming Calls**

Purpose: To receive calls into the practice and route them accordingly or take messages as appropriate
Equipment: Telephone, telephone message pad, writing utensil (pen or pencil), headset (if applicable)

Steps	Purpose
1. Gather the needed equipment.	Ensures that all materials are available and ready for use.
2. Answer the phone within two rings.	Demonstrates professionalism and courtesy to the caller.
3. Greet caller with proper identification (your name and the name of the office).	Demonstrates professionalism and courtesy to the caller.
4. Identify the nature or reason for the call in a timely manner.	Allows the call to be appropriately managed.
5. Triage the call appropriately.	Prompt identification of emergency calls is important for good patient care.
6. Communicate in a professional manner and with unhurried speech.	Demonstrates compassion and caring for the patient. An unhurried speech pattern is reassuring to the patient.
7. Clarify information as needed.	Prevents errors in communication.
8. Record the message on a message pad. Include name of caller, date, time, telephone number where the caller can be reached, description of the caller's concerns, and person to whom the message is routed.	Promotes good communication between you and the recipient of the message.

FOR DOCTOR Stephens	DATE 4/4/12	URGENT ☐
PATIENT Tommy Taylor	TIME 10 am	REFILL ☐
CALLER TEL. 312-462-5515	AGE 42	TEMP N/A
MEDICATION N/A		WT. N/A
MESSAGE *Per your instructions, pt. called to report improvement. He states he feels "a million times better."*		
PHARMACY / TELEPHONE N/A	ALLERGIES NKDA	RECEIVED BY LF, CMA

Step 8. Record the message.

Steps	Purpose
9. Give the caller an approximate time for a return call.	Provides reassurance to the patient that the call will be handled promptly and timely.
10. Ask the caller whether he or she has any additional questions or needs any other help.	Confirms that the patient's needs have been met.
11. Allow the caller to disconnect first.	Ensures that the caller has completed the communication.
12. Put the message in an assigned place.	Having a certain place assigned ensures that the call will be handled correctly and the intended recipient gets the information.
13. Complete the task within 10 minutes.	Ensures that the call is handled promptly and efficiently.
14. **AFF** Explain how you would respond to a patient who is obviously angry.	You must remain calm yourself or you will make the patient more angry. Keep your voice calm and at a low volume. Have the patient go to an area away from waiting patients and listen carefully to their issue. Above all, remain calm.

PSY PROCEDURE 5-2:   Calling Emergency Medical Services

Purpose: To initiate the 911 emergency system when a patient needs transport to another facility for emergency care
Equipment: Telephone, patient information, writing utensil (pen, pencil)

Steps	Reasons
1. Obtain the following information before dialing: patient's name, age, sex, nature of medical condition, type of service the physician is requesting, any special instructions or requests the physician may have, your location, and any special information for access.	Information is necessary for quick and correct dispatch of EMS personnel. Certain types of patients require special teams for transport.
2. Dial 911 or other EMS number.	The call cannot be placed if the number is not dialed correctly.
3. Calmly provide the dispatcher with the above information.	This allows information to be communicated quickly and professionally.
4. Answer the dispatcher's questions calmly and professionally.	Allows dispatcher to obtain any additional information and verify the message.
5. Follow the dispatcher's instructions, if applicable.	Following instructions provides good patient care.
6. End the call as per dispatcher instructions.	Ensures that all communication needs have been met.
7. Complete the task within 10 minutes.	Prompt access to EMS promotes good patient care and is essential for good outcomes.
8. **AFF** Explain how you would respond to a family member who is getting in the way of performing this task.	If feasible, ask the family member to step outside the exam room. If not, explain to the family member and the patient that you need them to let you do your work so you can get the patient transported as quickly and safely as possible.

PSY PROCEDURE 5-3:   Explain General Office Policies

Purpose: To instruct a new patient about office policies based on their individual needs and level of comprehension
Equipment: Patient's chart, office brochure

Steps	Purpose
1. Assess the patient's level of understanding.	Patients may have hearing difficulties, mental deficiencies, inability to read, etc.
2. Review important areas and highlight these in the office brochure.	Information about hours of operation, refill request procedures, etc. would be needed more than directions to the office, for example.
3. Ask the patient if he or she understands or has any questions.	Ensures that patient understood the information you provided and gives the patient an opportunity to clarify information or ask any additional questions.
4. Give the patient the brochure to take home.	Patients can read printed materials to refresh the memory.
5. Put in place a procedure for updating information and letting patients know of changes.	A printed announcement of changes in hours, availability, services, etc. will keep patients informed.
6. **AFF** Explain how you would instruct a hearing-impaired patient about office procedures.	Speak clearly in a normal volume. Face the patient when speaking to them. Do not exaggerate the movement of your mouth as you speak. Many hearing-impaired patients are lip readers. Be sure to give the patient complete information in writing as well. It is always helpful to have family members accompany the patient if possible.

Chapter Summary

- As the receptionist, you are the most visible and accessible representative of the medical practice. Duties and responsibilities of a receptionist vary among office settings.
- The key to being a good receptionist is to demonstrate tact and diplomacy in all interactions with patients. Providing a positive attitude will ease the patient's anxiety and ensure the best and most confident image of the practice is projected.
- Proper telephone etiquette and manners are essential for good patient care and to achieve effective communication among various health care providers. Triaging incoming calls is a skill that you must master if you are to be an effective receptionist.
- Excellent customer service is crucial to a successful medical practice.

Warm Ups | for Critical Thinking

1. How would you calm an irate patient on the telephone? Identify some phrases that you might use to calm the caller. What phrases may make the situation worse?
2. Assume you are working in an obstetrician's office. What kinds of educational videos might be appropriate for the waiting room? What if you were working in an orthopedic office or for a surgeon?
3. Describe how you would handle a patient who is vomiting in the waiting room.
4. Assume you are working for a pediatrician. A mother arrives carrying an 18-month-old child with symptoms of a respiratory illness. As per office policy, you direct her to sit in the sick child area. The mother refuses. What do you do?
5. A caller asks to speak to the office manager about a supply order on line 1, a patient is on line 2 complaining of chest pain, and line 3 is another patient needing a stronger pain medication. How would you handle these three callers?
6. A caller asks to speak to the physician directly. How would you respond?

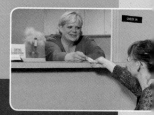

Outline

Learning Outcomes

Cognitive Domain

Note: AAMA/CAAHEP 2008 Standards are italicized.

1. Spell and define the key terms
2. *Discuss pros and cons of various types of appointment management systems for scheduling patient office visits, including manual and computerized scheduling*
3. *Describe scheduling guidelines*
4. Explain guidelines for scheduling appointments for new patients, return visits, inpatient admissions, and outpatient procedures
5. *Recognize office policies and protocols for handling appointments*
6. *Identify critical information required for scheduling patient admissions and/or procedures*

7. *Discuss referral process for patients in a managed care program*
8. List three ways to remind patients about appointments
9. Describe how to triage patient emergencies, acutely ill patients, and walk-in patients
10. Describe how to handle late patients
11. Explain what to do if the physician is delayed
12. Describe how to handle patients who miss their appointments
13. Describe how to handle appointment cancellations made by the office or by the patient

Psychomotor Domain

Note: AAMA/CAAHEP 2008 Standards are italicized.

1. *Manage appointment schedule, using established priorities*

a. Schedule an appointment for a new patient (Procedure 6-1)

b. Schedule an appointment for a return visit (Procedure 6-2)

2. *Schedule patient admissions and/or procedures*

a. Schedule an appointment for a referral to an outpatient facility (Procedure 6-3)

b. Arrange for admission to an inpatient facility (Procedure 6-4)
   - Verify eligibility for managed care services
   - Obtain precertification, including documentation
   - Apply third-party managed care policies and procedures
   - Apply third-party guidelines

3. *Use office hardware and software to maintain office systems*

Affective Domain

Note: AAMA/CAAHEP 2008 Standards are italicized.

1. *Implement time management principles to maintain effective office functions*

2. *Demonstrate empathy in communicating with patients, family and staff*

3. *Demonstrate sensitivity in communicating with both providers and patients*

4. *Communicate in language the patient can understand regarding managed care and insurance plans*

5. *Demonstrate recognition of the patient's level of understanding in communications*

ABHES Competencies

1. Schedule and manage appointments

2. Schedule inpatient and outpatient admissions

3. Be impartial and show empathy when dealing with patients

4. Apply third party guidelines

5. Obtain managed care referrals and pre-certification

6. Apply computer application skills using a variety of different electronic programs including both practice management software and EMR software

7. Communicate on the recipient's level of comprehension

8. Serve as liaison between physician and others

Key Terms

acute	constellation of symptoms	matrix	STAT
buffer	consultation	precertification	streaming
chronic		providers	wave scheduling system
clustering	double booking	referral	

Responsibility for scheduling and managing the flow of patient care in a medical office or clinic is one of the most important duties assigned to a medical assistant. As appointment manager, you make the first, last, and most durable impression on the patient and **providers**. Depending on your demeanor and actions, that impression can be favorable or unfavorable. A properly used appointment system helps maintain an efficient office. If improperly used, it can mean confusion and chaos; more important, it can waste precious time for the patient, the provider, and the staff.

To use the office facilities and the physician's availability most efficiently, determine which patients will be seen, when they will be seen, and how much time to allot to each of them, depending on their problems. Of course, every practice will have occasional delays and emergencies. Your responsibility is to manage all of this while maintaining a calm, efficient, and polite attitude.

COG Appointment Scheduling Systems

There are two systems of appointment scheduling for outpatient medical facilities: the manual system, which uses an appointment book, and a computerized scheduling system. The choice of systems will depend on the size of the practice, how many providers' schedules must be managed, and the preferences of the staff responsible for the daily schedule. Whether a medical office uses a manual or computerized system, many of the guidelines for effectively scheduling the workday discussed in this chapter are the same.

Manual Appointment Scheduling

Medical offices may choose to use a manual appointment scheduling system even if the other administrative functions in the office are computerized.

The Appointment Book

If your medical office uses a manual system of scheduled appointments for patient office visits, you will need an appointment book. An appointment book provides space for noting appointments for an entire year. It may have a single sheet for each day and a separate page for each provider or show an entire week on two facing pages. Some offices prefer an appointment book with pages showing only one day at a time; others may want to see a whole week at a glance. A different color page for each day may also be desired.

The more information required for scheduling, the larger the pages should be. Make sure the book has enough space for all pertinent information (e.g., patient's name, telephone number, reason for visit), is divided into time units appropriate for your practice (e.g., 10- or 15-minute intervals), can open flat on the desk where it will be used, and fits easily into its storage place when not in use.

Establishing a Matrix

Before you begin using the appointment book, you will have to set up a **matrix**. A matrix is established by crossing out times that providers are unavailable for patient visits (Fig. 6-1). For example, the physician may have a breakfast meeting and not be in the office until 10:00 a.m. This is indicated by crossing out the blocks from 8:00 to 10:00 a.m. Write in the reason for crossing off the space (e.g., vacation, meeting, hospital rounds). Some practices reserve specific times or even days for certain activities, such as physical examinations and surgery. Also, it is advisable to block off 15 to 30 minutes each morning and afternoon to accommodate emergencies, late arrivals, and other delays. Some physicians want their professional or personal obligations noted on the appointment schedule so that patients are not booked immediately before these times.

Once you have acquired and prepared an appointment book, it is not enough to schedule a time and date for a patient visit and hope everything will run smoothly. Before actually making an appointment, you should review the schedule carefully, evaluating the needs of each patient and considering the physician's preferences and availability of the office facilities. At the

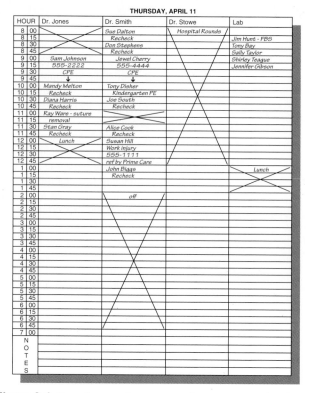

Figure 6-1 Sample page from manual appointment book.

beginning of each day, copies of the schedule should be distributed to all staff members. Along with the notations in a patient's chart, the pages of the appointment book provide documentation of a patient's visits and any changes, such as cancellations and rescheduled appointments. This provides further legal documentation to protect the physician and the patient in case of a dispute, as discussed in Chapter 2.

Computerized Appointment Scheduling

Medical management software designed to assist with administrative functions includes systems for appointment scheduling. Computerized scheduling often saves time. Information used to establish a matrix (e.g., hospital rounds 7:30–8:30, lunch 12:30–1:30) has to be entered only once.

Any medical office software will have an appointment toolbar that requires one click to add a patient, add to the waiting list, see a calendar, or search for available times. Many software packages offer an advanced search that defines the resources required for a certain type of appointment.

This quick method allows you to search for available appointment times. Typically, you enter the desired date, and the computer displays the schedule for that day, showing any available time slots. Another feature allows you to search the appointment database for the next available time slot. For example, a patient is

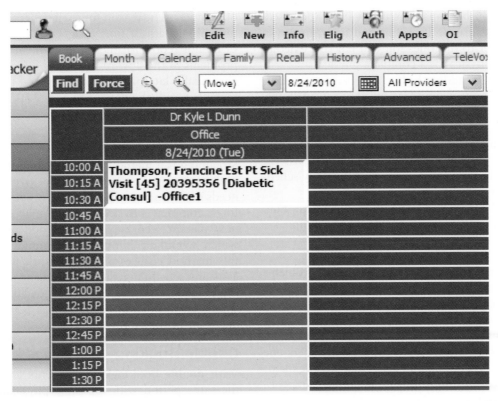

Figure 6-2 A computer-generated appointment schedule. Courtesy of Ingenix® CareTracker.™

instructed to return in 3 months and has a preference for the time of day. You can search for the first available afternoon appointment with that particular provider.

Depending on the specific software, you can also print numerous documents, such as the daily or weekly appointment schedule, appointment reminders, or billing slips. Once the daily schedule is printed, this important document is referred to as the daily activity sheet or the day sheet and is the guide for everyone involved in the flow of patient care. Figure 6-2 shows a computer-generated daily activity sheet.

An important advantage to computerized appointment scheduling is the easy access to billing information. For example, a patient may call for an appointment, and the medical assistant can inform the patient that he needs to pay his balance due of $32 when he comes in to be seen. Credit and collections are discussed in Chapter 12.

 CHECKPOINT QUESTION

1. What is the purpose of a matrix?

cog **Types of Scheduling**

Structured Appointments

Most medical offices use a system of structured or scheduled appointments for office visits. Each patient is assigned a time on the schedule and allotted a specific period for examination and treatment. Box 6-1 shows examples of time allotment. The advantages of this system include

good time management and optimum use of the office facility. Additionally, a daily schedule may be developed and charts may be prepared in advance of patient arrival.

A disadvantage of this system is that a patient may need more of the physician's time than you have scheduled. Therefore, it is important that you ask the proper questions at the time the appointment is made to anticipate the time needed. Such questions might include "Why do you need to see the doctor?" The patient's

---

BOX 6-1

HOW MUCH TIME DO I ALLOT?

Every outpatient medical facility has variables that determine the time allotted for each service. Factors like the number of providers, the number of examination rooms, and the size of the office must be considered when establishing the appointment scheduling guidelines. This partial list of typical outpatient services shows an estimate of the time needed for each.

Complete physical examination	1 hour
School physical	30 minutes
Recheck	15 minutes
Dressing change	10 minutes
Blood pressure check	5 minutes
Patient teaching	30 minutes–1 hour

reply will tell you how many issues will be addressed. "Do you have a form to be completed for your physical?" The answer to this question will tell you whether this is a school physical or a complete physical.

The practice of adding **buffer** time to the schedule gives extra time to accommodate emergencies, walk-ins, and other demands on the provider's daily time schedule that are not considered direct patient care. Such tasks include returning phone calls, reviewing records, and transcribing reports. For example, you may cross off 30 minutes at the beginning and end of the daily schedule to be used as a buffer.

Methods of scheduling patients include clustering, wave, modified wave, stream, and double booking.

Clustering

Clustering is grouping patients with similar problems or needs. For example, an obstetrics and gynecology practice may see all pregnant patients in the morning and other patients in the afternoon. A pediatrician may schedule vaccinations on certain days of the week. Special tests like sigmoidoscopies may be scheduled one morning a week. Advantages to clustering include maximum use of special equipment, ease in maintaining control of the schedule, the ability to provide many patients with information about their particular situation at the same time, and efficient use of employees' time.

Wave

Outpatient medical facilities may use the **wave scheduling system** or modify the wave system in ways that work for their particular specialty. With the wave system, several patients are scheduled the first 30 minutes of each hour. They are seen in the order that they arrive at the office. The second half of each hour is left open. This technique works well in large facilities with several departments giving medical care. For example, several patients may arrive for a 9:00 appointment, be seen by the physician, be sent to the laboratory for blood work, and return to the physician 20 minutes later. The physician has the second part of the hour to see these patients after their testing. That second half of each hour is used as a buffer or extra time that can be used for emergencies, walk-ins, returning phone calls, and tasks other than direct patient care. Modifications to this system may include seeing new patients who will have complete physical examinations on the hour with three or four rechecks scheduled on the half hour. For example, a 75-year-old man being seen for a complete physical would be scheduled at 9:00 a.m., with a 22-year-old being seen for a follow-up of strep throat and a 6-year-old being seen for recheck of an ear infection scheduled at 9:30 a.m.

Fixed Scheduling

Fixed scheduling is the most commonly used method. It divides each hour into increments of 15, 30, 45, or 60 minutes. The reason for each patient's visit will determine the length of time assigned. Patients who are late or do not report for their appointment can cause major problems in the flow of the day. It is helpful to schedule chronically late patients at the end of the day. Another tactic is to tell the patient to arrive 30 minutes prior to the time you schedule.

Streaming

Streaming is a method that helps minimize gaps in time and backups. Appointments are given based on the needs of the individual patient. If a patient is being seen for a complete physical, 1 hour may be allotted. The next patient seen may need a blood pressure recheck, which would be allotted a 15-minute slot. Although this method ensures a smooth work flow, the medical assistant scheduling the appointment must understand the procedures and guidelines for deciding the time that should be allotted. Box 6-1 outlines examples of services and their probable time allotments.

Double Booking

With **double booking**, two patients are scheduled for the same period with the same physician. This works well when patients are being sent for diagnostic testing because it leaves time to see both patients without keeping either one waiting unnecessarily.

Flexible Hours

Offices that operate with flexible hours are open at different times throughout the week. For example, Monday, Wednesday, and Friday office hours might be from 8 a.m. to 5 p.m., and Tuesday and Thursday office hours might be from 8 a.m. to 8 p.m. Some offices may also be open on Saturdays for all or part of the day. Patients still have scheduled appointments, but this greater range of available appointment times better accommodates work and family schedules. Your main challenge with flexible hours is to determine which patients really need to be scheduled for these special times. For example, Saturday appointments may be reserved only for patients whose work schedules do not permit weekday appointments. Flexible hours are most often used by clinics, group practices, and family physicians.

Open Hours

A medical office that operates with open hours for patient visits is open for specified hours during the day or evening. Patients may arrive at any time during those hours to be seen by the physician in the order of their arrival; there are no scheduled appointments. This system is commonly seen in emergency walk-in clinics and eliminates patient complaints such as "I had an appointment at 2 p.m. but had to wait until 3 p.m. to be seen." Open-hour scheduling, however, has some clear disadvantages:

- Effective time management is almost impossible.
- The facilities may be overloaded at some times and empty at other times.
- Charts must be pulled and prepared as each patient arrives.

So that patients are seen in the order in which they arrive, some offices use sign-in sheets. Some sign-in sheets require that patients record the reason for their visit. The use of sign-in sheets is discouraged under the Health Insurance Portability and Accountability Act of 1996 (HIPAA) regulations, as discussed in Chapter 8. Sign-in sheets are considered a breach of confidentiality, since patients signing the sheet can see the names and medical conditions of other patients.

 CHECKPOINT QUESTION

2. What are the three systems that can be used for scheduling patient office visits?

Factors That Affect Scheduling

Patients' Needs

People express their needs in varied ways. A patient might be feeling uncertainty, embarrassment, shyness, or fear. With a patient in an emotional state, even the slightest real or imagined miscommunication can lead to negative response from the patient. Be courteous and maintain your professionalism.

Before scheduling an appointment, you should determine:

- Why the patient wishes to see the physician
- How long the patient has had the symptoms
- Whether the problem is **acute** (abrupt onset) or **chronic** (longstanding)
- The most convenient time for the patient to come in (e.g., early morning or evenings)
- Any special transportation services the patient requires (community or hospital van services operate only during certain hours)
- Whether the patient needs to see other office staff
- Any third-party payers' constraints
- Receipt of necessary documentation for referrals when the patient is enrolled in a program that requires such documentation (third-party payers are discussed further in Chapter 14)

Control of the appointment schedule is your responsibility. Strive to accommodate a patient's requests whenever possible but not if it will overload the schedule. For example, if a patient requests a 2 p.m. appointment this Tuesday and you already have patients in that time slot, politely explain that you cannot schedule the appointment then unless you have a cancellation. You might offer a later time on Tuesday or on another day at 2 p.m. You can also ask if the patient wishes to be put on a move-up list to be notified if an earlier appointment opens up. In other words, you control the schedule. Do not let it control you. The entire medical office team depends on a well-managed schedule.

AFF ETHICAL TIP

Think Before You Speak

As discussed throughout the text, it is illegal and unethical to release patient information without the patient's consent. You may be breaching confidentiality without even realizing it. Consider this: You are a receptionist in a busy obstetrics/gynecology practice. A former classmate comes in for a pregnancy test. While you are making her return appointment, she tells you that the test was positive. Later, while having lunch at a nearby restaurant, you see her mother. You congratulate her on her new grandchild and quickly realize that she does not know about her daughter's pregnancy yet. You have just breached the patient's confidentiality.

What if the scenario had been like what follows? "Hi, Mrs. Roberts. What a conicidence; I just saw Susie this morning." Mrs. Roberts says, "Where did you see her?" You reply, "At work." You have just told Mrs. Roberts that her daughter was at an obstetrics/gynecology office. This innocent exchange is a serious violation of the Privacy Rule of HIPAA. Most employers consider this to be reason for immediate dismissal. Be careful.

Providers' Preferences and Needs

The management of the practice depends on the desires and requirements of the providers working in it. Providers in a medical practice may include the physician, nurse practitioner, or physician's assistant. Some providers often run behind schedule; others are extremely punctual. Recognize your providers' habits and communicate any problems to a supervisor. The physician may allow you to adjust the schedule to accommodate his or her habits. If you are employed to assist the physician with clinical duties (e.g., removing sutures, performing electrocardiograms, giving injections), the schedule can be adjusted to accommodate a larger number of patients while still allowing the provider enough time to give each patient personal attention.

As discussed earlier, the physician also needs time to receive and return telephone calls, review

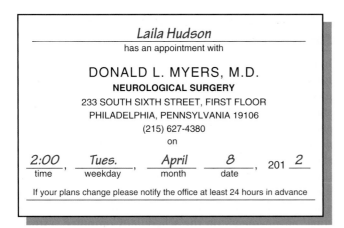

Laila Hudson
has an appointment with

DONALD L. MYERS, M.D.
NEUROLOGICAL SURGERY
233 SOUTH SIXTH STREET, FIRST FLOOR
PHILADELPHIA, PENNSYLVANIA 19106
(215) 627-4380
on

2:00	,	Tues.	,	April	8	, 201	2
time		weekday		month	date		

If your plans change please notify the office at least 24 hours in advance

Figure 6-4 Sample reminder postcard.

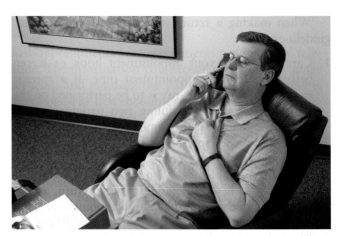

Figure 6-5 When a patient calls from home with a possible heart attack, you will call 911.

at 3:30 p.m." Unless the patient has a question, then say, "Thank you and goodbye." This reminder helps jog the patient's memory, and if the patient must cancel or reschedule an appointment, you will have time to fill the slot. Keep a list with the names and phone numbers of patients who have asked to be called or who need to be seen sooner than their next appointment. This list may be called a cancellation list, a waiting list, or a move-up list. Make a notation on the appointment schedule, such as confirmed, left message, or no answer. Figure 6-4 shows a sample appointment card.

Mailed Reminder Cards

Some offices send reminder cards instead of making phone calls. Reminder cards are also used to remind patients who could not be reached by phone that it is time to keep an upcoming scheduled appointment. These should be mailed at least a week before the date of the appointment. In addition, reminder cards are sent after a set period since a patient's last appointment. Reminder cards are often used to alert patients to the need for annual examinations (e.g., Pap smears, mammograms, prostate examinations).

To handle this kind of reminder, keep a supply of preprinted postcards in the office. The cards should have a simple one- or two-sentence message, such as, "According to our records, you are due for your annual physical. If you would kindly call the office, we will be glad to arrange an appointment for you." The physician's name, address, and telephone number should be printed on the card. Mail the card at the appropriate time. Most medical management software packages produce a list that can be used to alert you of the need for patient reminders.

 CHECKPOINT QUESTION

4. What are the three types of patient reminders?

Adapting the Schedule
Emergencies

When a patient calls with an emergency (Fig. 6-5), your first responsibility is to determine whether the problem can be treated in the office. The office should have a policy for evaluation of the situation. The word **STAT** is used in the medical field to indicate that something should be done immediately (Box 6-2). You also should have a list of appropriate questions to ask the patient, such as "Are you having chest pain? Are you having difficulty breathing? How long have you had the symptoms?" (Box 6-3). When several symptoms occur together, they may indicate a particular problem. This

---

BOX 6-2

WHEN DOES THE PATIENT NEED TO BE SEEN *NOW*?

When the patient calls with any of the following complaints:

- Shortness of breath
- Severe chest pain
- Uncontrollable bleeding
- Large open wounds
- Potential accidental poisoning
- Bleeding in a pregnant patient
- Injury to a pregnant patient
- Shock
- Serious burns
- Severe bleeding
- Any symptoms of internal bleeding (dark, tarry stools; discoloration of the skin)

Note: Remember to check with the physician for proper procedures concerning triage.

WHEN A PATIENT COULD BE HAVING A HEART ATTACK

When a patient calls complaining of the following constellation of symptoms, you should assume that this is a potential heart attack:

- Shortness of breath
- Chest pain
- Arm or neck pain
- Nausea and/or vomiting

Just one of these symptoms alone may not indicate a cardiac event, but when there is more than one, you should be alert to the fact that this may be a heart attack. Studies have shown that, in women, early symptoms of a heart attack are different from those in men. These symptoms include jaw, neck, and back pain and severe fatigue. Keep this in mind when questioning the patient. Call 911 and stay on the line with the patient. Do not advise the patient to drive to the hospital. Follow office policies for such an emergency.

group of complaints is referred to as a **constellation of symptoms.** One group of symptoms found to indicate a certain disorder is severe right lower quadrant pain, nausea, and fever. A physician who sees this constellation of symptoms considers appendicitis.

Patients Who Are Acutely Ill

Patients who are acutely ill often have serious, although not life-threatening, conditions. These patients need to be seen as soon as possible but not necessarily on that same day. Obtain as much information about the patient's medical problem as you can so your message to the physician will allow him or her to decide how soon the patient should be seen. Place the chart with a note in the location selected by the physician, and tell the patient you will call back as soon as the physician makes a decision.

Walk-in Patients

Walk-in patients are those who arrive at the office without a scheduled appointment and expect to see the physician that day. Typically, the physician will have a set protocol, or prescribed list of steps, for handling such situations. In general, you must first determine the reason for the walk-in. Patients with medical emergencies need to be seen immediately. Other patients can be asked to have a seat in the waiting room while you inform the physician of the patient's presence. The physician can then make the decision to see the patient or not.

If the patient is to be seen, explain that you will work him or her into the schedule as soon as possible for a brief examination. When the patient leaves the office, you might apologize for the delay and then ask the patient to schedule an appointment for the next visit.

If the physician decides not to see a walk-in patient, you will have to ask the patient to schedule an appointment and to return later.

Late Patients

Patients who are late cause problems in the schedule. You should gently but firmly apologize for any delay but tell the patient, "You were late, and Dr. Wooten is seeing another patient now. The doctor should be able to see you in about 15 minutes." Patients who are routinely late should be politely advised that "According to our office policy, patients who are more than 15 minutes late will have to be rescheduled." Some offices have found that scheduling the habitually late patient at the end of the day is helpful. In addition, ask patients to call the office if they know ahead of time that they are going to be late.

Physician Delays

Of course, sometimes the physician calls in to say he or she has been delayed and will be in the office later. If office hours have not yet begun, call patients with appointments scheduled early, and give them the option of coming in later in the day or rescheduling the appointment for another day. If patients are waiting in the office, inform them immediately if the physician will be delayed. For example, you might say, "Dr. Franklin has been delayed and will probably be 20 to 30 minutes late. Would you like to wait, or would you prefer to reschedule for another time?" Always keep your patients informed; most people will understand if they know you have not ignored or forgotten them. Most patients appreciate the fact that the physician would also be available to them in an emergency. If you reschedule an appointment, note in the patient's chart the reason for the cancellation or rescheduling.

Missed Appointments

A missed appointment, or no-show, occurs when a patient neglects to keep an appointment and does not notify the office. When this happens, call the patient to try to determine why the appointment was missed and to reschedule for another time. If you are unable to reach the patient by telephone, send a card asking the patient to call the office to reschedule. Note in the patient's chart the missed appointment and that you have either rescheduled the appointment or mailed a card to schedule another appointment. Even if the facility does not routinely remind patients of appointments, be sure to call and remind habitually late patients the day before the appointment.

BOX 6-4

CHARTING EXAMPLE

05/12/12–1530

Mrs. Parrish was called regarding missing scheduled appointment for today at 9:30 a.m. Patient said she forgot about the appointment. Appointment was rescheduled for 05/14/12 at 10:00 a.m. Patient was advised of the need to have regular prenatal checkups. Patient verbalized understanding. Dr. Wong was notified that appointment was missed and rescheduled.—Tamara Dorsett, RMA

Continued failure to keep appointments should be brought to the attention of the physician, who may want to call the patient personally (particularly if the patient is seriously ill) or send a letter expressing concern for the patient's welfare. In extreme cases, the physician may choose to terminate the physician–patient relationship. See Chapter 2 for the proper procedure for this action. Notations of all actions and copies of any letters sent to the patient should become a permanent part of the individual's medical record. Box 6-4 is an example of a chart note.

COG Cancellations

Cancellations by the Office

You may have to cancel a patient's appointment if the physician is ill, has an emergency, or has personal time off. Patients who must be rescheduled need not be told the specific reason for the physician's absence. These cancellations should be noted in the patient's medical record.

When you have advance notice, write a letter to patients with appointments you must cancel, indicating that the physician will be away from the office but will return by a certain date. Patients should be alerted to cancellations a week before their appointments. Ask the patient to call the office to reschedule. If you have to cancel on the day of the appointment, call the patient and explain. For example, you might say, "Dr. Flora has been called out of the office unexpectedly. Would it be convenient to reschedule your appointment for sometime next week?" If the patient arrives at the office before you can contact him or her, apologize and politely explain the situation. Most patients will be understanding. When a physician is unavailable for an extended period, another physician must cover the practice or be on call. Everyone in the office should have a list of names and addresses of on-call physicians, and you should give this information to your patients, according to your office policy. When a locum tenens, or substitute physician, is employed, the office appointments will not be interrupted (see Chapter 2).

 AFF LEGAL TIP

DOCUMENT, DOCUMENT, DOCUMENT!

When a patient does not show up for his or her appointment, you must make an entry in the chart. Because your physician has a legal contract with the patient, he or she has an obligation to treat the patient as long and as often as necessary. If the patient does not report for scheduled appointments, the patient is breaking the contract. This would be an important factor in a court cases involving a physician being sued for abandonment. The chart is the physician's defense. Being diligent with documentation is not optional.
Example:
  10/07/12. Mr. Quinn did not report for his appointment at 10:00 a.m. today. I called him at 11:00 a.m., and he stated that he did not want to reschedule. He says he is doing fine and will call next week to reschedule.—Tracy Amaral, CMA

Cancellations by the Patient

When a patient cancels an appointment, ask the reason for the cancellation and mark it on your appointment schedule and in the patient's chart. Offer to reschedule at another time. If the patient is being seen for a continuing problem, be sure he or she understands the necessity for the follow-up visit. If the patient wants to call back for an appointment, make a note to yourself to check on the call-back in a few days. If a patient cancels appointments frequently, bring this to the physician's attention.

If a patient cancels an appointment and you have a full schedule, no action is needed. If your schedule is light, however, refer to your move-up list to try to fill the vacancy.

COG Making Appointments for Patients in Other Facilities

Referrals and Consultations

When the provider requests assistance from another physician in **consultation**, makes a **referral** to another physician, or sends a patient to another facility for testing, make certain that the referral meets the requirements of any third-party payers. Managed care companies like health management organizations have strict requirements regarding **precertification** and documentation for referrals to specialists and other facilities. If the patient's third-party payer requires a referral form, you will need to complete it with the referral approval number that you must obtain from the insurance company. Figure 6-6

LSW HEALTH

REFERRAL FORM

This form must be completed in full or treatment of the patient may be delayed.
ALL INFORMATION IS STRICTLY CONFIDENTIAL AND WILL BE HELD BY THE AREA HEALTH SERVICE.

PATIENT DETAILS: Interpreter Required: YES / NO

TITLE SURNAME GIVEN NAME

MEDICARE NUMBER HEALTH CARD NO

ADDRESS DOB

POST CODE

HOME TEL

COUNTRY OF BIRTH MOBILE

FIRST LANGUAGE SPOKEN BUS TEL

GENERAL MEDICAL PRACTITIONER NAME:	CONTACT TEL:
MEDICAL SPECIALIST NAME:	CONTACT TEL:

Referred to: Enclosures Medical Documents: Yes☐ No☐ Specialists Reports: Yes☐ No☐

Specialty:

History and Reason for referral:

Significant Medical History: (include any relevant access issues or special requirements)

(Signature) (Printed Name) (Date)

REFERRING CLINICIAN:

Provider Name: Provider No:

Address:

Telephone: Fax: Email:

Figure 6-6 Sample referral form.

is a sample referral form (see Chapter 13). Be sure the physician you are calling is on the preferred provider list for the patient's insurance company. Patients should be given a choice when being referred to a specialist.

When calling another physician's office for an appointment for your patient (Procedure 6-3), provide the following information:

- Physician's name and telephone number
- Patient's name, address, and telephone number
- Reason for the referral
- Degree of urgency
- Insurance information

Record in the patient's chart the time and date of the call and the person who received your call. Tell the person you are calling that you wish to be notified if your patient does not keep the appointment. If this occurs, be sure to tell the physician and enter this information in the patient's record.

Write the name, address, and telephone number of the referral doctor on your office stationery and include the date and time of the appointment. Give or mail this information to your patient. The patient may call the referring physician to make his or her own appointment. If this is the situation, ask the patient to call you with the appointment date and document it in the chart.

Diagnostic Testing

Sometimes, patients are sent for diagnostic testing or treatment at another facility. Such testing includes laboratory tests, radiology, computed tomography, magnetic resonance imaging, and nuclear medicine studies. These appointments are usually made while the patient is still in the office. Before scheduling, determine the exact test or tests the physician requires and how soon the results are needed. (Be sure to indicate to the facility if the results are needed immediately, or STAT.) Also, check with the patient for any time restrictions he or she may have. Give the facility the patient's name, address, telephone number, the exact test or tests required, and any other special instructions from the physician. Give the patient a laboratory or x-ray referral slip with the time and date of the appointment and the name, address, and telephone number of the outside facility.

Some laboratory studies or x-ray tests require advance preparation by the patient. Give your patient a written and verbal explanation of the required preparation, and be sure he or she understands the importance of following the instructions. On the patient's chart, note the name of the outside facility and the date and time of the appointment. Also set a reminder on your appointment schedule to be sure the test results are received as requested (see Procedure 6-3).

Surgery

You also assist with the scheduling of procedures in a hospital operating room or an outpatient surgical facility. Determine the patient's need for precertification with the insurance carrier. You may have to call the number on the back of the patient's insurance card for a precertification number. Call the participating facility chosen by the patient and specify the time and date the physician has requested. The operating facility will need to know the exact procedure, the amount of time needed, the type of anesthesia required, and any other special instructions your physician may have. The facility will also need the patient's name, age, address, telephone number, insurance information, and the precertification number if required.

If the hospital has supplied your office with preadmission forms, give a copy to the patient and make sure he or she understands the need to complete and return the form in a timely manner. Follow the policies of the surgical facility regarding preadmission testing, which may include laboratory studies, x-rays, or autologous blood donation (donation of a person's own blood in advance). Write down all appointment dates, times, and locations for the patient and be certain he or she understands where to go and when.

Finally, note in the patient's record the name of the operating facility and the date and time the surgery is scheduled. You may also need to arrange for hospital admission by providing the same information to the hospital admitting department (Procedure 6-4).

CHECKPOINT QUESTION

5. What information should be readily available when calling to schedule a patient for surgery in another facility?

COG When the Appointment Schedule Does Not Work

No appointment schedule runs smoothly all the time, and an occasional glitch is to be expected. If, however, you find that your schedule is chaotic nearly every day, you should determine the cause. Evaluate the schedule over time, generally 2 to 3 months. For example, make a list of all patients seen, their arrival times, the amount of time they spent with the physician, the time they left, and the amount of time needed to perform each examination or treatment. Since the work flow of the office affects every staff member, involve all employees in your study.

Office meetings are an ideal way to identify scheduling problems. Your evaluation may reveal that many of your patients are arriving late or that you have not allotted enough time for certain procedures. Sometimes, a habitually delayed physician is the problem. You may find that too many staff people are making appointments. If this is the case, you can assign only one staff person to handle all scheduling. Some problems may never be completely solved. If they are identified, however, you can often make adjustments to avoid causing frustration for both patients and office personnel.

MEDIA MENU

- **Student Resources on thePoint**
  - **Video: Scheduling an Appointment for a New Patient (Procedure 6-1)**
  - **Video: Scheduling an Appointment for a Return Patient (Procedure 6-2)**
  - **Video: Making an Appointment for a Referral to an Outpatient Facility (Procedure 6-3)**
  - **Video: Arranging for Admission to an Inpatient Facility (Procedure 6-4)**
  - **CMA/RMA Certification Exam Review**

SPANISH TERMINOLOGY

español

¿A qué se debe su visita?
Why do you need to see the doctor?

¿Desde cuando se siente mal?
How long has this been going on?

¿Prefiere la cita por la mañana o par la tarde?
Would you prefer morning or afternoon?

Llamo para recordarle de su cita.
I am calling to remind you of your appointment.

Le voy a dar una cita para que vea al doctor nuevamente.
I will give you an appointment to return to see the doctor.

Para su proxima visita, por favor traiga su tarjeta del seguro médico y todas las medicinas que esta tomando.
Please bring your insurance card and medicine bottles with you for your next appointment.

Dias de las semana Days of the week	**La una y media** 1:30
Domingo Sunday	**Las dos en punto** 2:00
Lunes Monday	**Son las dos y media** 2:30
Martes Tuesday	**Tres en punto** 3:00
Miércoles Wednesday	**Son las tres y media** 3:30
Jueves Thursday	**Las siete en punto** 7:00
Viernes Friday	**Son las siete y media** 7:30
Sábado Saturday	**Ocho en punto** 8:00
Las horas del día Times of the day	**Son las ocho y media** 8:30
Mañana Morning	**Nueve en punto** 9:00
Tarde Afternoon	**Son las nueve y media** 9:30
Mediodía Noon	**Son las diez y cuarto** 10:15
Noche Night	**Once y cuarenta y cinco** 11:45
La una One o'clock	

PSY PROCEDURE 6-1: **Making an Appointment for a New Patient**

Purpose: To secure an allotted time for a patient who is new to your facility to see the provider
Equipment: Patient's demographic information, patient's chief complaint, appointment book or computer with appointment software

Steps	Reasons
1. Obtain as much information as possible from the patient, such as: • Full name and correct spelling • Mailing address (not all offices require this) • Day and evening telephone numbers • Reason for the visit • Name of the referring person	To stay on schedule, you must allow enough time for the appointment. This information will help determine appointment needs and save time at the first visit.
2. Determine the patient's chief complaint or the reason for seeing the physician.	The reason for the visit will determine the time allotment, use of special rooms or equipment, etc.
3. Explain the payment policy of the practice. Most offices require payment at the time of an initial visit.	Patients must understand this policy if they are to follow it. Instruct patients to bring all pertinent insurance information.
4. Be sure patients know your office location; give directions if needed. You may also want to give patients an idea of how long they can expect to be at the office.	Helps patients arrive on time and lets them concisely budget their time.
5. To avoid violating confidentiality, ask the patient if it is permissible to call at home or at work.	HIPAA's Privacy Rule prohibits leaving messages on an answering machine or giving any information to another individual who has not been named by the patient.
6. Before ending the call, confirm the time and date of the appointment. Say, "Thank you for calling, Mr. Brown. We look forward to seeing you on Tuesday, December 10, at 2 p.m."	Repeating the appointment time will ensure that effective communication has taken place and increase the likelihood that the patient will be there on time.
7. Always check your appointment book to be sure that you have placed the appointment on the correct day in the right time slot.	Failure to record every appointment in the proper location can cause overbooking, frustrated physicians and staff, and irate patients.
8. If the patient was referred by another physician, you may need to call that physician's office before the appointment for copies of laboratory work, radiology, pathology reports, and so on. Give this information to the physician prior to the patient's appointment.	Remember, the patient must give authorization to release medical documents (see Chapter 9).
9. **AFF** Explain how you would respond in a situation in which a patient does NOT give permission to phone him or her at work.	Make sure that information is recorded prominently so all will know. Do not call the patient at work under any circumstances. Call only the number the patient gave you permission to call.

PSY PROCEDURE 6-2: **Making an Appointment for an Established Patient**

Purpose: To secure an allotted time for a patient who is returning to your office as an established patient
Equipment: Appointment book or computer with appointment software, appointment card

Steps	Reasons
1. Determine what will be done at the return visit. Check your appointment book or computer system before offering an appointment.	If a specific examination, test, or scan is to be performed, you will want to avoid scheduling two patients for the same examination at the same time.
2. Offer the patient a specific time and date. Avoid asking the patient when he or she would like to return, as this can cause indecision.	Give the patient a choice, and if neither time is convenient, offer another specific time and date. Giving a patient a choice is good practice. "Mrs. Chang, we can see you next Tuesday, the 15th, at 3:30 p.m., or Wednesday, the 16th, at 9:00 a.m."
3. Write the patient's name and telephone number in the appointment book or enter it in the computer.	Writing the phone number in the appointment book or making a notation in the computer will give you a quick reference if you need to call the patient to change the appointment.
4. Transfer the pertinent information to an appointment card and give it to the patient. Repeat aloud the appointment day, date, and time to the patient as you hand over the card (see Fig. 6-4).	Repeating the information reinforces the patient's memory and helps ensure that the appointment will be kept.
5. Double-check your book or computer to be sure you have not made an error.	Errors in appointments waste the patient's, staff's, and physician's time.
6. Whether in person or on the phone, end your conversation with a pleasant word and a smile.	A smile always feels good to a patient who may be apprehensive about needing to return to the doctor.
7. **AFF** Explain how you would respond to a patient who insists on coming for a return appointment at a time when the doctor is in surgery.	Explain that the doctors have certain hours that they see patients, but he/she is welcome to see another provider in the practice.

PSY PROCEDURE 6-3: **Making an Appointment for a Referral to an Outpatient Facility**

Purpose: To secure an allotted time for a patient who needs to be seen in another facility
Equipment: Patient's chart with demographic information; physician's order for services needed by the patient and reason for the services; patient's insurance card with referral information, referral form, and directions to office

Steps	Reasons
1. Make certain that the requirements of any third-party payers are met.	Some third-party payers require that referrals be precertified. Pre-existing conditions may not be covered for referral. Most companies require that only the patient's primary care physician or gatekeeper make referrals. It is important to research each situation. Telephone numbers for precertification and questions will be printed on the back of the insurance card.
2. Refer to the preferred provider list for the patient's insurance company. Allow the patient to choose a provider from the list.	Managed care companies have strict requirements for precertification and documentation for referrals (see Chapter 13). If there is more than one provider with the same qualifications, the patient should always be given a choice.
3. Have the following information available when you make the call: • Physician's name and telephone number • Patient's name, address, and telephone number • Reason for the call • Degree of urgency • Whether the patient is being sent for consultation or referral	The referred or consulting physician's office needs to know these things to serve the patient well.
4. Record in the patient's chart the time and date of the call and the name of the person who received your call.	This is necessary for proper documentation of the patient's care.
5. Tell the person you are calling that you wish to be notified if your patient does not keep the appointment. If this occurs, be sure to tell your physician and enter this information in the patient's record.	Anyone in the office who needs this information will have it.
6. Write down the name, address, and telephone number of the doctor you are referring your patient to and include the date and time of the appointment. Give or mail this information to your patient. Be certain that the information is complete, accurate, and easy to read.	It is important that the patient keeps his or her appointment. The physician is responsible for the patient's care and should know if the appointment is not kept.
7. If the patient is to call the referring physician to make the appointment, ask the patient to call you with the appointment date, and then document this in the chart.	Recording the appointment information in the patient's chart completes the transaction and proves that the physician's order was carried out.
8. **AFF** Explain how you would handle the following situation: There are two physicians listed for a certain specialty in a patient's managed care's preferred provider list. The patient asks you who she should choose.	You could alternate the physicians each time this situation arises. You want to avoid any appearance of favoritism for one physician over another.

PSY PROCEDURE 6-4: **Arranging for Admission to an Inpatient Facility**

Purpose: To arrange admission to an inpatient facility providing all necessary information and to provide instructions to the patient

Equipment: Physician's order with diagnosis, patient's chart with demographic information, contact information for inpatient facility

Steps	Reasons
1. Determine the place that the patient and/or physician wants the admission arranged.	Physicians may have privileges at one hospital or several hospitals. The patient's insurance carrier may have a preferred facility list as well.
2. Gather information for the other facility, including demographic and insurance information.	Having the patient's demographic and insurance information handy avoids delays.
3. Determine any precertification requirements. If needed, locate contact information on the back of the insurance card and call the insurance carrier to obtain a precertification number.	Most insurance carriers must be notified in advance of an admission to an inpatient facility. You will be given a precertification number that must be given to the hospital admissions department. This number will follow the patient through the claims later filed for that admission.
4. Obtain from the physician the diagnosis and exact needs of the patient for an admission.	The hospital admissions department will need the patient's exact diagnosis. They will also need to know of any special requirements, such as a private room, isolation, etc.
5. Call the admissions department of the inpatient facility and give information from Step 2.	The admissions department handles all preliminary information, insurance information, etc. before assigning the patient a room.
6. Obtain instructions for the patient and call or give the patient instructions and information.	Patients should be given complete information in writing if possible. Patients may be afraid and emotional when they are being admitted to a hospital. Be sure they understand their instructions.
7. Provide the patient with the physician's orders for his or her hospital stay, including diet, medications, bed rest, etc.	If the patient is not at your office, the physician must call in this information. Most hospitals prefer that patients bring this information.
8. Document time, place, etc. in patient's chart, including any precertification requirements completed.	Any appointments made for the patient must be documented in the patient's chart. This provides the information to anyone in the office who needs it.
9. **AFF** Explain how you would respond to a patient who is visibly shaken about finding that he is being admitted to the hospital.	Remain calm yourself. Be patient and do not rush the patient, if possible. Reassure the patient that he will receive excellent care. Be careful not to make promises of any outcomes.

- The outpatient medical facility can be chaotic without an efficient appointment system. Moving patients through the facility while treating each person equally and thoroughly is one of the biggest challenges in the medical office.
- It is difficult for a busy practice to run smoothly all of the time. You need structure, but you must be flexible. Available times, equipment and room usage, and personnel coverage must be considered when finding just the right formula for a well-run and efficient office.
- The goals of the outpatient medical facility are to provide quality patient care and maintain financial stability. To reach those goals, an office must have a plan for the efficient scheduling and carrying out of the daily activities.
- Appointment scheduling systems include manual systems using appointment books and computerized systems that render helpful reports and daily activity sheets. The size of a practice, the number of physicians, the types of services, and so on are considered when establishing an appointment scheduling system.
- Sick patients calling to make appointments should be given priority, and there are established guidelines for determining the urgency of a patient's problem. Other functions, such as phone calls, reviewing records, and lunch breaks, are also scheduled into the daily activities of the office.
- An established protocol or list of steps should be in place to handle pharmaceutical representatives and other visitors to the office. As the medical assistant at the front desk, you will be one of the most important factors in the daily operation of the outpatient medical facility.
- As a medical assistant, you will make appointments, document encounters with patients that deal with appointments, and make referrals to other health care facilities. Learning the issues involved in successful appointment scheduling will help you make sure your facility runs smoothly.

Warm Ups   for Critical Thinking

1. Assume that you are the office manager in a physician's office. Create a policy and procedure for scheduling patients.
2. Sign-in sheets can cause a breach in patient confidentiality. What other methods could you use that would limit the potential for invasion of patient privacy?
3. You notice that patients typically wait 30 to 45 minutes past their scheduled appointment times because of the physician. How would you approach a physician who chronically runs late?

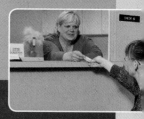

CHAPTER

7

Written Communications

Learning Outcomes

Cognitive Domain

Note: AAMA/CAAHEP 2008 Standards are italicized.

1. Spell and define the key terms
2. *Recognize elements of fundamental writing skills*
3. Discuss the basic guidelines for grammar, punctuation, and spelling in medical writing
4. *Organize technical information and summaries*
5. Discuss the 11 key components of a business letter
6. Describe the process of writing a memorandum
7. List the items that must be included in an agenda
8. Identify the items that must be included when typing minutes
9. Cite the various services available for sending written information
10. Discuss the various mailing options
11. Identify the types of incoming written communication seen in a physician's office
12. Explain the guidelines for opening and sorting mail
13. *Discuss applications of electronic technology in effective communication*

Psychomotor Domain

Note: AAMA/CAAHEP 2008 Standards are italicized.

1. *Compose a professional/business letter (Procedure 7-1)*
2. Open and sort mail (Procedure 7-2)
3. *Document patient care*
4. *Report relevant information to others succinctly and accurately*

Affective Domain

Note: AAMA/CAAHEP 2008 Standards are italicized.

1. *Use language/verbal skills that enable patient's understanding*
2. *Demonstrate empathy in communicating with patients, family, and staff*
3. *Demonstrate sensitivity appropriate to the message being delivered*
4. *Demonstrate recognition of the patient's level of understanding in communications*

ABHES Competencies

1. Perform fundamental writing skills including correct grammar, spelling, and formatting

techniques when writing prescriptions, documenting medical records, etc.
2. Apply electronic technology
3. Adapt communications to individual's ability to understand
4. Respond to and initiate written communications
5. Utilize electronic technology to receive, organize, prioritize, and transmit information
6. Use correct grammar, spelling, and formatting techniques in written word

Key Terms

agenda	enclosure	margin	semiblock
annotation	font	memorandum	template
BiCaps	full block	proofread	
block	intercaps	salutation	

Good written communication skills are important for success. In the medical office, written communication is generated in several forms, such as reports (Table 7-1) and letters. Medical assistants commonly compose collection letters, patient reminders, and notifications of test results. You may also have an opportunity to produce memoranda, agendas, and minutes for meetings. Another important form of written communication is the handwritten entry in a patient's medical record. No matter which form it takes, your written communication must be clear, concise, and correct. Poorly written documents reflect negatively on the physician's practice and on you. Written communication may be sent or received through facsimile machines, electronic mail, delivery services, or United States postal service. As discussed throughout this text, the Health Insurance Portability and Accountability Act of 1996 (HIPAA) Privacy Rule protects the confidentiality of all medical communication. Sending and receiving written communication according to the rules of confidentiality are also discussed. This chapter discusses guidelines for composing letters, writing memoranda, and composing agendas and minutes with proper grammar, spelling, and punctuation.

COG Guidelines for Producing Professional and Medical Documents

Basic Grammar and Punctuation Guidelines

Professional writing requires that you follow the appropriate rules of grammar and punctuation. Box 7-1 provides a helpful list of key rules you will need to know.

Basic Spelling Guidelines

Good spelling skills take time to acquire. Box 7-2 lists basic tips for spelling. Many words sound exactly alike but are spelled differently and have different meanings. Be very careful with these words. Which of the following sentences has a spelling error?

- Wound cultures were taken from the left lower leg site.
- Wound cultures were taken from the left lower leg cite.

TABLE 7-1   Medical Reports

Hospital (inpatient) documents and medical office (outpatient) documents are different. You need to become familiar with the reports generated in a hospital because they become a part of the office chart and are needed for patient care, coding insurance claims, etc. Appendix F contains samples of typical reports generated in a hospital or inpatient setting.

Medical Office Documents	Hospital Documents
The most common documents generated in a medical office are: • history and physical examination (H&P) reports • consultation reports • progress reports • diagnostic test reports (if the practice offers diagnostic tests) Other types of documents in outpatient facilities include: • reports of minor surgical procedures • legal abstracts • general office correspondence	Documents generated in the hospital setting include: • H&Ps • consultation reports • radiology and pathology reports • transfer summaries • discharge and death summaries • autopsy reports

BOX 7-1

BASIC GRAMMAR AND PUNCTUATION TIPS

Punctuation
- Period (.)—Used at end of sentences and following some abbreviations.
- Comma (,)—Used to separate words or phrases that are part of a series of three or more. The final comma before the "and" may be omitted. A comma can also be used after a long introductory clause or to separate independent clauses joined by "and," "but," "yet," "or," and "nor."
- Semicolon (;)—Used to separate a long list of items in a series and to separate independent clauses not joined by a conjunction (e.g., and, but, or).
- Colon (:)—Used to introduce a series of items, to follow formal salutations, and to separate the hours from minutes indicating time.
- Apostrophe (')—Used to denote omissions of letters and to denote the possessive case of nouns.
- Quotation marks (" ")—Used to set off spoken dialogue, some titles (e.g., journal articles, newspaper articles, television and radio program episodes), and words used in a special way (Table 7-2).
- Parentheses [( )]—Used to indicate a part of a sentence that is not part of the main sentence but is essential for the meaning of the sentence. Also used to enclose a number, for confirmation, that is spelled out in a sentence.
- Ellipsis (…)—Used in place of a period to indicate a prolonged continuation of a conversation or list. Also used to display individual items or to connect phrases that are loosely connected.
- Diagonal (/)—Used in abbreviations (c/o), dates (2003/2004), fractions (3/4), and to indicate two or more options (AM/FM).

Sentence Structure
- Avoid long, run-on sentences.
- A verb must always agree with its subject in number and person.
- Ensure that the proper pronoun (he or she) is used.
- Adjectives should be used when they add an important message. Don't overuse adjectives or adverbs. Remember, double negatives used in one sentence make the sentence positive.

Capitalization
- Capitalize the first word in a sentence, proper nouns, the pronoun "I", book titles, and known geographical names.
- Names of persons, holidays, and trademark items should be capitalized.

BOX 7-1 *(continued)*

TABLE **7-2**	The Use of Other Punctuation with Quotation Marks
Rule	**Example**
Place commas and periods inside quotation marks.	"Your bill," explained the patient, "has not come in the mail."
Place colons and semicolons outside quotation marks.	She said, "The doctor told me to come back on Friday"; however, he has no openings.
Place other punctuation inside quotation marks only if they belong in the quotation.	The student asked, "Is that going to be on the test?"
Place commas and periods outside quotation marks when used with single letters or single words.	Even though she earned an "A", she felt it was not her best work.

The first sentence is correct. Site and cite sound alike, and both are spelled correctly, but in the second sentence, the wrong word was used.

Spell check in word processing programs can be a great asset, but it has limitations. Medical terminology spell check software should be added to your computer and be updated frequently. You can add medical terms into your computer's spell check dictionary, but make sure that any word you add is spelled correctly! Spell checks can never be 100% stocked with all the needed terms, especially in the medical profession, as new technologies, medications, and treatments arise daily.

Remember, spell check will not recognize words that are spelled correctly but misused. Even if you use spell check, you should proofread your document for other errors.

For example, the following sentence would pass spell check but is incorrect.

- The patient has inflammation of the prostrate.

Prostrate is an adjective that means face down. "The patient was in a prostrate position." The patient has inflammation of the *prostate*, the male sex gland.

- The physician received a plague.
- The physician received a plaque.

There is a big difference between plaque (commemorative item) and plague (bacterial disease)! These types of errors occur as a result of poor word usage and poor spelling. Box 7-3 lists some commonly used medical words that can easily be misspelled or misused.

Accuracy

Many of the medical documents or letters that you will write contain information that requires precision,

BOX 7-2

BASIC SPELLING TIPS

When in doubt about the spelling of a word, always use a dictionary or a spell check. Keep in mind that a computer spell check will check for spelling but will not alert you to inappropriate word usage.

Remember this rhyme: I comes before e, except after c, or when sounded like a as in neighbor and weigh. Examples: achieve, receive. (The exceptions are either, neither, weird, leisure, and conscience.)

- Words ending in -ie drop the e and change the i to y before adding -ing. Examples: die, dying; lie, lying.
- Words ending in -o that are preceded by a vowel are made plural by adding s. Example: studio, studios; trio, trios. Words ending in o that are preceded by a consonant form the plural by adding es. Examples: potato, potatoes; hero, heroes.
- Words ending in -y preceded by a vowel form the plural by adding s. Examples: attorney, attorneys; day, days. For words ending in -y that are preceded by a consonant, change the y to i and add es. Examples: berry, berries; lady, ladies.
- The final consonant of a one-syllable word is doubled before adding a suffix beginning with a vowel. Examples: run, running; pin, pinning. If the final consonant is preceded by another

(continued)

is used, with the abbreviation following in parentheses. For example, "The patient had a coronary artery bypass graft (CABG) in 1987." Become familiar with the abbreviations and symbols that are used where you work. Appendix D lists the most common abbreviations.

Plural and Possessive

Converting words to plural or possessive form can be tricky in English. Most medical terms have a Latin or Greek origin and have their own set of rules for pluralization. Box 7-4 shows the rules for pluralizing most medical terms. When writing in a medical chart, you should be accurate because mistakes can cause confusion. It is best to avoid contractions. For example, "The patient's coming in Monday to be taught to give herself allergy injections. This will require the patient's undivided attention." The contraction in the first sentence should be written out. The second sentence shows the proper usage of the apostrophe.

To show possession, use an apostrophe and add an S to the word: "The patient's appointment is tomorrow." To show possession in a plural word, place the apostrophe after the S: "The medical assistants' credentials are verified before they are hired."

It is common in the medical world to hear possessive units of time: "The patient will return in 2 weeks' time." or "Tuesday's patients will have to be rescheduled."

Numbers

In general, numbers one to nine should be spelled out, except when used with units of measurement (e.g., 5 mg), and numbers 10 and over may be expressed as a numeral. When several numbers are used in a sentence, this ruled is ignored in order to maintain consistency. All numbers in the sentence should be written in the same form. For example, "There are 21 students in the 2-year medical assisting program."

Here are some important tips you will need to remember about numbers:

- Numbers referring to an obstetrical patient's medical history are not written out: "The patient is a gravida 3, para 2." Do not convert these numbers.
- Watch decimal point placement. There is a huge difference in medication between 12.5 mg and 1.25 mg.
- Double-check that you have not transposed numbers. For example, you typed, "The patient's red blood cell count was 5.1," but it was actually 1.5. A red blood cell count of 1.5 is incompatible with life.
- Roman numerals should never be changed to words. For example, "lead II of the patient's electrocardiogram" should never be changed to "lead two of the patient's electrocardiogram."

BOX 7-4

RULES FOR PLURALIZING MEDICAL TERMS

A add an E	bulla becomes bullae
UM changes to A	ovum becomes ova
US changes to I	bronchus becomes bronchi
ON changes to A	phenomenon becomes phenomena
IS changes to ES or IDES	testis becomes testes, epididymis becomes epididymides
AX or IX: change the X to C and add ES	thorax becomes thoraces
EX changes to ICES	index becomes indices
EN: drop the EN and add INA	lumen becomes lumina
MA changes to MATA	carcinoma becomes carcinomata
NX or YNX change to NGES	phalanx becomes phalanges, larynx becomes larynges

---

- Many health care professionals use military time. Time that is written in military style does not have to be changed if the recipient of the letter is familiar with it (doctors, nurses). If the letter is going to a patient or other person who may not be able to interpret it, however, either convert the time or express the standard time in parenthesis; for example, "The patient's next appointment is at 1430 hours (2:30 p.m.)." No colons are used in military time.
- Temperatures must always have the correct symbol for Celsius or Fahrenheit included (98.6°F or 37°C).
- Telephone numbers should include the area code in parentheses or followed by a hyphen, then the number with a hyphen. Add extensions to the number by placing a comma after the last digit of the number, then type Ext. and the number: (800) 555-0000, Ext. 6480. Periods may replace hyphens and parentheses: 800.555.0000.

CHECKPOINT QUESTION

2. Why should all numbers in a sentence be written in the same way regardless of the rule?

COG Professional Letter Development

Professional writing is different from writing letters to your friends or family members. The goal of professional writing is to get information communicated in a concise, accurate, and comprehensible manner. Slang or idiomatic terms that are commonly used in writing letters to friends are not appropriate for business letters. For example, "Drop by and say hi" is not suitable for a professional letter, even if you know the recipient personally.

Writing effective business letters is a skill that requires practice and careful attention to detail. To write a professional business letter, you must:

- Understand the components of a letter
- Use the correct letter format
- Ensure that the message is clear, concise, and accurate

Word processing has replaced the typewriter for written correspondence and medical reports. Documents can be saved and retrieved, and editing applications make it easy to produce professional documents. Form letters can be used and correspondence merged with a mailing list to make communicating with patients easy and efficient. Grammar and spell check applications mark errors by underlining the incorrect item in green or red. Figure 7-1 shows a letter generated in Microsoft Word.

These skills are described in the following sections.

Components of a Letter

A typical business letter has 11 components. We will explore each one, beginning at the top of the page. For easy reference, Figure 7-2 displays a sample business letter with these components marked.

1. *Letterhead.* The letterhead consists of the name of the practice or physician, address, telephone number, fax number, and sometimes the company logo. The letterhead is often embossed in color and centered on the top of the page. The letterhead may also be preset into a **template**. (Templates are discussed later in the chapter.)

2. *Date.* The date includes the month, day, and year. It should be positioned two to four spaces below the letterhead. The date must be typed on only one line, and abbreviations should not be used.

3. *Inside address.* The inside address refers to the name and address of the person to whom the letter is being sent. A nine-digit zip code should be used if available. The inside address is placed two spaces down from the date unless the letter is being mailed with a window envelope and it will not be aligned correctly. Never abbreviate city or town names. States can be abbreviated. (See Appendix C for a list of abbreviations approved by the postal service.) Never abbreviate business titles (e.g., President, Chief Executive Officer). Here are some other points to remember:

- If the letter is going to a business, type the name of the addressee, followed by his or her title, the

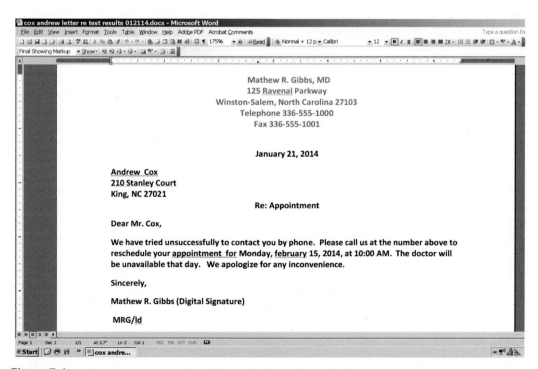

Figure 7-1 A document generated in Microsoft Word. Note the four errors marked by spell and grammar check. The letter uses a digital signature line supplied with the software license.

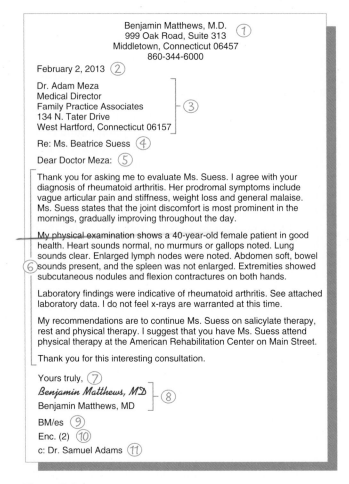

Benjamin Matthews, M.D. ①
999 Oak Road, Suite 313
Middletown, Connecticut 06457
860-344-6000

February 2, 2013 ②

Dr. Adam Meza
Medical Director
Family Practice Associates ③
134 N. Tater Drive
West Hartford, Connecticut 06157

Re: Ms. Beatrice Suess ④

Dear Doctor Meza: ⑤

Thank you for asking me to evaluate Ms. Suess. I agree with your diagnosis of rheumatoid arthritis. Her prodromal symptoms include vague articular pain and stiffness, weight loss and general malaise. Ms. Suess states that the joint discomfort is most prominent in the mornings, gradually improving throughout the day.

My physical examination shows a 40-year-old female patient in good health. Heart sounds normal, no murmurs or gallops noted. Lung sounds clear. Enlarged lymph nodes were noted. Abdomen soft, bowel ⑥ sounds present, and the spleen was not enlarged. Extremities showed subcutaneous nodules and flexion contractures on both hands.

Laboratory findings were indicative of rheumatoid arthritis. See attached laboratory data. I do not feel x-rays are warranted at this time.

My recommendations are to continue Ms. Suess on salicylate therapy, rest and physical therapy. I suggest that you have Ms. Suess attend physical therapy at the American Rehabilitation Center on Main Street.

Thank you for this interesting consultation.

Yours truly, ⑦
Benjamin Matthews, MD ⑧
Benjamin Matthews, MD

BM/es ⑨
Enc. (2) ⑩
c: Dr. Samuel Adams ⑪

Figure 7-2 Components of a business letter. This letter is done in full block format and contains the following elements: (1) letterhead, (2) date, (3) inside address, (4) subject line, (5) salutation, (6) body, (7) closing, (8) signature and typed name, (9) identification line, (10) enclosure, and (11) copy.

name of the business on the next line, and then the address.

- If the letter is being addressed to two or more people at different addresses, type the individual address block one line space under the other or place the addresses side by side.
- If the letter is going to two people at the same address but with different last names, type the woman's name on the first line, man's name on the second line, then the address. If the sexes are the same, do them in alphabetical order, followed by the address.

4. *Subject line.* The subject line, an optional component, is used to state the intent of a letter or to indicate what the letter is regarding. It is placed on the third line below the inside address and is written as Re: (an abbreviation for regarding) followed by the subject. For example, Re: Blood tests.

5. *Salutation.* The **salutation** is the greeting of the letter. It is placed two spaces down from the inside address

or the subject line. Capitalize the first letter of each word in the phrase, and end the phrase with a colon. It is permissible to eliminate the salutation if the letter is informal or if a subject line has been used. When writing to a physician, write out the word doctor. Here are some recommendations when writing salutations:

- If the letter is going to one person and the gender is known, write "Dear Mr. Rogers."
- If the letter is going to one person and the gender is *not* known, write "Dear Pat Smith" (use the person's first name).
- If the letter is going to a woman and a man with different last names, always address the woman first: "Dear Ms. Ray and Mr. Oscar."
- If the letter is going to several people, place them in alphabetical order: "Dear Mr. Andersen, Mr. Cats, Ms. Dart, and Mr. Raymond."
- To Whom It May Concern, Dear Sir, or Dear Madam should not be used.

6. *Body of the letter.* The body of the letter contains the message. It should be single-spaced with double spacing between the paragraphs. Here are some guidelines for writing the body of the letter:

- If the letter is more than one page long, try to avoid dividing a paragraph at the end of a page. If you must, leave at least two sentences at the bottom of the first page. Use the widow and orphan control feature of your word processor program to prevent orphan lines from appearing.
- Tables and graphs should not be broken. They should appear on one page only.
- Web addresses and e-mail addresses should fit on one line and never be continued to another page.
- If the letter is more than one page long, page numbers should be used.
- Use a bulleted format to highlight key points for the reader. For example, "The possible side effects of this medication are:" (then list them vertically with a bullet symbol).
- The letterhead is used only on the first page of the letter. The second page should be the same quality paper as the letterhead. Start the second page with a continuation line (name of person the letter is going to and the date of the letter). Continue the letter two lines down from the continuation line. Your **margins** must be the same as those on page 1. Most templates type the continuation line for you.

7. *Closing.* The closing concludes the letter. Some common closings are: Sincerely, Yours truly, Regards, Respectfully, and Cordially yours. Only the first word is capitalized, and a comma follows the phrase. Closings are placed two spaces down

from the end of the letter. Never put the closing alone on a page.

8. *Signature and typed name.* The name of the person sending the document is typed four spaces below the closing, with the person's title typed directly below. The physician will read and sign the letter above the typed name. If you are instructed to sign the letter, sign the physician's name followed by a slash mark and your name, e.g., Susan James, MD/ Raymond Smith, RMA.

9. *Identification line.* The identification line, an optional component, indicates who dictated the letter and who wrote it. It consists of abbreviations only. The initials of the person who dictated the letter are capitalized (generally the physician); the initials of the writer of the letter are in lowercase (generally these will be yours). The identification line can also be called the *reference line.* The dictator can sign off on the document electronically by using a digital signature provided in the word processing software. In the letter in Figure 7-1, a digital signature is used.

10. *Enclosure.* An **enclosure** is something that is included with a letter. It is abbreviated Enc. and is placed two spaces down from the identification line. The number of documents included is placed in parentheses; if only one document is included, just the abbreviation Enc. is used.

11. *Copy.* The abbreviation c is used to indicate that a duplicate letter has been sent. It is typed two spaces below the enclosure line. Usually, letters are copied to managers, supervisors, or to the physician who requested that the given information be dispersed.

Letter Formats

There are three basic types of letter formats: **full block, semiblock,** and **block.** Office policy or the physician preferences will dictate which format you use. Full block is shown in Figure 7-2, which shows the components of a business letter. The elements of the block letter are seen in Figure 7-3, and the semiblock format is seen in Figure 7-4. Semiblock is also referred to as *modified block.*

Composing a Business Letter

To create a professional business letter, follow these three steps: preparation, composition, and editing. Box 7-5 gives you some guidelines for starting to write a letter.

CHECKPOINT QUESTION

3. Whose address is typed as the inside address? What is the purpose of the salutation? What is the purpose of the identification line?

William Erikson, MD
Storrs Family Practice
22 Maple Avenue
Storrs, Connecticut 06268

August 15, 2012

Ms. Karen Roberts
Office Manager
ABC Copier
Fifth Avenue
Storrs, Connecticut 06268

Dear Ms. Roberts:

We are pleased to announce that we have selected your firm to meet our copying needs for 2013.

Please forward a contract to us, including the stipulations that were previously discussed. After reviewing the contract, I will contact you to arrange for a date and time for a staff orientation session on using the new copier.

I look forward to working with you and ABC Copier.

Sincerely,

Jenny Jacobs, RMA

WE/jj

c: William Erikson, M.D.

Figure 7-3 Sample block letter.

Elizabeth Jones, M.D.
750 East Street, Suite 205
Hialeah, Florida 33013
305-311-2666

June 12, 2013

Margaret Trent
18 Cambridge Street
Hialeah, Florida 33013

Dear Ms. Trent:

As per our phone conversation, your blood glucose level remains elevated. It is essential that we stabilize your blood sugar level.

In order to achieve normal blood sugar levels, you must follow the enclosed diet. A meeting with a Registered Dietitian can be arranged for you to discuss any dietary concerns you may have.

I am also enclosing patient education instructions for the use of a glucometer. You must test your blood sugar every morning and keep a diary of your results. Glucometers can be purchased from any pharmacy. If you need assistance in using the glucometer, please contact Raymond Smith, CMA, at 555-6423.

Presently, I do not wish to prescribe any medications. If we are unable to get your blood sugar under control, I will prescribe an oral diabetic medication.

Please call my office and schedule an appointment for the week of June 20 for a blood draw and a follow-up visit.

Sincerely,

Elizabeth Jones, M.D.

EJ/rs

enc. (2)

Figure 7-4 Sample semiblock letter.

PSY BOX 7-5

HOW TO START WRITING A LETTER

By determining the answers to these four questions, you can better prepare the message of your letter.

1. Who is my reader?

It is very important that you use proper gender identification. Be especially careful with names that can be used for males or females (e.g., Sam, Kelly, Ronnie, Alex, Tracy). Determine the reader's comprehension level. Letters to physicians will be more technical and will use medical terminology. Letters to patients will be less technical and use medical terminology sparingly.

2. What do I want my reader to do?

This is your call to action; make it clear and specific. For example, you might write, "Please complete the enclosed insurance form (two pages). Be sure to include all necessary information and sign your name. Place the form in the enclosed envelope, and return it to our office by June 15, 2003." Avoid using "at your earliest convenience"; include a date for the required action. If possible, include a response mechanism, such as a self-addressed, stamped envelope.

3. What do I want to say?

Briefly list the necessary information. To help you remember all of the necessary information, ask yourself who, what, where, when, why, and how.

4. How will I organize my message?

Here are three basic ways that you can organize your message:

- Chronological: Discuss items in a sequential manner, beginning with the earliest date and proceeding to the most recent date. For example, when discussing the physician's career, list his or her earlier experiences before the most recent career achievements.
- Problem oriented: Let the reader know about a specific problem and provide instructions for correcting the problem. For example, if a patient's blood work came back with abnormal findings, a letter would be sent identifying the problem (e.g., low hematocrit) and advising the patient on the possible causes, treatments, and follow-up procedures.
- Comparison: Evaluate the effectiveness of two or more items. For example, as an office manager, you may have to write to the physician comparing two service contracts or two sample computer software packages.

Composition

The goal of composition is to ensure that your message is transmitted clearly, concisely, and accurately to your reader. As you did during preparation, focus on the message, not on the mechanics.

A clear message ensures that your reader knows precisely what is expected; an unclear message leaves room for doubt.

Unclear: Please contact me.
Clear: Please contact me by Thursday, October 1.
Unclear: You need to make an appointment for blood work.
Clear: Call Temple Hospital laboratories (555-4010) and make an appointment for a blood glucose test on March 13.

A concise message is short and to the point. Wordy phrases with many adjectives should not be used.

Not concise: Please enclose a check in an envelope for exactly $50.
Concise: Please enclose a $50 check.

An accurate message includes the correct date, time, figures, and information. Inaccurate messages cause delays and confusion and can lead to poor public relations.

Editing

After you have composed the letter, edit it for both grammatical errors and factual information. Editing is a key step in making your letter a success. Editing entails two steps: proofreading and corrections.

Proofreading

Whenever possible, have a colleague **proofread** (read text and check for accuracy) your letter and provide constructive criticism. Be sure to maintain confidentiality. If you are using a computer, consider printing out a hard copy of your document for proofreading; some individuals find it difficult to proofread a document on the computer screen. Check for the following items:

- Accuracy of all information
- Clarity and conciseness
- Grammar
- Spelling
- Punctuation
- Paragraphs appropriate in length and limited to one subject
- Capitalization
- Logical organization and flow

Use proofreader marks (Box 7-6) to speed up the editing process. These are standard marks used to indicate corrections. You should become familiar with the basic marks.

BOX 7-6

STANDARD PROOFREADER MARKS

ℨ or ⌿ or ⌐ delete; take it out

⌒ close up; print as o ne word

ℨ delete and closse up

∧ or > or ⋏ caret; insert here ⁀(something

\# insert a space

eq \# space evenly where indicated

stet let marked text stand as set

tr transpoes; change order the

/ used to separate two or more marks and often as a concluding stroke at the end of an insertion

[set farther to the left

] set farther to the right

⌒ set ae or fl as ligatures æ or fl

= straighten alignment

|| straighten or align

✗ imperfect or broken character

☐ indent or insert em quad space

⊓ begin a new paragraph

(SP) spell out (set 5 lbs. as five pounds)

cap set in capitals (CAPITALS)

sm cap or s.c. set in small capitals (SMALL CAPITALS)

lc set in lowercase (lowercase)

ital set in italic (*italic*)

rom set in roman (roman)

bf set in boldface (**boldface**)

= or -/ or ⌒ or |ᴴ| hypen

|⅟ₙ| or en or |ɴ| en dash (1965–72)

⅟ₘ or em or |ᴹ| em—or long—dash

∨ superscript or superior (∨² as in π r²)

∧ subscript or inferior (∧₂ as in H₂O)

◇ or ✕ centered (◇ for a centered dot in *p* • *q*)

∧ comma

∨ apostrophe

⊙ period

; or ;/ semicolon

: or ⊙ colon

⌄⌄ or ∨∨ quotation marks

(/) parentheses

[/] brackets

OK/? query to author: has this been set as intended

↓ or ↲¹ push down a ▮ work-up

↺¹ turn over an inverted letter

wf¹ wrong font; a character of the wrong size or esp. style

¹ The last three symbols are unlikely to be needed in making proofs of photocomposed matter.

4. What is the purpose of proofreading?

Corrections

After making corrections, print a final copy of the letter. Remember, a computer spell check should be used with caution because it highlights misspelled words but not incorrectly used words.

Types of Business Letters

You will be asked to create and type various letters. Letters that you write will be sent to patients, insurance companies, other health care providers, pharmaceutical companies, and various businesses. Here are some common types of letters that you may write:

- Letters welcoming new patients to the practice
- Letters to patients regarding their test results
- Consultation reports to other health care professionals
- Workers' compensation letters verifying the patient's injury or treatment
- Justification or explanation of treatments to insurance companies
- Cover letters for transferring patients' records to another practice
- Clarification or explanation to patients regarding fees or billing concerns
- Thank you letters to sales representatives
- Physician changes for on-call schedules (generally sent to the hospital and covering physicians)
- Announcements of new services, hours, or office location changes

COG Memorandum Development

A **memorandum** (often called a memo) is for communication within the office or with another department only; it is never sent to patients. It is less formal than a letter and is generally used for brief announcements.

Components of a Memorandum

A memorandum contains the standard elements in the following list. Use these guidelines to complete each element. Figure 7-5 shows a sample memorandum.

1. *Heading.* The word "Memorandum" is typed across the top of the page.
2. *Date.* Use the same rules for letters when typing the date for memorandums.
3. *To.* List the names of all recipients in either alphabetic or hierarchic order. If the memorandum is going to a particular group (e.g., all department managers, all employees), it can be addressed to the group.

Franklin Dermatology Center
123 Main Street
Rockfall, Kansas
913-755-2600

Memorandum

To: All Medical Assistants
From: Patty Stricker, Office Manager
Date: 12/03/12
Re: Holiday time

Please notify me by December 10 of any requests you have for taking time off during Christmas or New Year's. Remember that holiday requests will be based on seniority. The office will be closed at noon on December 24. The office will be closed on the 25th and reopen on the 26th. The office will also close on December 31st at noon. The office will be closed on January 1, reopening on the 2nd.

If you have any questions, please e-mail me.

Figure 7-5 Sample memorandum.

4. *From.* List the name and title of the person sending the memorandum.
5. *Subject.* Insert a brief phrase describing the purpose of the memorandum.
6. *Body.* Write the message of the memorandum here.
7. *Copy (c).* Use the same rules as for letters when sending duplicate copies of memorandums.

Salutations and closings are not used in memorandums. All lines in a memorandum are justified left, and 1-inch margins are used. Writing a memorandum entails the same steps (preparation, composition, editing) as writing a business letter. The memorandum should be read and initialed by the physician before it is distributed. Your computer software will have a memorandum template.

 CHECKPOINT QUESTION

5. What are memorandums used for?

Composing Agendas and Minutes

Two other forms of written communication are agendas and minutes.

Agendas

The purpose of an **agenda** is to outline briefly the topics to be discussed at a meeting. It allows the meeting participants to prepare any necessary reports before the meeting and to anticipate questions. Agendas usually begin with a call to order, followed by a review of previous meeting minutes, old business updates, and then new business. Adjournment is the last item on the agenda. The format and amount of detail included in an agenda is determined by the type of group that is meeting. Figure 7-6 shows an appropriate format for the meeting of a professional or civic organization. Your

Forsyth-Stokes-Davie Chapter of Medical Assistants
Winston-Salem NC
Meeting Agenda
September 13, 2013

Welcome
President
Introductions
Members
Introduction of Speaker
Program Committee Chair
Speaker
Roberta Williams, BSN, OSHA Update
Call to Order
President
Reading of the Minutes of October Mtg.
Secretary
Officers' Reports
Committee Reports
Membership Campaign
New Business
Announcements
Newsletter Deadline Dec. 1
Adjournment

Figure 7-6 Sample meeting agenda.

physician may take a leadership role in an organization, and you would be asked to prepare an agenda for the meetings.

Minutes

The minutes of a meeting outline the actions of the group. Members may need to refer back to the minutes of a previous meeting. In organizations with officers, the secretary takes notes and/or records the meeting. For other meetings such as committee or board meetings, someone is assigned the task of preparing the minutes. You should type the minutes of a meeting as soon as possible. Record only motions, seconds, and the results of a vote. You may include a brief discussion of the motions, but do not include unrelated items, opinions, or individual members' statements. The minutes of a meeting become an important document in the association's history. Include the following information:

- List of members present
- List of members absent
- Date and time the meeting was called to order
- Statement regarding the acceptance of the previous minutes

- Motions made and the name of the person making the motion.
- Brief report of discussion
- Results of voting, whether the motion passed or not
- List of reports that were submitted
- Date and time of the next meeting
- Adjournment time
- Signature of the person who prepared the minutes and the chairperson's signature

AFF ETHICAL TIP

Be Careful What You Record in the Minutes

Remember, you are recording the happenings of a meeting that will stay on record for years. The minutes of a meeting should not include personal opinions or any information that is not relevant to the *business* of the group. The purpose of minutes is to record the *actions* that took place at the meeting, not this:

Tracy Amaral made a motion to have a bake sale for the scholarship fund. Anna Hylton seconded the motion. Discussion followed: Tracy told the group not to tell Rebecca about the bake sale. Judy reminded the group about Rebecca's ginger cookies that broke Shelby's tooth that time. Everybody got a good laugh. The motion passed.

A more appropriate entry is as follows:

A motion was made by Tracy Amaral to hold a bake sale on November 2nd at the community college from 7:00 a.m. until 3 p.m. with proceeds going to the scholarship fund. The motion was seconded by Anna Hylton. Discussion followed. The motion passed.

COG Sending Written Communication

After the document has been written, proofread, and signed, it is ready for you to send it to its receiver. Fold the letter in thirds, and place it in an envelope. Most professional letters are sent through the postal service. Other types of written communications are sent through facsimile machines or by electronic mail. Here are two key steps to remember when sending any type of written communication:

- All attempts must be made to ensure patient confidentiality. The outside of envelopes should be marked confidential when the correspondence contains information about a patient. Send letters only to known or confirmed addresses.

- Return addresses must be used so that mail can be returned if the recipient is no longer at the given address.

Facsimile Machines

Facsimile, or fax, machines allow the medical office to send and receive printed material over a phone line. These machines offer a convenient and cost-effective way to transmit records, orders, prescriptions, test results, and other materials that require quick receipt. Always use a cover sheet (Fig. 7-7) when sending papers through a fax machine. At minimum, a cover sheet should have the following information:

- Name, address, telephone, and fax number of the physician's practice
- Name of the intended receiver of the fax
- Number of pages being sent, counting the cover sheet
- Telephone number of the fax machine of the intended recipient
- Date and time the fax was sent
- Confidentiality statement (e.g., "The information in the facsimile message and any accompanying documents is confidential. This information is intended only for use by the individual or entity name above.

Cardiology Associates
Maria Sefferin, MD
897 Bayou Drive
Philadelphia, PA
215-112-9999

facsimile transmittal

To:	Fax:
From:	Date:
Re:	Pages:
CC:	

☐ Urgent ☐ For Review ☐ Please Comment ☐ Please Reply ☐ Please Recycle

Comments:

CONFIDENTIAL INFORMATION

The information in the facsimile message and any accompanying documents is confidential. This information is intended only for use by the individual or entity name above. If you are not the intended recipient of this information you are hereby notified that any disclosure, copying or distribution of this information is strictly prohibited. Please notify the sender immediately by telephone.

Figure 7-7 Sample fax cover sheet.

If you are not the intended recipient of this information, you are hereby notified that any disclosure, copying, or distribution of this information is strictly prohibited. Please notify the sender immediately by telephone.").

When you receive a fax, forward it to the appropriate person. The fax machine should be checked regularly throughout the day, and all items should be sorted quickly.

Sometimes when you fax a given letter, the fax machine may be busy, or the number dialed may be busy. If the number is busy, it is not acceptable to leave the fax papers in the machine for redial unless you are sure that no one else will have access to that document. Never leave documents unattended.

Electronic Mail

Electronic mail, or e-mail, allows computer-to-computer communication, whether within the same facility or anywhere throughout the world. The communication occurs through a modem. Each computer must be linked to an online service provider. Chapter 9 discusses electronic mail in more detail. Here are a few things you should remember about sending letters via electronic mail:

- Confidentiality cannot be guaranteed.
- Follow the usual steps of preparation, composition, and editing.
- You can attach letters to an e-mail by clicking on the file attachment icon, locating the letter, and inserting it. It is always a good idea to open the attachment to make sure that you are attaching the correct letter or version.

United States Postal Service

Written communication is commonly sent via the United States Postal Service (USPS). Envelopes must be correctly prepared so that the optical character readers (OCR) used by the USPS can sort the mail quickly and efficiently. The OCR reads the envelope, scanning for information. The OCR scans all envelopes using these margins: 1/2 inch on either side and 5/8 inch from the top or bottom of the envelope. Addresses or notations outside of these margins will not be read.

Addressing Envelopes

The standard business envelope is no. 10. USPS regulations state that the minimal size of an envelope is 3 1/2 × 5 inches. It must be rectangular and no less than 0.007 inch thick. The standard no. 10 business envelope is 4 1/8 × 9 1/2 inches.

The requirements for addressing an envelope are necessary because the postal service uses OCRs, which quickly and efficiently sort the mail. As the mail travels through the scanning devices, it is sorted electronically.

The return address is placed in the upper left hand corner. It should not exceed five lines. The return address

is typed with the same guidelines as for letters and is single spaced. Often, medical offices have the return address preprinted on the envelope.

The recipient's address is typed 12 spaces down from the top and centered on the face of the envelope. All words of the address should be capitalized. Only postal abbreviations for states should be used, and no punctuation is used between the postal abbreviation and the zip code. All addresses must include the five-digit zip code; whenever possible, the four-digit expanded zip code should also be used. The expanded zip code allows the USPS to sort and route the mail faster and more accurately. Envelopes should not be handwritten, as this does not portray a professional image. The entire address should not exceed five lines. Your software may allow you to insert a USPS PostNet bar code. This is generally inserted two to three lines below the address. This bar code accelerates USPS sorting. Always check your software to make sure it is certified by the USPS.

Special notations such as "confidential" or "personal" are placed on the left-hand side of the envelope two lines below the return address. Notations for hand canceling and special delivery are made in the upper right-hand corner of the envelope below the postage. Nothing should be printed in the right lower corner of the envelope because the USPS uses that space for its bar codes. Figure 7-8 displays a properly addressed envelope.

Here are some additional things to remember regarding envelopes:

- Be sure that graphics or logos do not impede the OCR's ability to read the address.
- Do not use fancy **fonts** that may impede the OCR's ability to read the address.
- A minimum of eight-point type is recommended by the USPS.
- USE ALL CAPS.
- Do not use dark envelopes.
- White or tan envelope with black type is preferred.
- Do not use the # sign; if it cannot be avoided, leave one space between the # sign and the number (this is a USPS recommendation).
- If you are using an envelope with a window frame, there should be an eighth-inch clearance around the address.

```
PIEDMONT INTERNAL MEDICINE
1050 S MAIN STREET
ASHEBORO NC 26092-1050


            SEAMSTER JANITORIAL SERVICE
            P O BOX 5030
            RALEIGH NC 25532-5030
```

Figure 7-8 Sample envelope.

CHECKPOINT QUESTION

6. What does an optical character reader do?

Affixing Postage

Proper postage must be affixed to the envelope by a stamp, permit imprint, or a postage meter machine. Postage meter machines are in-house machines that are regulated by the USPS. They contain a prepaid amount of postage and can imprint the postage stamp either directly on the envelope or onto an adhesive tape that is applied to the envelope. Some machines weigh, stuff, and seal the envelopes. The date on the postage machine must be changed daily, and the ink roller must be kept full.

The physician may opt to use the USPS permit imprint program. In this case, you take the mail, sealed and ready to be sent, to the post office. The postal clerk passes your letters through the USPS machine, and a permit stamp is placed on the envelope. The postal clerk deducts the postage charges from your prepaid account. The advantages to this system are that it saves time and does not require the office to care for the postal meter machine.

United States Postal Service Mailing Options

Mail can be sent in a variety of ways based on its urgency and value. The following is a brief description of the services offered by the USPS:

- Express mail, the fastest service, ensures delivery of your package by the next day (by noon in most areas). Express mail is delivered 7 days a week. Express mail is automatically insured for $500. Additional insurance is available.
- Priority mail, the second fastest service, offers 2-day delivery to most destinations. The maximum weight is 70 pounds, and the maximum size is 108 inches combined length and girth. The rate is based on the weight of the package. You can purchase up to $5,000 of insurance for packages.
- First-class mail is the service used for sending standard mail (letters and postcards) weighing up to 13 ounces. Mail weighing more than 13 ounces will be considered priority mail.
- Standard mail (A) is used by companies to mail books and catalogs. Standard mail (B) is used to mail packages weighing more than 1 pound. The maximum weight is 70 pounds, and the maximum measurement is 130 inches combined length and girth.
- Postal rates, fees, and services are subject to change. You must stay abreast of the latest information. Use the USPS Web site for additional information and updates.

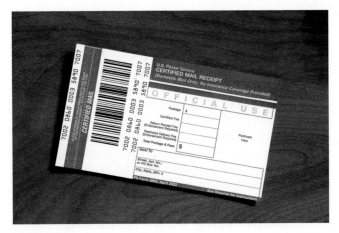

Figure 7-9 Certified mail receipt.

United States Postal Service Special Services

A certificate of mailing is used to prove that a document was mailed. No record is kept at the post office. It does not provide proof that the letter was received by the addressee.

Certified mail provides a mailing receipt and a record of the mailing at the local post office (Fig. 7-9). This service is available only for first-class and priority mail. Return receipts can be purchased in conjunction with this. Return receipts are used to prove that the recipient received the document (Fig. 7-10).

Registered mail provides the most protection for valuables. It is available only for priority and first-class mail. The maximum insurance that can be obtained is $25,000. This service can be combined with return receipts. International rates are available from your local post office. Type the address as discussed earlier, and type the name of the country on the last line without abbreviations (Japan, Korea). All physician offices should have a supply of express and priority mail envelopes along with a current fee schedule.

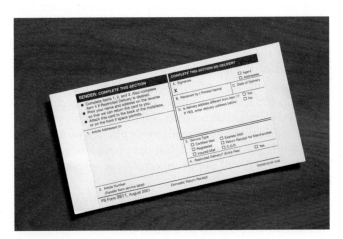

Figure 7-10 Return receipt.

Other Delivery Options

Many other companies specialize in document and package delivery, particularly with next-day or second-day delivery services. Examples of these companies include Airborne Express, Federal Express, and United Parcel Service (UPS). Use the company with which the physician has an account. Fees vary, so you may have to contact each company for prices and available services. These companies offer services such as tracking, pick-up services, money back guarantees, and proof of delivery. The tracking service can be done through their Web sites.

COG Receiving and Handling Incoming Mail

Part of the daily routine for a medical assistant is handling the incoming mail. Sort the mail quickly and promptly to ensure efficient functioning of the office.

Types of Incoming Mail

Many types of mail are received daily in a physician's office:

- Advertisements
- Bills for office services
- Consultation letters
- Hospital communications and newsletters
- Laboratory and radiographic reports
- Office supply magazines
- Patient correspondence
- Payments from insurance companies and patients
- Professional journals
- Literature from professional organizations
- Samples (drugs, laboratory test kits)
- Waiting room magazines

Opening and Sorting Mail

Each physician will have an individual policy on which mail you should open and how you should process it. Any mail marked urgent should be handled first, followed by mail about patient-related issues. Promotional materials should be handled last. Some physicians will have you sort, file, and respond to mail without their review. In some practices, however, all mail is placed in a special file folder and handled only by the physician or office manager. Procedure 7-2 outlines the steps for opening and sorting the mail. Most physicians will open and handle their own e-mail. If the physician is on vacation, he or she will apply an auto reply response to his or her e-mail address.

When the physician is away, personal mail is placed on his or her desk and left for the physician to handle. Mail that pertains to patient care issues should be

opened and handled appropriately. Ask your supervisor if you are unsure which pieces of mail you should open. If the mail requires an urgent response, the covering physician should be contacted unless otherwise directed. Mail should never be allowed to accumulate in outside mailboxes because patient information is confidential.

 CHECKPOINT QUESTION

7. What mail must be opened first?

Annotation

Some physicians request that letters be annotated. **Annotation** involves reading a document and highlighting the key points. If the letter is very detailed, a summary of the key points should be written in the margins. The summary should be factual and not editorialized.

 MEDIA MENU

Purpose: To construct a clear and concise business letter using proper grammar and punctuation
Equipment: Computer with word processing software, 8 1/2 × 11 white paper, no. 10–sized envelope
Scenario: Type a letter from Dr. Tom Chandler (1200 West Main Street, Suite 103, Danberry, VA 24451) to patient James Heffernan (1010 Chestnut Street, Danberry, VA 24451). The letter is in reference to the denial of his insurance claim by Unique Comprehensive Medical Benefits. The denial letter, dated May 28th of the current year, states that the procedure planned by Dr. Chandler has been deemed as medically unnecessary. The letter should inform Mr. Heffernan of his insurance company's decision. Dr. Chandler instructs you to advise the patient that he has every intention of writing a letter to appeal this decision.

Steps	Reasons
1. Move the cursor down two lines below the letterhead and enter today's date, flush right.	Use the date that the letter was dictated or constructed by the sender, not the date it was typed.
2. Flush left, move the cursor down two lines and enter the inside address using the name and address of the person to whom you are writing.	Check the incoming correspondence or directory for the exact spelling of the name of the recipient.
3. Double space and type the salutation followed by a colon.	Using a proper salutation and colon denotes professionalism.
4. Enter a reference line.	At a glance, the reader will know what or who the letter is about. Those filing the letter have a quick reference as well.
5. Double space between paragraphs.	This is block letter style.
6. Double space and flush right, enter the complimentary close.	The close should be professional in a business letter. "Later," would not be an appropriate closing.
7. Move cursor down four spaces and enter the sender's name.	This leaves space for the sender's signature.
8. Double space and enter initials of the sender in all caps.	Reference initials let the sender and recipient know who composed and dictated the letter.
9. Enter a slash and your initials in lowercase letters.	Lowercase initials indicate the person who typed the letter. If necessary, that person can be identified in case of error, omission of enclosures, etc.
10. Enter c: and the names of those who get copies of the letter.	In the days of carbon paper and typewriters, cc: meant carbon copy. Using a single c: is now acceptable to indicate that a copy of this letter was also sent to the person listed.
11. Enter Enc: and the number and description of each enclosed sheet.	If there are enclosures, the reader can see what the sender intended to be included in the envelope with the letter. These enclosures may or may not be mentioned in the body of the letter.
12. Print on letterhead.	Letterhead gives the correspondence a professional look. If no letterhead is available, you may construct it using the name, address, and phone number of the sender.
13. Proofread the letter.	This is the most important step in this procedure. No matter how well written a letter is, errors indicate a lack of professionalism.
14. Attach the letter to the patient's chart.	When the sender of the letter receives the letter for signature, he or she may need to refer back to the information used to compose the letter.
15. Submit to the sender of the letter for review and signature.	The sender should review the letter carefully. It is the sender who is ultimately responsible for the content and condition of the correspondence.
16. Make a copy of the letter for the patient's chart.	Medical documentation guidelines require you to keep copies of every transaction and communication with or on behalf of a patient.
17. Address envelopes using all caps and no punctuation.	In order for the USPS OCR equipment to read an envelope, it should be typed in all capital letters or written in block with no punctuation.
18. **AFF** Explain how you would respond in this situation: your physician reviews the letter you prepared and asks you to insert a comma where you know a comma is not required.	Respectfully tell the physician that your resources do not suggest a comma in this instance. You may even show him the resource.

PSY PROCEDURE 7-2:   Opening and Sorting Incoming Mail

Purpose: To efficiently and accurately open and sort mail to be distributed to the appropriate persons in the office
Equipment: Letter opener, paper clips, directional tabs, date stamp

Steps	Reasons
1. Gather the necessary equipment.	An efficient medical assistant has his or her tools at his or her fingertips.
2. Open all letters and check for enclosures.	If the letter states that enclosures were sent but they are not in the envelope, contact the sender and request them. Indicate on the letter that the enclosures were missing and the name of the person you contacted.
3. Paper clip enclosures to the letter.	Paper clipping enclosures to a letter reduces the chance of misplacing.
4. Date-stamp each item.	Stamping each piece of correspondence with the date it was opened gives more authenticity to a letter. It also lets the reader know when action should be taken.
5. Sort the mail into categories and deal with it appropriately. Generally, you should handle the following types of mail as noted: *Correspondence regarding a patient:* **a.** Use a paper clip to attach letters, test results, etc. to the patient's chart. **b.** Place the chart in a pile for the physician to review. *Payments and other checks:* **a.** Record promptly all insurance payments and checks and deposit them according to office policy. **b.** Account for all drug samples and appropriately log them into the sample book.	Using these guidelines helps ensure the proper handling of all incoming mail.
6. Dispose of miscellaneous advertisements unless otherwise directed.	Dispose of items only when instructed to do so by the recipient of the mail. Your idea of junk mail and the recipient's may be different.
7. Distribute the mail to the appropriate staff members. For example, mail might be for the physician, nurse manager, office manager, billing clerk, or other personnel.	Take care that the appropriate person gets each piece of mail. Many times, a letter has the name of someone who is not really the person in the office who should get this type of information. Determine the right person to receive the correspondence.
8. **AFF** Explain how you would handle a letter marked "Personal and confidential."	Do not open the letter. Place it on the top of the addressee's stack of mail.

- As a medical assistant, you need excellent written communication skills.
- Careful attention to detail is essential.
- Medical information is crucial to patient care and must be prepared with proper grammar, punctuation, and spelling.
- You will write letters, memorandums, and other correspondence with patients, physicians, and businesses.
- After preparing your document, you must be able to select the appropriate service for mailing your letters.
- Medical information is confidential and must be handled according to HIPAA guidelines
- Your primary goal with all written communication is to get your message across in a clear, concise, and accurate manner.

Warm Ups for Critical Thinking

1. Create a business letter. Include all the components and use the full block format. Print your unedited copy and, using proofreader marks, indicate your corrections. Make the corrections and reprint a final copy. Ask your instructor to review both copies.
2. Write 10 sentences using terms from Box 7-3. Use some terms correctly and others incorrectly. Exchange your sentences with another student. Correct your peer's sentences.
3. Collect five pieces of mail that you have received at home. What method of affixing postage did they use? Go to your local USPS office. Obtain either a priority mail or express mail envelope. Correctly address the envelope.
4. Suppose the physician told you to read his e-mails while he was on vacation. In doing so, you come across a personal piece of information that you know he would not want you to see. How would you handle it? Would you tell anyone that you saw it? Would you question the physician about it?

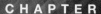

Health Information Management and Protection

Learning Outcomes

Cognitive Domain

Note: AAMA/CAAHEP 2008 Standards are italicized.

1. Spell and define the key terms
2. Explain the requirements of the Health Insurance Portability and Accountability Act relating to the sharing and saving of personal and protected health information
3. *Identify types of records common to the health care setting*
4. Describe standard and electronic health record systems
5. Explain the process for releasing medical records to third-party payers and individual patients
6. *Discuss principles of using an electronic medical record*
7. *Describe various types of content maintained in a patient's medical record*
8. *Identify systems for organizing medical records*
9. Explain how to make an entry in a patient's medical record, using abbreviations when appropriate
10. Explain how to make a correction in a standard and electronic health record
11. *Discuss pros and cons of various filing methods*
12. *Describe indexing rules*
13. *Discuss filing procedures*
14. *Identify both equipment and supplies needed for filing medical records*
15. Explain the guidelines of sound policies for record retention

16. Describe the proper disposal of paper and electronic protected health information
17. *Explore issue of confidentiality as it applies to the medical assistant*
18. *Describe the implications of HIPAA for the medical assistant in various medical settings*

Psychomotor Domain

Note: AAMA/CAAHEP 2008 Standards are italicized.

1. *Establish, organize, and maintain a patient's medical record (Procedure 8-1)*
2. *File a medical record (Procedure 8-2)*
3. *Maintain organization by filing*
4. *Respond to issues of confidentiality*
5. *Apply HIPAA rules in regard to privacy/release of information*
6. *Apply local, state, and federal health care legislation and regulation appropriate to the medical assisting practice setting*

Affective Domain

Note: AAMA/CAAHEP 2008 Standards are italicized.

1. *Demonstrate sensitivity to patient rights*
2. *Demonstrate awareness of the consequences of not working within the legal scope of practice*
3. *Recognize the importance of local, state, and federal legislation and regulations in the practice setting*

ABHES Competencies

1. Perform basic clerical functions
2. Prepare and maintain medical records
3. Receive, organize, prioritize, and transmit information expediently
4. Apply electronic technology
5. Institute federal and state guidelines when releasing medical records or information
6. Efficiently maintain and understand different types of medical correspondence and medical reports

Key Terms

alphabetic filing	electronic health records (EHR)	numeric filing	reverse chronological order
chief complaint	flow sheet	present illness	SOAP
chronological order	medical history forms	problem-oriented medical record (POMR)	subject filing
clearinghouse	microfiche		workers' compensation
covered entity	microfilm	protected health information (PHI)	
cross-reference	narrative		
demographic data			

COG Medical records have a vital role in ensuring quality patient care. The health care industry's move to the electronic management of patient information is now being mandated by the federal government. Government incentives are making it easier for physicians to digitize their operations. The outpatient medical facility in today's world may be in any phase of computerization depending on geographic location, availability of funds, and personal preferences of the physicians and owners. Whether information is maintained on paper or in electronic form, proper management of the information requires adherence to certain legal, moral, and ethical standards. If these standards are disregarded, a breach of contract between patient and physician may occur, exposing the patient to potential embarrassment or harm and making the physician vulnerable to fines and/or lawsuits (see Chapter 2).

A thorough and accurate medical record furnishes documented evidence of the patient's evaluation, treatment, change in condition, and communication with the physician and staff. Medical records have many other uses as well, including research, quality assurance, and patient education. Information gathered from medical records aids the government in planning for future health care needs and protecting the health of the public. In 1996, the Health Insurance Portability and Accountability Act (HIPAA) was enacted to provide consumers with greater access to health care insurance, to protect the privacy of health care data, and to promote more standardization and efficiency in the health care industry.

COG The Health Insurance Portability and Accountability Act of 1996

Congress addressed the need for reform in the health care industry by passing HIPAA. The act includes five "titles." The titles of HIPAA and their subject matter are outlined in Table 8-1.

HIPAA's goals include:

- Simplifying the health insurance claims process and speeding up the process of reimbursement
- Providing greater access to health care insurance when individuals change employers
- Addressing issues dealing with funds set up by employers to pay for health care costs
- Requiring ease of electronic transmissions by establishing a Standard Unique Employer Identifier, which provides complete but coded information about the holder of the code.
- Protection of communication of health information between physicians and insurance companies

In addition to these issues addressed by HIPAA, the rapid advancement of technology in medical information maintenance caused the need for strict regulations to keep electronically transmitted and stored **protected health information (PHI)** safe from unauthorized releases. Confidentiality has always been required in the medical world, but each state had its own laws regarding the exchange of medical information. HIPAA also addresses important new issues that arose after medical facilities became computerized. The use of the internet brought concerns about hackers obtaining personal health information.

Physician offices must also take appropriate steps to ensure that any company they are associated with also follows HIPAA regulations. Physician offices often have a variety of business partnerships that help keep the office flowing professionally and effectively. Some examples of business partnerships are cleaning services, document-shredding companies, laboratory and specimen transport personnel, temporary staffing agencies, and educational facilities. Contracts among physicians and their business partners should reflect that the business adheres to HIPAA regulations. For example, for The Joint Commission to meet HIPAA regulations and ensure security and privacy of patient information during the site visit, health care settings being surveyed must sign a business associate agreement prior to inspection. Students completing externships are also required to sign confidentiality agreements.

TABLE 8-1	Titles of HIPAA
Title	**Action**
Title I, Health Insurance Access, Portability, and Renewal	Amended the Employee Retirement Income Security Act of 1974 (ERISA) and the Public Health Act.
	Changed the rules about pre-existing condition exclusions by insurance companies.
	Prohibited discrimination based on health status by insurance companies.
Title II, Preventing Health Care Fraud and Abuse	Is concerned with how health care providers interact with the insurance network. Includes the Privacy Rule.
	Prevents fraud and abuse in the delivery of and payment for health care.
	Improves the Medicare program and others.
	Establishes standards and requirements for all electronic transmission of certain health information.
Title III, Tax-Related Provisions	Deals with MSAs (Medical Savings Accounts).
	Consumers deposit money into the account and withdraw it as needed for medical bills only.
	The money deposited is tax free.
	Concerned with how employers handle these funds.
Title IV, Group Health Plan Requirements	Amends earlier legislation regarding group insurance.
	Allows people to carry the same health insurance coverage to a new job.
	Avoids starting over again with waiting periods for pre-existing conditions.
	Costs are high without employer's contribution.
Title V, Revenue Offsets	Changes to the Internal Revenue Code of 1986 to generate more revenue to offset the HIPAA-required costs.

Covered Entities

HIPAA uses the language "**covered entity**" to describe those who must adhere to these regulations. A covered entity is defined as health insurance plans, health care **clearinghouses** (entities that receive, review, send, and manage insurance claims for physicians), and health care providers who use electronic billing, funds transfers, and **electronic health records (EHR)**. In some instances, HIPAA identifies covered entities as those meeting the criteria above with more than 25 employees. Civil and criminal penalties are set by the federal act, but each state has enacted regulations governing insurance companies. Covered entities are subject to individual state laws, but if state and federal laws are different, you must follow the strictest laws. In the medical office, you will be concerned with the administrative simplification and privacy rules.

Administrative Simplification

There are four parts to HIPAA's Administrative Simplification section. They include electronic transactions, privacy requirements, security requirements, and national identifier requirements.

The HIPAA Officer

Each health care provider must have certain policies in place to comply with the rulings. In most cases, as long as reasonable care is taken to comply with the intent of the ruling and that effort is documented, providers are considered compliant with HIPAA. HIPAA requires that at least one employee be designated as the HIPAA Officer and one as a Privacy Officer. This requirement varies with the size of the practice or business. The HIPAA Officer coordinates and oversees the various aspects of compliance. Covered entities are subject to inspections by representatives of the Centers for Medicaid and Medicare Services (CMS). Any audits would be coordinated through the HIPAA officer. The Privacy Officer keeps track of who has access to protected health information. The responsibilities of these employees are listed in Box 8-1. These duties should be listed on the job descriptions of these appointed employees.

HIPAA's Forms

The Notice of Privacy Practices must be provided to patients at the first office visit (Fig. 8-1). HIPAA also requires you to obtain patients' written acknowledgement that notice has been received and file the acknowledgement in the patient record. A patient's refusal to sign the acknowledgement should be documented and filed in the patient record. A sample Notice of Privacy Practices can be downloaded and tailored to reflect your practice's policies and your state's privacy laws. State

> ### BOX 8-1
>
> ## RESPONSIBILITIES OF A HIPAA OFFICER
>
> 1. Assess, establish, and review policies and procedures to ensure continuous HIPAA compliance.
> 2. Coordinate mandatory training of employees including specific rules and regulations, reporting any event that might compromise the protection of information, explanation of privacy issues, etc. For example, proper log in and log off procedures.
> 3. Monitor the access to health information by periodically checking for security threats or gaps when changes occur in equipment or software.
> 4. Ensure sound practices by the human resources department as employees leave the workforce or move from one department to another. Passwords and access to certain information should be adjusted as employees change responsibilities according to the minimum necessary information needed as stated in the privacy rule. For example, does the appointment secretary need access to the entire chart in order to schedule an appointment?
> 5. Maintain the integrity of the system by ensuring data and information have not been altered or destroyed in an unauthorized manner by designing and monitoring tracking reports.

privacy laws should continue to be followed if they are more stringent than the HIPAA regulations.

The following information is required to be included in the Notice of Privacy Policies:

- How the covered entity may use and disclose protected health information about an individual
- The individual's rights with respect to the information and how he or she may exercise these rights, including how to make a complaint to the physician's office
- The physician's office's legal duties with respect to information, including a statement that the covered entity is required by law to maintain the privacy of protected health information
- Whom patients can contact for further information about the office's privacy policies

Although not specifically required by HIPAA, it is recommended that you use a Patient Consent Form in your practice. A consent form specifies methods by which a patient agrees to let your practice use his or her protected information for routine treatment, payment, or health care operations (TPO) purposes. Should a patient complain that his or her privacy rights have been violated, a consent

Southern Arundel OBGYN
3008 Pryson Avenue, Severn, Maryland 21140
Privacy Official: Jessica Pyrtle, CMA
Telephone: 410-966-2100

Authorization for Use or Disclosure of Health Information

Patient Name: _____
[print or type]

Patient's Date of Birth: _____ Patient's Identification/Chart No.: _____

I hereby authorize the use and disclosure of individually identifiable health information relating to me as described below:

Specific Description of the Information to be Used or Disclosed Including (If Practicable) the Dates of Service(s) Related to Such Information: _____

_____

The above information will be called "Authorized Information" throughout the rest of this form.

Persons or Class of Persons Authorized to Make the Use or Disclosure of Authorized Information:

_____

_____

Persons or Class of Persons to Whom the Use or Disclosure of Authorized Information May be Made:

_____

_____

Authorized Information will be used and/or disclosed for the following purposes:
[ ] At the request of the individual (check box if applicable)
[ ] Other (*Please list each purpose of the use(s) or disclosure(s) in the space provided.*):

_____

_____

- I understand that if the person or entity receiving Authorized Information is not a health plan or health care provider covered by federal privacy regulations, the authorized information may be re-disclosed by the recipient and may no longer be protected by federal or state law.

- I understand that I may revoke this authorization at any time by notifying _____ [NAME OF PRACTICE] in writing. However, if I choose to do so, I understand that my revocation will not affect any actions taken by
_____
[NAME OF PRACTICE] before receiving my revocation.

- I understand that I may refuse to sign this authorization and that my refusal to sign in no way affects my treatment, payment, enrollment in a health plan, or eligibility for benefits.

  [ALTERNATIVE, IF APPLICABLE: I understand that _____ [NAME OF PRACTICE] may require me to sign an authorization prior to receiving research-related treatment or treatment solely for the purpose of creating health information for another party and that _____ [NAME OF PRACTICE] will not provide such research-related treatment unless I provide this authorization. **NOTE:** If this provision is applicable, the third party for whom the information is being created must be listed under "Persons or Class of Persons to Whom the Use or Disclosure of Authorized Information May be Made." Also, the purpose for which the information is to be created and disclosed must be listed under "Authorized Information will be Used or Disclosed for the Following Purposes."

- [FOR MARKETING AUTHORIZATIONS ONLY, IF APPLICABLE] I understand that the person or entity I am authorizing to use and/or disclose Authorized Information for marketing purposes may receive either direct or indirect compensation for doing so.

This authorization expires at the earlier of _____ **OR the date the following event occurs:** _____

_____
[describe event or write "not applicable"]

Signature of Patient or Patient's Personal Representative: _____ Date: _____

For Personal Representative of the Patient (if applicable): _____

Print Name of Personal Representative: _____

Describe Personal Representative Relationship/Authority to Act for the Individual (parent, guardian, etc.): _____

Figure 8-1 A sample Notice of Privacy Practices required by HIPAA.

I, _____, give my
permission for _____ to
release information generated in my medical record
between the dates of _____
and _____ to _____.

Signature _____ Date _____
Witness _____ Date _____

Or

I, _____, give my
permission for _____ to release
information in my medical record regarding the care
and treatment of _____
to _____.

Signature _____ Date _____
Witness _____ Date _____

Figure 8-2 A proper authorization for release of information.

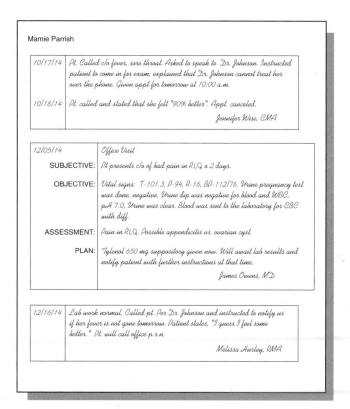

Mamie Parrish

10/17/14	Pt. Called c/o fever, sore throat. Asked to speak to Dr. Johnson. Instructed patient to come in for exam; explained that Dr. Johnson cannot treat her over the phone. Given appt for tomorrow at 10:00 a.m.
10/18/14	Pt. called and stated that she felt "90% better". Appt. canceled.
	Jennifer Wise, CMA

12/05/14	Office Visit
SUBJECTIVE:	Pt presents c/o of bad pain in RLQ x 2 days.
OBJECTIVE:	Vital signs: T-101.3, P-94, R-16, BP-112/76. Urine pregnancy test was done, negative. Urine dip was negative for blood and WBC, pH 7.0. Urine was clear. Blood was sent to the laboratory for CBC with diff.
ASSESSMENT:	Pain in RLQ. Possible appendicitis vs. ovarian cyst.
PLAN:	Tylenol 650 mg suppository given now. Will await lab results and notify patient with further instructions at that time.
	James Owens, MD

| 12/16/14 | Lab work normal. Called pt. Per Dr. Johnson and instructed to notify us if her fever is not gone tomorrow. Patient states, "I guess I feel some better." Pt. will call office p.r.n. |
| | Melissa Hurley, RMA |

Figure 8-3 Sample page from patient's chart.

form may afford you an extra measure of protection if your practice is investigated for HIPAA noncompliance.

HIPAA privacy regulations do not require you to obtain patients' consent to use their PHI for routine disclosures such as those related to TPO. However, the regulations do mandate that you obtain written patient consent before releasing their information for any reason other than TPO (e.g., disclosure of psychotherapy notes). To comply, you'll need to identify situations in your practice where special authorization is needed and develop an authorization form for patients to sign. A signed copy or documentation of the patient's refusal to sign should be retained in the patient record. Figures 8-1 through 8-3 show samples of the necessary forms.

Releasing Medical Records

The protection of personal information is crucial to the privacy of patients. Although the physical medical record legally belongs to the physician, the information belongs to the patient. Any release of records must first be authorized by the patient or the patient's legal guardian. When releasing a medical record, provide a copy only. *Never* release the original medical record except in limited circumstances.

Insurance companies, lawyers, other health care practitioners, and patients themselves may request copies of medical records. All requests should be made in writing, stating the patient's name, address, and social security number, and must contain the patient's *original* signature authorizing the release of records. Never release information over the telephone. You will have no way of verifying that the person with whom you are speaking is actually the person who has authorization.

State laws allow facilities to charge a fee for copying the medical record. The American Medical Association (AMA) published guidelines for physicians to ensure ethical business practices. They recommend a reasonable fee for reproduction of records to be no more than $1 per page or $100 for the entire record, whichever is less. If the record is less than 10 pages, the office may charge up to $10 to cover postage and miscellaneous costs associated with the retrieval process. Laws may vary from state to state.

HIPAA's Privacy Rule

HIPAA provides protection of the sharing of what is referred to as PHI. PHI is any information that can be linked to a specific person. A diagnosis alone without a full name is not identifiable, but a first and last name associated with a diagnosis is identifiable; therefore, it is protected health information. For example, the Centers for Disease Control and Prevention (CDC) publishes information to cite statistics about communicable diseases. Since the names of the people who have been diagnosed with the diseases are not published, this information is not protected.

The privacy rule establishes safeguards to protect the confidentiality of medical information. Covered entities must:

- Share health information for health purposes only
- Provide the minimum amount of information necessary
- Adopt written privacy procedures
- Designate a Privacy Officer
- Train employees

 ETHICAL TIP

HIPAA Says Patients Have Rights

Through HIPAA, the federal government recognizes that it is ethical to give patients certain rights. HIPAA protects the rights of patients by allowing them to:

- Ask to see and get a copy of their health records
- Have corrections added to their health information
- Receive a notice that tells them how their health information may be used and shared
- Decide if they want to give permission before their health information can be used or shared for certain purposes such as for marketing
- Get a report on when and why their health information was shared for certain purposes
- File a complaint with the provider or health insurer if they believe their rights have been denied or their health information is not being protected
- File a complaint with the U.S. government

Patients can learn about their rights, including how to file a complaint, from the Web site at http://www.hhs.gov/ocr/privacy/hipaa/understanding/consumers/index.html or by calling 1-866-627-7748.

CHECKPOINT QUESTION

1. What is the purpose of HIPAA?

COG **Releasing Records to Patients**

As discussed previously, releasing medical records is an important part of any medical facility. When patients request copies of their own records, the doctor makes the decision about what to copy. Patients aged 17 years and under cannot get copies of their own medical records without a signed consent from a parent or legal guardian, except for emancipated minors. However, they may obtain certain services independently (check your state's

law regarding treatment of minors); in such cases, under the law, you are not permitted to contact the parent or guardian. Some states allow minors to seek treatment for sexually transmitted diseases and birth control without parental knowledge or consent. Sometimes, the parent or guardian may still be billed for these services without the bill being itemized. The billing statement should include only the treatment dates and amount due.

 LEGAL TIP

SUBPOENA DUCES TECUM

An original record may be released when it is subpoenaed by a court of law. In such situations, the physician may wish to have the judge sign a document stating that he or she will temporarily take charge of the medical record. This signed document should be filed in the medical office until the record is returned. To further ensure the record's safety, a staff member can transport the original record to court on the day it is requested and then return the record at the end of the court session that day. As soon as it is known that a record will be part of a court case, the record should be kept in a locked cabinet. When the court orders that a record be submitted to the court at a given date and time, the legal order is termed *subpoena duces tecum*.

 LEGAL TIP

ABBREVIATIONS? WHEN IN DOUBT, SPELL IT OUT

The Joint Commission is charged with monitoring and accrediting inpatient and outpatient medical facilities. Recent changes in standards regarding some ambiguous handwritten abbreviations reflect the growing feeling that many commonly used abbreviations are overused, used incorrectly, open to interpretation, or easily confused with another abbreviation. For instance, the abbreviation BS might stand for bowel sounds, breath sounds, or blood sugar. In addition to requiring facilities to keep a list of acceptable abbreviations used in the facility, The Joint Commission issues a "Do Not Use" list that can be found at http://www.jointcommission.org. Even though some abbreviations can be confusing and should not be used, many continue to be used. Appendix D has a general list of commonly used abbreviations. The Joint Commission is covered in more detail in Chapter 10.

Proper Authorization

You must follow certain guidelines even with a signed release form (see Fig. 8-3). The authorization form must give the patient the opportunity to limit the information to be released. Patients may release only information relating to a specific disorder, or they may specify a time limit. They may not, however, ask that the physician leave out information pertinent to the situation.

References to mental health diagnoses or treatments, drug or alcohol abuse, HIV, AIDS, or any other sexually transmitted disease may not be released without specific mention on the signed authorization form. If it is not specifically requested by the patient, when you are copying the record, place a piece of blank white paper over any such areas of information. Never white-out these areas on the original document or mention what these blank areas included.

Protected health information can be shared with proper authorization by the patient. By signing an appropriate authorization, the patient gives permission for the health care provider to share their personal health information with anyone they designate. The form must include the name of the person to receive the information, the name of the provider releasing the information, and the dates of service and/or certain conditions covered by the authorization. It is recommended that there also be a witness signature. Figure 8-3 is a sample of a proper authorization form.

 CHECKPOINT QUESTION

2. What is required for a legal disclosure of a patient's HIV status?

Legally Required Disclosures

As previously discussed in Chapter 2, in certain situations, the law requires reporting information to particular authorities. Requirements for reporting vary among states.

As with most laws, there are exceptions to the privacy rule. Certain information is crucial to the patient, needed for the protection of the public, or involves criminal activity and is released without the patient's permission. Such disclosures include:

- Vital statistics
- Child and elder abuse or maltreatment
- Emergency circumstances
- Identification of body of deceased person
- Cause of death
- Public health needs, such as communicable diseases
- Research
- Judicial and administrative proceedings
- Law enforcement concerns such as violent criminal activities
- Activities related to national defense and security

 CHECKPOINT QUESTION

3. Why is some information released without a patient's permission?

 AFF PATIENT EDUCATION

PROTECT YOUR PATIENTS BY TEACHING THEM TO READ WHAT THEY ARE SIGNING

Many patients feel inadequate when it comes to understanding the intricacies of the laws that are designed to protect them. Patients are often ready to sign a form handed to them without even reading it. Patients trust and depend on their health care provider to protect their rights to privacy. Whatever form, authorization, or consent the patient is handed should be accompanied by a verbal explanation of what they are signing.

For example, legal experts advise that some forms designed for patients to give their authorization to release their personal information are too general and are not even considered legally binding. Proper authorization should include the elements in Figure 8-2. Patients should understand that it would be improper to sign a form like this:

I, _____, give my permission for the release of my medical records.

Signature: _____.

This blanket permission opens patients up to the possibility of any and all of their information being shared with anyone at anytime. Each time patients need or want their information to be released, they must sign a new authorization outlining the specific information to be released by who and to whom. Help them understand the importance of knowing what they are signing, and tell them to ask questions if they need any clarification.

COG Standard Medical Records

Even though our expanding technology gives today's medical office the ability to store health information in electronic form, the migration to a paperless environment has been slow. Outpatient medical offices that are not electronic accumulate mounds of paper every day. A medical facility has a variety of options for standard or manual record keeping. The best systems are those that have been tried, revised, and revised again. No matter how the records are stored, make sure that the information is:

- Easily retrievable
- Kept in an orderly manner

- Assistance with clinical decision making—Alerts, reminders, and patient care recommendations give providers valuable information at their fingertips.
- Improved communication—Easy access to information enhances communication among medical office staff, as well as with patients and other health care entities.
- Support for administrative, financial, and operational functions—Electronic health records assist with storage of patient **demographic data**, appointment scheduling, insurance billing and coding (see next section), accounting procedures, and inventory and supply tracking, among other tasks. EHR may even help increase revenue by (eventually) allowing the practice to eliminate the file room and turn the extra space into exam rooms or office space. EHR also reduces medical transcription costs.

Electronic health records do have some disadvantages, however, including cost, potential software or hardware damage or failure, and the need for in-depth staff training. The task of inputting data from hundreds or thousands of charts into the computer is time consuming but must be done before the system is used. Sometimes, in the beginning stages, implementing EHR can actually reduce physician and staff productivity instead of increasing it. But over time, the benefits should outweigh the drawbacks.

COG Billing and Coding Using Electronic Health Records

In later chapters, you will learn the world of coding. Selecting the various levels of patient visits to the office is based on many factors. Physicians must choose the level based on the amount of information gathered, the extent of the physical examination performed, and the level of decision making the patient's care required. Many EHR software companies include drop-down lists and preset menus to help providers select the appropriate code based on the information entered for that visit. This is an important feature because every office that accepts Medicare and/or Medicaid is subject to government audits. These audits are designed to verify that the level of office visit charged to the patient is consistent with the criteria outlined by the CMS. If discrepancies are found, the office may be fined. Software that assists with these coding issues can have many benefits, such as avoiding returned claims, preventing insurance fraud, decreasing staff data entry errors, reducing the possibility of an audit, and increasing revenue through streamlined and timely billing processes.

The Medical Assistant's Role

As a medical assistant, you have the same roles and responsibilities related to EHR as with paper records.

The difference is that you will perform more of your regular tasks using the computer. Two of your main responsibilities are data collection and patient care. Electronic health records allow you to quickly and accurately record chart notes, look up test results, call in medication orders, and so on. With computers in exam rooms, no time is wasted looking for missing patient data; records are easily stored and retrieved. EHR may also help you gather more complete patient information by prompting you to ask questions that might otherwise be missed before allowing you to move on to the next screen. Tools such as tickler messages can also remind you to provide patient teaching on topics such as vaccines, yearly checkups, blood pressure checks, mammograms, and so on.

Medical assistants can also provide assurance to patients about the safety and security of their health information. In order to comply with HIPAA, electronic health record systems have built-in features to decrease the risk of stolen or misused data. These safeguards include password protections, electronic firewalls that block access by unauthorized users, audit trails that can track who accessed a record and when, data encryption, and more. By explaining the privacy safeguards integrated into EHR, you promote patient confidence in the medical practice. (See Electronic Health Record Security section for more details about EHR security.)

 AFF WHAT IF?

What if the EHR system goes down due to a power outage?

If the lights go out, return to the old paper system, and then input the data when the electricity comes back on again. Use backup reports and schedules that were printed ahead of time. Backup tapes should be done at the end of every workday to save information in case a problem occurs. Always have contingency plans for data backup, disaster recovery, or other emergencies ready to be implemented if needed.

Electronic Health Record Security

AMA and many risk management companies have published guidelines for the EHR. Following are suggestions and guidelines based on HIPAA's requirements for practices using computers to transfer or store patient information. Experts advise physicians and office managers considering software programs to look for the following capabilities:

- User-friendly commands that allow users to move easily within the system.

- Spell check and free text fields for inserting corrections and late entries. The electronic record is corrected by using the same rules as in the standard record. Entries are not deleted but corrected, with an explanation to avoid the appearance of hiding information.
- Security levels to limit entry to all functions. For example, a receptionist does not need access to the physician's personal taxes.
- A system, including encryption, to repel hackers. Evidence shows that persons with access to technology can invade patients' records stored on computer databases. This is a breach of confidentiality and is illegal.

To maintain security, facilities are urged to do the following:

- Keep all computer backup disks in a safe place away from the practice.
- Store disks in a bank safe-deposit box.
- Use passwords with characters other than letters and encrypt the passwords.
- Change log-in codes and passwords every 30 days.
- Prepare a backup plan for use when the computer system is down.
- Turn terminals away from areas where information may be seen by patients.
- Keep the fax machines and printers that receive personal medical information in a private place.
- Ensure that each user is restricted to the information needed to do his or her job.
- Train employees on confidentiality and each person's responsibility to adhere to HIPAA's Privacy Rule.
- Design a written confidentiality policy that employees sign.
- Conduct routine audits that produce a trail of each employee's movement through the EHR system.
- Include disciplinary measures for breaches of confidentiality.

Providers may use a handheld personal data device (PDA), laptop, electronic notebook, or personal computer (PC) in central areas or examination rooms. The same security measures apply to these items. Patients should not have access to computer screens in the examination room. The physician should take care in keeping a personal data system, just as he or she protects the prescription pad. The personal data devices and laptops, may contain the entire *Physicians' Desk Reference*, giving the provider information needed for prescribing drugs at the fingertips. Other applications of such portable devices include downloading patient education materials and documenting and transferring information about patient encounters when the office is closed. In this era of paperless medical offices, care must be taken to protect the privacy of the patient as carefully as in the world of paper.

COG Medical Record Organization

Information in the paper medical record is usually organized in a standard chart order and placed in a specially designed folder. The order in which documents are placed in the medical record depends on the physician's preference. As mentioned earlier, the demographic information is kept separate from the clinical information. The clinical portion of the medical record is organized in either a source-oriented or a problem-oriented format. In source-oriented medical records, all similar categories or sources of information are grouped together. The typical groupings:

- Billing and insurance information
- Physician orders
- Progress notes
- Laboratory results
- Radiographic results (magnetic resonance imaging, computed tomography, ultrasound)
- Patient education

All documentation in these categories is placed in **reverse chronological order**; that is, the most recent documents are placed on top of previous sheets.

Provider Encounters

Whether the patient is new or established or seen by a physician assistant, nurse practitioner, or physician, the visit must be documented. It may be handwritten, typed, or entered into a computer, but in any event, it must be recorded. In the paperless office, you will complete the information gathered at the patient's visit by choosing items from a drop-down box that appears when you click on a particular field.

Some offices record new patients' encounters in the history and physical format. Visits of established patients returning for follow-up are documented in a different format. Although some offices use the same format for new and established patients, the most common formats used to document each established patient encounter are narrative, SOAP, and POMR.

Narrative Format

Some providers document visits in the narrative form. **Narrative** is the oldest documentation form and the least structured. It is simply a paragraph indicating the contact with the patient, what was done for the patient, and the outcome of any action. In the sample page shown in Figure 8-3, the chart entries made are in narrative format.

SOAP Format

The **SOAP** (subjective-objective-assessment-plan) format is one of the most common methods for documenting

SOAP METHOD TO DOCUMENT PATIENT INFORMATION

Jennifer Mosley states that her daughter, Marcia, has been vomiting all night. She also states that Marcia had diarrhea for 2 days before her appointment and has only eaten crackers and bananas since 6:00 p.m. last night. Dr. Gibson's notes indicate that Marcia has lost 3 pounds since her last visit and that she appears pale, weak, and slightly dehydrated. He suspects a viral infection.

Dr. Gibson ordered a stool culture along with a complete blood count (CBC) with differential. He prescribed the BRAT (bananas, rice, applesauce, and toast) diet and suggested that Mrs. Mosley give Marcia Imodium A-D for the next 48 hours. He also told Mrs. Mosley to call the office if Marcia's symptoms worsen and to bring her back for a recheck if the symptoms are not cleared up by the end of the week.

S: According to the patient's mother, the patient has been vomiting all night and has had diarrhea for the past 2 days. She has eaten only crackers and bananas since 6:00 p.m. the night before.

O: Patient appears pale, weak, and slightly dehydrated and has lost 3 pounds since her last visit.

A: Possible viral infection.

P: Stool culture, CBC with differential, BRAT diet, and Imodium for the next 48 hours. Call office if symptoms worsen; return to office if patient not well by the end of the week.

patient visits. The *subjective* component is a statement of what the patient says. Whenever possible, actual quotations by the patient should be used. The *objective* component is what is observed about the patient when the medical assistant begins the assessment and when the provider does the examination. The *assessment* portion is a phrase stating the impression of what is wrong or the patient's diagnosis. If a final diagnosis cannot be made yet, the provider lists possible disorders to be ruled out, called the differential diagnosis. The *plan* is a list of interventions that are to be carried out. In Box 8-3, the second note is written in the SOAP format.

POMR Format

The **problem-oriented medical record (POMR)** lists each problem of the patient, usually at the beginning of

the folder, and references each problem with a number throughout the folder. This method was developed by Dr. Lawrence Weed and is a common method of compiling information because of its logical flow and the ease with which information can be reviewed. In group practices where patients may be seen by more than one physician, the POMR format makes it easier to track the patient's treatment and progress. For instance, if Mr. Jones has hypertension and hyperglycemia, each diagnosis will be assigned a problem number as soon as the diagnosis is made:

2/4/9 #1. Hypertension
2/4/9 #2. Hyperglycemia

At each subsequent visit made by Mr. Jones, these problems will be referenced by these numbers. If a problem develops and is resolved, the problem number will be terminated by a single strikethrough with a date beside it or by adding an X to a heading that indicates resolution of problems. Chronic problems, such as hypertension and hyperglycemia, will be retained by number for as long as the patient remains with the practice. These may be divided by headings of acute and chronic or short-term and long-term for convenience.

POMR documents are divided into four components:

1. *Database.* This contains the following:
   • Chief complaint (Fig. 8-4 shows charting for a chief complaint and history of present illness)
   • Present illness
   • Patient profile
   • Review of systems
   • Physical examination
   • Laboratory reports
2. *Problem list.* This includes every problem the patient has that requires evaluation, including social, demographic, medical, and surgical problems. (Demographic problems relate to statistical characteristics of certain populations.)

Jamie Williams	
08/18/14	*Office Visit*
Vitals:	*BP 110/68, P 80, T 98.6*
CC:	*Patient states: "I hurt my left arm when I fell off my horse yesterday." Has been taking Tylenol with some relief.*
HISTORY OF PRESENT ILLNESS:	*Patient's left arm is edematous. Deformity noted. Left radial pulse present. Able to move fingers on left hand. Nail beds on left hand pink and warm to touch.*
	Tonya Swain, RMA

Figure 8-4 Charting a chief complaint and history of present illness.

3. *Treatment plan.* This includes management, additional workups that may be necessary, and therapy.
4. *Progress notes.* These are structured notes corresponding to each problem.

CHECKPOINT QUESTION

5. What are three common formats used to document patient–provider encounters?

Documentation Forms

Using printed forms and flow sheets in the medical record saves space and time and allows for easy retrieval of information. They are usually customized to meet the needs of the individual practice. Some forms, like vaccination records, are required by federal law. In the paperless office, these forms are completed by the patient and transferred to the patient's electronic record by data entry, and then the completed form is shredded.

Medical History Forms

Medical history forms are commonly used to gather information from the patient before the visit with the physician (see Chapter 18, Fig. 18-1). Some medical offices mail these forms to new patients and have them bring the completed form to their visit. This gives the patient the opportunity to concentrate on the questions, gather information about the family history, and give a more complete history. Whether the patient brings the completed form or fills out the history form in the office, you will review the information with the patient to clarify any questions and add additional information gathered in the interview. Specialty practices use forms designed to gather the type of information they will need to manage the patient's care. For example, an orthopedist's history form might include fields for prior orthopedic injuries, accident information, and physical therapy visits.

Flow Sheets

The **flow sheet** is designed to limit the need for long, handwritten care notes by allowing information to be recorded in either graphic or table form. Generally, flow sheets are designed for a given task. Color-coded sheets for medication administration, vital signs, pediatric growth charts, and so on eliminate the need to read through the pages of a chart to retrieve information. For example, if the physician asks you what the baby weighed 3 months ago, you find the pink growth chart, which saves time and frustration. An advantage of using electronic health records is the capability of converting such information to charts, graphs, and flow sheets. In an electronic health record, clicking an icon for a growth chart takes you to a screen that allows you to enter the information. The software transfers the numbers to a

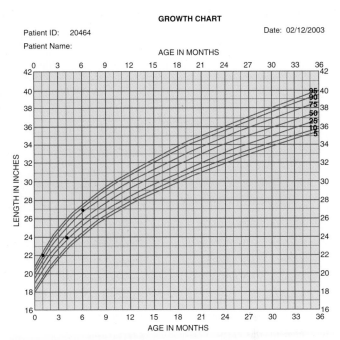

Figure 8-5 Growth chart from electronic health records.

graph. Figure 8-5 shows the growth chart that appears on the screen. When you refill a patient's daily blood pressure medication, you enter the information into the computer record, and it is transferred to the medication record. The record of all entries related to the patient's medications can then be easily retrieved by clicking on the medication icon. Figure 8-6 is an example of a medication flow sheet from a fictitious patient's electronic chart.

Progress Notes

Progress notes are statements about various aspects of patient care. The entries in Figure 8-4 are typical progress notes. Some facilities use a lined piece of paper with two columns. The left column is used to document the date and time, and the right column is used to write the note. Others use a plain or lined piece of paper without columns. The progress notes will reflect each encounter with the patient chronologically, whether by phone, by e-mail, or in person. In the electronic health record, you will record vital signs, information given by the patient, etc. The results of lab work done in one area of a practice can be entered into the computer. The computer screen in the examination room will then display the results. This immediate availability makes patient care more efficient and convenient for the physician and the patient. No matter what form is used for documenting, you must always include the date, time, your signature, and your credential. The electronic health record has a feature that allows you to assign your signature electronically. A typical user message might say "press enter to sign."

Ardmore Family Practice, P.A.
2805 Lyndhurst Avenue
Winston-Salem, NC 27103
PHONE: 336-659-0076
FAX: 336-659-0272

Patient: MICHAEL FIELDS

Date: 02-12-2014 9:06 AM

MEDICATIONS

Date	Drug Name	Strength/Form	Dispense	Refill	Sig	Last Dose/ Disc Date	Status
1/28/14	SINGULAIR	10 MG TABS	5	0	1 PO BID		NEW
1/28/14	ZITHROMAX	200 MG/5ML SUSR	5	0	1 P.O Q DAY		NEW
1/22/14	ACCUPRIL	10 MG TABS	34	4	1 PO QD	1/28/14	CONTINUE
1/22/14	ADVIL	200 MG TABS	1	1	1/2 Q A.M.	1/25/14	NEW
1/22/14	ALTACE	5 MG CAPS	60	5	ONE TWICE DAILY	1/28/14	CONTINUE
1/22/14	MACROBID	100 MG CAPS	14	0	1 PO BID	1/28/14	CONTINUE
8/26/13	ALTACE	5 MG CAPS	60	5	ONE TWICE DAILY		CONTINUE
8/7/13	PRECOSE	25 MG CAPS	60	0	1/2 B.I.D.	10/5/13	NEW
5/2/12	ACCUPRIL	10 MG TABS	34	4	1 PO QD		NEW
5/2/12	ACCUPRIL	20 MG TABS	30	0	1 PO QD		NEW
5/2/12	ACCUPRIL	40 MG TABS	30	5	1 PO QD		NEW
4/25/12	ACCUPRIL	20 MG TABS	30	0	1 PO QD	4/25/12	NEW
4/25/12	ACCUPRIL	40 MG TABS	30	5	1 PO QD		NEW
4/25/12	MACROBID	100 MG TABS	14	0	1 PO BID	5/1/12	NEW
3/2/12	ACIPHEX 20 MG	TABS	30	6	1 PO QD		NEW
3/2/12	ACTOS 30 MG	TABS	30	2	1 PO QD		NEW
1/23/12	ENTEX PSE	120-600 MG TB12	45	0	1 PO BID		NEW
1/23/12	NASONEX	50 MCG/ACT SUSP	1	3	2 SPRAYS EACH NOSTRIL QD		NEW
8/24/10	ADALAT CC	60 MG TBCR	34	5	1 PO QD	8/24/10	NEW
7/8/10	NITROGLYCERIN	0.4 MG/DOSE AERS	100	1	1 TAB SL Q 5 MIN X 3, IF CHEST PAIN PERS	7/8/10	NEW
6/26/10	CLARITIN	10 MG TABS	30	5	ONE EVERY MORNING		NEW
6/23/10	CELEBREX 100 MG	CAPS	90	3	1 PO Q AM AND 2 PO Q PM		NEW
6/3/10	GLUCOPHAGE	850 MG TABS	90	6	ONE 3 TIMES DAILY	6/3/10	NEW
6/3/10	HYTRIN	5 MG CAPS	30	6	ONE EVERY DAY	6/3/10	NEW

Figure 8-6 Medication administration flow sheet.

CHECKPOINT QUESTION

6. List three advantages of using flow sheets in a medical chart.

COG Medical Record Entries

Proper medical record entries are necessary for efficient communication and for legal considerations. The medical record allows health care practitioners to communicate among themselves and therefore provide the best care possible for the patient. Good communication fosters continuity of patient care.

The medical record is a legal document that can be subpoenaed in a malpractice suit. If the documentation is accurate, timely, and legible, it can help win a lawsuit or prevent one altogether. If the documentation is messy, inaccurate, or improperly done, however, it can raise questions that might cause the practice to lose a malpractice suit. Figure 8-7 is a charting example that shows the difference between a well-written chart note and one that leaves what really happened in question. It has been said that if it is not documented, it was not done. The reality is that it is very difficult to prove what was done if the patient information is incomplete. Therefore, all patient procedures, assessments, interventions, evaluations, teachings, and communications must be documented. Box 8-4 lists guidelines for documenting in patients' medical records.

Charting Communications with Patients

As discussed earlier, in addition to documenting patient visits to the facility, other encounters and communications may occur and should become a part of the permanent record. To ensure continuity of care and patient safety, charts should contain a progress sheet or some sort of tool to record each communication with a patient. Actions taken by the physician or employees as directed by the physician on behalf of the patient should be charted. For example, when a prescription is phoned

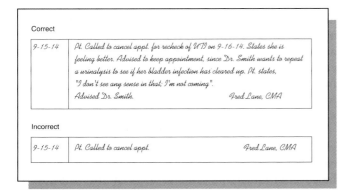

Figure 8-7 Charting example showing correct and incorrect entries.

BOX 8-4

DOCUMENTATION GUIDELINES

1. Make sure you know the office policy regarding charting. Find out who is allowed to write in the chart and the procedures for doing so.
2. Make sure you have the correct patient chart. If the patient's name is common, ask for a birth date or social security number as a double check.
3. Document in ink.
4. Sign your complete name and credential.
5. Always record the date of each entry. Some outpatient facilities record the time as well. Using military time will eliminate the need to use AM and PM (Fig. 8-8)
6. Write legibly. Printing is more legible than cursive writing.
7. Check spelling, especially medical terms, before entering them into the chart. Chapter 7 offers help with spelling.
8. Use only abbreviations that are accepted by your facility. Because abbreviations can cause confusion and errors in patient care, the use of certain handwritten abbreviations has been prohibited by The Joint Commission. (See Legal Tip: Abbreviations? When in Doubt, Spell It Out.)
9. When charting the patient's statements, use quotation marks to signify the patient's own words. For example, "My head is killing me."
10. Do not attempt to make a diagnosis. For example, if the patient says, "My throat is sore," do not write pharyngitis. It is not within the scope of your training to diagnose.

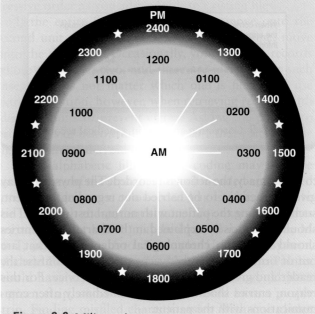

Figure 8-8 Military time.

(continued)

BOX 8-5

INDEXING RULES FOR ALPHABETIC FILING

When filing records alphabetically, use these indexing rules to help you decide the placement of each record. Indexing rules apply whether you use the title of the record's contents or a person's name.

File by name according to last name, first name, and middle initial, and treat each letter in the name as a separate unit. For example, Jamey L. Crowell should be filed as Crowell, Jamey L. and should come before Crowell, Jamie L.

- Make sure professional initials are placed after a full name. John P. Bonnet, D.O., should be filed as Bonnet, John P., D.O.
- Treat hyphenated names as one unit. Bernadette M. Ryan-Nardone should be filed as Ryan-Nardone, Bernadette M. not as Nardone, Bernadette M. Ryan.
- File abbreviated names as if they were spelled out. Finnigan, Wm. should be filed as Finnigan, William, and St. James should be filed as Saint James.
- File last names beginning with Mac and Mc in regular order or grouped together, depending on your preference, but be consistent with either approach.
- File a married woman's record by using her own first name. Helen Johnston (Mrs. Kevin Johnston) should be filed as Johnston, Helen, not as Johnston, Kevin Mrs.
- Jr. and Sr. should be used in indexing and labeling the record. Many times, a father and son are patients at the same facility.
- When names are identical, use the next unit, such as birth dates or the mother's maiden name. Use Durham, Iran (2-4-94) and Durham, Iran (4-5-45).
- Disregard apostrophes.
- Disregard articles (a, the), conjunctions (and, or), and prepositions (in, of) in filing. File *The Cat in the Hat* under Cat in Hat.
- Treat letters in a company name as separate units. For ASM, Inc., "A" is the first unit, "S" is the second unit, and "M" is the third unit.

Numeric Filing

Numeric filing uses digits, usually six. The digits are typically run together but read as three groups of two digits. For example, the record filed as 324478 is read as 32, 44, 78. Commas are not placed or

any separation used when applying the labels to the tabbed edge of the file folder. The records are placed in numeric order without concern for duplication, which may sometimes happen with the alphabetic system. If you use this technique, it is called straight digit filing because you are reading the number straight out from left to right.

Sometimes, the file label will look the same, 324478, but will be read in the reverse order: 78, 44, 32. This technique is called terminal digit filing; that is, the groups of numbers are read in pairs from right to left. Be careful not to mix the two filing systems. If using both techniques within your office, be sure to keep them separate by changing the folder color or some other means to prevent errors. The chart is filed by using the last pairs of digits.

Numeric filing plays an important role in the medical office. With HIPAA's Privacy Rule requirements, the use of numeric filing makes sense. When this technique is used, it is important to keep a **cross-reference** in a secure area, away from patient areas, listing the numeric code and the name of the patient. Such a reference is called a master patient index. This way, a limited number of people know who the patient is, which maintains privacy. Boxes 8-6 and 8-7 describe how to file patient records alphabetically or numerically.

BOX 8-6

ALPHABETIC FILING EXAMPLES

The following patient records are to be filed alphabetically:

Mary P. Martin
Floyd D. Huey, Sr.
Susan Bailey
Ellen P. Parrish
Karen Hart
Susan Roberts-Hill
Amy Dalton
Amy Roberson
Clayton A. Parker, MD
Mrs. John Moser (Donna)

The correct order is:

Susan Bailey
Amy Dalton
Karen Hart
Floyd D. Huey, Sr.
Mary P. Martin
Donna Moser
Clayton A. Parker
Ellen P. Parrish
Amy Roberson
Susan Roberts-Hill

BOX 8-7

NUMERIC FILING EXAMPLES

The following patient records are to be filed numerically:

Ramsey, LeRoy	213456
Flora, Curtis	334387
King, Sharon	979779
Moore, Cathy	321138

In straight digit filing, the proper order is:

213456
321138
334387
979779

In terminal digit filing, the proper order is:

321138
213456
979779
334387

With files in which one or two groups of numbers are the same numbers, you refer to the second or third groups of numbers. For example, in straight digit filing (reading from left to right) the number 003491 comes before 004592. The first group of numbers (00) is the same for both files, so you determine the order of filing by the second group of numbers; in this case, 34 comes before 45.

In terminal digit filing (reading from right to left), 456128 would come before 926128. The first two groups of numbers (28 and 61) are the same for both files, so you go to the third group of numbers; in this case, 45 comes before 92.

Other Filing Systems

The medical office keeps files other than patient records. An office manager keeps files on employees, insurance policies, accounts payable, and so on. For this type of filing, systems include **subject filing**, in which documents are arranged alphabetically according to subject (e.g., insurance, medications, referrals); geographic filing, in which documents are grouped alphabetically according to locations, such as state, county, or city; and chronological filing, in which documents are grouped in the order of their date.

A well-kept, complete, and accurate medical record and the ability to quickly retrieve information are reflections of the quality and efficiency of the medical facility in which they are generated.

CHECKPOINT QUESTION

10. What are the two main filing systems? Briefly describe each.

COG Storing Health Information

Whether a facility uses an electronic form, a manual system, or a combination of both, the records used in the delivery of health care must be stored safely and privately. A goal of a good system includes easy retrieval of the information. Logical organization and policies that ensure that information is safe, secure, and easily accessed make for an efficient medical office.

Electronic Data Storage

The paperless medical office must consider storage of data other than using paper and folders. HIPAA's Administrative Simplification section addresses the issues involved in storing electronically generated transmissions and storage. Backup copies of computerized records must be made daily and stored in a safe, fireproof location. Security experts advise storing backup disks off site. HIPAA mandates that offices establish a disaster plan that includes emergency storage of data and security and safety of that data. Any computer infrastructure should allow for chart availability in a disaster situation. A medical office may choose to outsource the off-site storage of their data. Health information stored off site may be classified as "hot," which means the records are accessible and usable. A storage backup would need activation for use. The speed of computer technology and government involvement promises changes and new practices. In order to optimize efficiency, you must keep abreast of these new regulations and technologies.

Storage of Standard Medical Records

Medical offices use a variety of storage methods for active files that are used on a daily basis. Shelf files are stationary shelves. Shelving units are stacked on each other or placed side by side. These shelves may also be custom-ordered to the width you need. Records are stored horizontally, and labels are read from the side. Figure 8-10 shows an example of shelving units.

Drawer files are a type of filing cabinet. The drawer pulls out for easy access and visibility of all records. This type of filing system allows you easier access to all sides of files, which can help in searches for missing files that may have been pushed to the back or behind other files. Drawer files also allow easier filing because you can read from above the files, rather than squatting to read the labels from the sides as you work your way down to the lower shelves. A disadvantage is that these files take up a great deal of space.

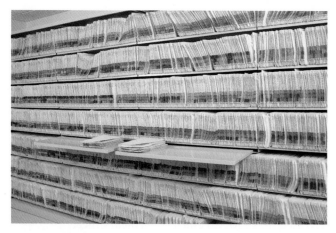

Figure 8-10 File cabinets.

Rotary circular or lateral files allow records to be stored in units that either spin in a circle or stack one behind the other, enabling you to rotate different units to the front. This system allows for maximum use of office space and is suggested for a medical office with large quantities of records to be stored. With shelf or drawer units, more wall space is needed to spread out each unit, but with rotary files, less wall space is needed.

Classification of Medical Records

For the purpose of storing records, they may be classified in three categories: active, inactive, or closed. Active records are those of patients who have been seen within the past few years. The exact amount of time is designated within each practice; it usually ranges from 1 to 5 years. Keep these records in the most accessible storage spot available because you will be using them regularly.

Inactive records are those of patients who have not been treated in the office for a set time. Most offices consider files inactive after 2 to 3 years. You will still keep inactive records in the office, but they do not have to be as accessible as the active files. Usually, they are placed on bottom shelves to eliminate constant bending when reaching for active files, or they may be stored in another room within the office. They can be stored in the office in an out-of-the-way area, such as a basement or attic. They may even be kept in the physician's home. This practice is permitted because the records belong to the physician, but it is not recommended because, at any time, the office staff may need access to these records. "Inactive" patients have not formally terminated their contact with the physician, but they have either not needed the physician's services or have not informed the office regarding a move, change in physician, or death.

Closed records are those of patients who have terminated their relationship with the physician. Reasons for such termination might include the patient moving, termination of physician–patient relationship by letter, no further treatment necessary, or death of the patient.

Many practices use **microfilm** or **microfiche** to store closed records. Microfilm and microfiche are ways to photograph documents and store them in a reduced form. Microfilm, a popular method for storing large volumes of records, particularly in hospitals and clinics, uses a photographic process that develops medical records in miniature on film. Information is stored on cards holding single film frames or in reels or strips for projection on compact electric viewers placed at convenient office locations. The cost of the equipment is declining, making this a more practical method for storing and retrieving inactive files.

Microfiche is a miniature photographic system that stores rows of images in reduced size on cards with clear plastic sleeves rather than on film strips. Information can be handled manually, examined on a viewer that enlarges the record, or reproduced as hard copy on a high-speed photocopier. A standard microfiche card holds more than 60 pages of information. The microfiche process allows 3200 papers to be reduced to fit on a single 4- to 6-inch transparency.

Medical Record Retention

As discussed in Chapter 2, the statute of limitations is the legal time limit set for filing suit against an alleged wrongdoer. The time limit varies from state to state. You must observe the statute of limitations in your particular state to know how long medical and business records should be kept in storage.

It is recommended that medical records be stored permanently because, in some states, malpractice lawsuits can be filed within 2 years of the date of discovery of the alleged malpractice. The statute of limitations for minors is extended until the child reaches legal age in every state; the time given past the legal age varies, however.

When a health care provider's practice ends, either from retirement or death, notice to all patients with records stored in the facility is required. This notice can be in the form of a letter to each patient and/or a newspaper notification advising patients of the closing of the practice and giving them a reasonable length of time in which to pick up their records. Since the facility no longer exists, you may release the original record to the patients. As discussed previously, the record itself belongs to the facility, but the information in the record belongs to the patient. Since the facility no longer exists, it is felt that the record now belongs to the patient. Retiring physicians or the families of deceased physicians may ask a colleague to maintain storage of any patient records that are not claimed. This location should be given to the patients in their written notification. Of course, the statute of limitations for legal action and the need for these records should be taken into consideration. Most risk management experts advise that the records should be kept in some form forever, but this is not always feasible. At the least, every reasonable attempt should be made to notify patients and disseminate the information maintained by the retiring or deceased physician.

 AFF WHAT IF?

You work in a family practice office where your physician treats many children. How long should you keep the children's records? The statute of limitations in your state is 3 years from the date of the last treatment.

By law, when a physician treats an adult, the record should be kept until the statute of limitations expires. A minor has the right to bring suit against a health care provider when he becomes of legal age. Therefore, the minor's records should be kept at least 3 years past the 18th birthday.

COG Disposal of Medical Records

Before a paper medical record is destroyed, the owner of the information should be given the opportunity to pick up the record. If this is not possible, and/or the record will not be needed for continuity of care in the future, then the record can be destroyed. Paper medical records should *never* be placed in a regular trash can or a dumpster. There are cases of companies being fined for illegally discarding medical records in dumpsters. These records contained patient names, birth dates, social security numbers, and other protected health information.

Before protected medical records can be thrown out, they should be shredded or burned. Many medical facilities outsource this task to a record disposal company. Keep small trash cans labeled "TO BE SHREDDED" at each work station to encourage employees to comply.

Electronic PHI is less likely to require disposal. However, if your office uses any type of removable or portable electronic media such as floppy disks, CDs, or flash drives, be sure to erase, delete, or reformat any information that is no longer needed. Be sure to remove information from the hard drive of computers that are no longer in use or being sold in such a way that prevents the data from being recovered. Box 8-8 is the position statement of the North Carolina Medical Society. It is designed to assist physicians in adopting medical record retention and disposal practices.

CHECKPOINT QUESTION

11. What is the primary basis for deciding how long a record should be kept?

BOX 8-8

NORTH CAROLINA MEDICAL BOARD'S POSITION STATEMENT

The North Carolina Medical Board supports and adopts the following language of Section 7.05 of the American Medical Association's current Code of Medical Ethics regarding the retention of medical records by physicians.

7.05: Retention of Medical Records

Physicians have an obligation to retain patient records which may reasonably be of value to a patient. The following guidelines are offered to assist physicians in meeting their ethical and legal obligations:

1. Medical considerations are the primary basis for deciding how long to retain medical records. For example, operative notes and chemotherapy records should always be part of the patient's chart. In deciding whether to keep certain parts of the record, an appropriate criterion is whether a physician would want the information if he or she were seeing the patient for the first time.
2. If a particular record no longer needs to be kept for medical reasons, the physician should check state laws to see if there is a requirement that records be kept for a minimum length of time. Most states will not have such a provision. If they do, it will be part of the statutory code or state licensing board.
3. In all cases, medical records should be kept for at least as long as the length of time of the statute of limitations for medical malpractice claims. The statute of limitations may be three or more years, depending on the state law. State medical associations and insurance carriers are the best resources for this information.
4. Whatever the statute of limitations, a physician should measure time from the last professional contact with the patient.
5. If a patient is a minor, the statute of limitations for medical malpractice claims may not apply until the patient reaches the age of majority.
6. Immunization records always must be kept.
7. The records of any patient covered by Medicare or Medicaid must be kept at least five years.
8. In order to preserve confidentiality when discarding old records, all documents should be destroyed.
9. Before discarding old records, patients should be given an opportunity to claim the records or have them sent to another physician, if it is feasible to give them the opportunity.

(continued)

BOX 8-8 *(continued)*

Please Note:

a. North Carolina has no statute relating specifically to the retention of medical records.

b. Several North Carolina statutes relate to time limitations for the filing of malpractice actions. Legal advice should be sought regarding such limitations.

(Adopted 5/98)

Reprinted with permission from NC Medical Society.

español SPANISH TERMINOLOGY

Vamos a necesitar copias de su historial médico de su médico anterior.

We will need copies of your medical records from your previous doctor.

Al firmar aquí, usted nos da permiso de compartir su información medica con su compañía de seguro.

By signing here, you are giving us permission to share your medical information with your insurance company.

MEDIA MENU

- **Student Resources on thePoint**
  - **CMA/RMA Certification Exam Review**
- **Internet Resources**

U.S. Department of Health and Human Services, CMS, HIPAA—General Information
http://www.cms.gov/HIPAAGenInfo

U.S. Department of Health and Human Services, CMS, National Provider Identifier Standard
http://www.cms.gov/NationalProvIdentStand

American Health Information Management Association
http://www.ahima.org

Health Level Seven (HL7)
http://www.hl7.org

Certification Commission for Health Information Technology
http://www.cchit.org

Office of the National Coordinator for Health Information Technology
http://www.hhs.gov/healthit/hithca.html

PSY PROCEDURE 8-1: **Establishing, Organizing, and Maintaining a Medical File**

Purpose: To create a file that will organize and save a patient's medical information, including records of transactions and interactions with the office and its staff

Equipment: File folder, metal fasteners, hole punch, five divider sheets with tabs, title, year, and alphabetic or numeric labels

Steps	Reasons
1. Decide the name of the file (a patient's name, company name, or name of the type of information to be stored).	Properly naming a file allows for easy retrieval.
2. Type a label with the title *in unit order* (e.g., Lynn, Laila S., *not* Laila S. Lynn).	Typing the label in unit order helps avoid filing errors.
3. Place the label along the tabbed edge of the folder so that the title extends out beyond the folder itself. (Tabs can be either the length of the folder or tabbed in various in various positions, such as left, center, and right.)	This ensures easy readability when the folder is in a storage cabinet.

Step 3. Place label along tabbed edge of folder.

Steps	Reasons
4. Place a year label along the top edge of the tab before the label with the title. This will be changed each year the patient has been seen. *Note:* Do not automatically replace these labels at the start of a new year; remove the old year and replace with a new one only when the patient comes in for the first visit of the new year.	Doing this makes removing inactive files more time efficient. At the beginning of each new year, you can easily spot the records that are years beyond your storage time limit in the active file area. Doing this also can help you locate inactive files if patients return years later. (By determining the last year the patient was seen, you can narrow your search to files with a matching year label.)
5. Place the appropriate alphabetic or numeric labels below the title.	This aids in accurate filing and retrieval.

(continued)

Steps	Reasons
6. Apply any additional labels that your office may decide to use.	Labels noting special information (e.g., insurance, drug allergies, advanced directives) act as quick and easy reminders.

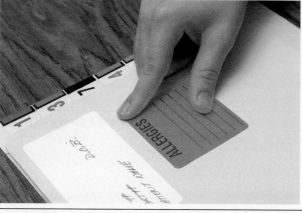

Step 6. Apply additional labels as needed.

Steps	Reasons
7. Punch holes and insert demographic and financial information using top fasteners across the top.	General information should not be intermingled with clinical information.

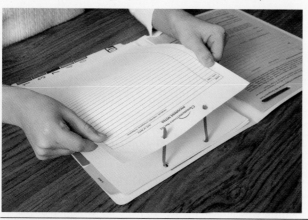

Step 7. Punch holes and insert pages in chart.

Steps	Reasons
8. Make tabs for: Ex. H&P, Progress Notes, Medication Log, Correspondence, and Test Results.	This will allow quick and easy retrieval of specific information.
9. Place pages behind appropriate tabs.	Misplacing charts or sheets out of charts creates big problems for everyone.
10. **AFF** Explain what you would do when you receive a revised copy correcting an error on a document already in a patient's chart.	Attach the revised document to the old one. The new one should be marked "revised" and placed on top of the old one. In an electronic record, the new document should be scanned into the patient's record and the old document can be deleted. In other words, you are replacing the document altogether.

PSY PROCEDURE 8-2: Filing Medical Records/Maintain Organization by Filing

Purpose: To place medical information in a designated location that will facilitate easy retrieval and the safety of the record

Equipment: Simulated patient file folder, several single sheets to be filed in the chart, file cabinet with other files

Steps	Purpose
1. Double-check spelling of names on the chart and any single sheets to be placed in the folder.	You can never be too careful with patient identification.
2. Condition any single sheets, etc.	Removing staples, paper clips, and tape will keep paper from getting torn.
3. Place sheets behind proper tab in the chart.	Organizing documents and placing tabs allows for easy retrieval of specific information.
4. Remove out guide.	The out guide will serve as a double-check for the proper placement of the chart.
5. Place the folder between the two appropriate existing folders, taking care to place the folder between the two charts.	It is easy to accidentally place a folder within a folder.
6. Scan color coding to ensure none of the charts in that section are out of order.	Color-coded tabs enable you to spot a misfiled chart easily.
7. **AFF** Explain what you would do when you find a chart out of order.	If a chart is out of order, the efficiency of patient care is affected. At the least, it should be mentioned at the next office meeting.

- Medical records are not only a means of communication among health care providers but also are legal documents depicting the quality of patient care.
- HIPAA ensures confidentiality of all medical information. The patient's privacy must be protected at all times.
- You must adhere to strict guidelines when sharing protected health information electronically and releasing any information in patients' medical records.
- You must use sound practices when entering information into a patient's chart.

- To ensure efficient recording and retrieval, you must be familiar with the varied documentation forms as well as the different kinds of filing systems.
- The system of storage of medical information used by a provider must ensure the safety, security, and confidentiality of the patient's protected health information.
- You must follow sound guidelines regarding the retention and disposal of records in order to safeguard the patient's rights to their personal medical information.
- The quality, use, and care of the medical record are reflections of the quality of the medical facility itself.

Warm Ups for Critical Thinking

1. Interview a fellow student with a hypothetical illness. Document the visit with the chief complaint.
2. Compare and contrast alphabetic filing with numeric filling. Which system do you think works better? Explain your response.
3. Role play with a fellow student who is requesting his or her medical records for a new doctor. Construct a proper authorization for release of information form and have the "patient" complete it.

4. Write an office policy for maintaining confidentiality with electronic modalities, such as fax machines, printers, laptops, and computer screens.
5. You work for an orthopedist who is retiring in 3 months. He asks you to construct a letter to be sent to all of the patients informing them of his retirement and instructing them to come in and pick up their records. List the hours the office will be open and the deadline for picking up the records. Include in the letter the location of the records after that deadline.

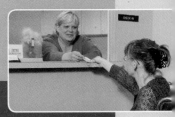

Outline

Learning Outcomes

Cognitive Domain

*Note: AAMA/CAAHEP 2008 Standards are
italicized.*

1. Spell and define the key words
2. Identify the basic computer components
3. *Discuss the importance of routine mainte-
    nance of office equipment*
4. Explain the basics of connecting to the
    Internet
5. Discuss the safety concerns for online
    searching
6. Describe how to use a search engine
7. List sites that can be used by professionals
    and sites geared for patients
8. Describe the benefits of an intranet and
    explain how it differs from the Internet
9. Describe the various types of clinical soft-
    ware that might be used in a physician's
    office

10. Describe the various types of administrative
    software that might be used in a physician's
    office
11. *Discuss applications of electronic technol-
    ogy in effective communication*
12. Describe the considerations for purchasing a
    computer
13. Describe various training options
14. Discuss the adoption of electronic health
    records
15. Describe the steps in making the transition
    from paper to electronic records
16. Discuss the ethics related to computer access

Affective Domain

*Note: AAMA/CAAHEP 2008 Standards are
italicized.*

1. *Apply ethical behaviors, including honesty
    and integrity in performance of medical
    assisting practice*

Psychomotor Domain

Note: AAMA/CAAHEP 2008 Standards are italicized.

1. Care for and maintain computer hardware (Procedure 9-1)
2. Use the Internet to access information related to the medical office (Procedure 9-2)
3. *Use office hardware and software to maintain office systems*
4. *Execute data management using electronic health care records such as the EMR*
5. *Use office hardware and software to maintain office systems*

ABHES Competencies

1. Apply electronic technology
2. Receive, organize, prioritize, and transmit information expediently
3. Locate information and resources for patients and employers
4. Apply computer application skills using variety of different electronic programs including both practice management software and EMR software

Key Terms

cookies	Ethernet	literary search	virtual
downloading	Internet	search engine	
encryption	intranet	virus	

Computers play a major role in the physician's office. Computers are used for both clinical and administrative applications. A few examples of administrative applications are appointment scheduling, billing, staff scheduling, and insurance filings. Clinical software programs are used for many areas, such as reading laboratory and radiology reports and helping the physician to prescribe medications. Computers promote communication among health care professionals and provide access to new treatment options. You will need excellent computer skills to work as a medical assistant. This chapter will help you to improve your existing skills. It provides a basic review of computer components. You will learn how the Internet is used in health care settings and some precautions. Various medical software applications will also be discussed. You will learn about training options and governmental regulations associated with electronic health records.

COG The Computer

A computer system is roughly divided into two areas, hardware and peripherals.

Hardware

Computer hardware consists of seven key elements (Fig. 9-1). Here is a review of their parts:

- *Central processing unit.* The central processing unit (CPU), or microprocessor, is the circuitry imprinted on a silicon chip that processes information. The CPU consists of a variety of electronic and magnetic cells. These cells read, analyze, and process data and instruct the computer how to operate a given program. All CPUs function basically the same way, but chips differ dramatically in capabilities and speeds. Your CPU has many ports to connect the printer, mouse, and speakers. At minimum, it has two serial ports, one parallel port, and two universal serial bus (USB) ports. Serial ports are used for items like modems; parallel ports are used for connecting printers and backup drives to the CPU; and USB ports allow the computer to connect with various instruments.
- *Keyboard.* The keyboard is the primary means by which information is entered into the computer. Besides the typical letter and number keys, you will find special function keys that provide increased capabilities. Examples of special function keys are Alt, Ctrl, Insert, and Esc. Each of these keys has a specific function that is determined by the software program. These functions may include searching for and replacing words, moving blocks of text, indenting or centering text, and spell checking.
- *Monitor.* Monitors, also called the visual display terminals, come in various sizes and qualities. The quality

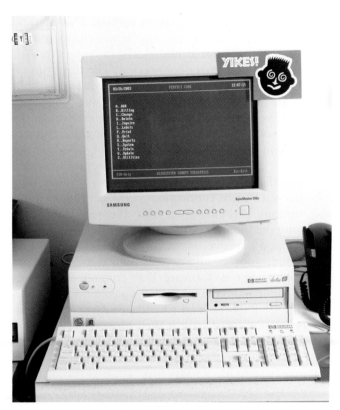

Figure 9-1 The computer consists of the CPU, keyboard, monitor, hard drive, printer, and secondary storage systems. Additional peripherals include the mouse, battery backup, and modems.

of the image is based on the DPIs (dots per inch). The more DPIs there are, the clearer the picture. There are adjustment dials for brightness and contrast. Flat-panel LCD monitors are popular and provide the most protection from unauthorized eyes.

- *Hard drive.* The hard drive provides storage for programs, data, and files. The capacity of a hard drive (i.e., the quantity of program and data it can hold) is measured in megabytes or gigabytes. Originally, hard drives could hold 5 MB (equivalent to about 2,000 typed pages), but today they have much more capacity.

- *Printer.* The printer transfers information to paper (hard copy). Printers use various technologies, operate at various speeds, and print in either black or color. The printer allows you to generate bills, print letters, and produce a daily schedule. The most commonly used printer is a laser printer, which focuses a laser beam to form images that are transferred to paper electrostatically.

- *Scanner.* A scanner allows you to take a picture or report and read it into the computer. In offices with no paper charts, you scan laboratory reports, radiology reports, discharge summaries, letters, and any other paper documents into a patient's file. This is also helpful when a new patient arrives with reports from

a previous physician. Patient education materials can also be scanned into the computer and then adjusted to meet the needs of your office. Keep in mind that you need to adhere to copyright laws.

- *Secondary storage systems.* All computers have multiple methods for saving data. Examples include floppy diskettes, compact disks, digital video disks, and zip drives. Cartridges are used by hospital for large storage systems. When saving any type of data, remember that good organization skills are essential. Name your files appropriately and place files in properly identified folders. Most computers have preset timing systems that automatically save data. Check your default setting and readjust as needed.

 CHECKPOINT QUESTION

1. What do the CPU cells do?

Peripherals

Computers can have many peripheral connections. Three key computer peripherals that you need to know are:

- *Mouse.* The mouse can be used to control the cursor on the display screen. Although you cannot type in characters using the mouse, you can move or delete individual characters, words, or entire blocks of text with it. The track ball is an alternative to a mouse. Your finger rotates the ball to move the pointer. It takes less space than a mouse and is used based on personal preference.

- *Battery backup.* A battery backup allows the computer system to function in the event of a power failure. Batteries come in various sizes depending on the size of your computer and the amount of work to be done during a power failure.

- *Modem.* A modem is a communication device that connects your computer with other computers, including the Internet, online services such as bulletin boards, and electronic mail systems. The faster the modem is, the faster the transmission. Modems may be connected through cable systems or through the telephone. Digital subscriber line (DSL) is the preferred method. To use a cable or DSL connection, your computer must have an **Ethernet** port or an Ethernet interface card. Ethernet is a type of networking technology for local area networks; coaxial cable carries radiofrequency signals between computers at a rate of 10 megabits per second.

 CHECKPOINT QUESTION

2. What is an Ethernet, and why should your computer have an Ethernet port or Ethernet interface card?

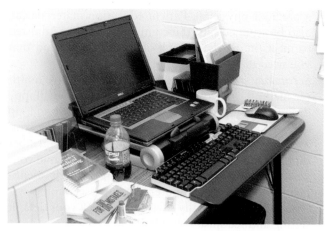

Figure 9-2 A messy desk can be a disaster for the hardware components of a computer.

Care and Maintenance of the System and Equipment

As with any piece of equipment in the medical office, it is necessary to maintain your computer on a regular basis. Some maintenance agreements require that a service representative clean and inspect the system on a regular basis. Each employee should take the responsibility of taking care of the equipment in an office. A computer and its accessories will last longer and perform better with care and maintenance. Most equipment in a medical office is very expensive. Its accuracy is crucial. Imagine the inefficiency that would be created if a physician's office could not make copies or receive faxes because of equipment failure. Just as the human body performs better with health maintenance, computer hardware and other equipment and machinery perform better when care and maintenance are carried out. A messy desk (Fig. 9-2) can be a disaster for the hardware components of a computer. Procedure 9-1 outlines the general care guidelines for a computer.

COG Internet Basics

Most physicians' offices can connect to the **Internet**. The Internet is used for both clinical and administrative reasons. The first thing you need to know is how to get your computer connected.

Getting Started and Connected

The Internet is used for access to the World Wide Web (WWW) and for electronic mail (e-mail). To get connected, you will need an Internet connection company and appropriate Internet software.

There are three ways that your computer can connect to the Internet. One is an Internet service provider (ISP). The ISP is a company that connects your computer's modem to the Internet through the phone line. It is often called a dial-up service. This method provides the slowest service but is the cheapest. The second option is your cable television company. This system provides a faster connection. The third option is a DSL. This is the fastest connection but is not available in all areas. DSL is the most expensive connection system. If you need to download large files through the Internet, you should use either a DSL or cable connection. If you are having trouble accessing the Internet because of either slow service or connection troubles, speak to the physician or office manager to determine whether a different connection or ISP is needed. Wireless options are emerging, and the technology for accessing the Internet without a land line will continue to grow and improve.

Second, your computer will need a Web browser. A Web browser is software that communicates with your computer and the Internet. Two common examples are Internet Explorer and Mozilla Firefox. Most computers are preloaded with a Web browser. Clicking on the Web browser icon makes the actual connection to the Internet. Depending on how your system is set up, you may have to use a password.

 CHECKPOINT QUESTION

3. Which two types of Internet connections are recommended for downloading large files?

Security of Electronically Shared Personal Health Information

As previously discussed, the federal government regulates the sharing and storage of protected health information. The Health Insurance Portability and Accountability Act of 1996 (HIPAA) legislation mandates that, when a health care provider and health plan transmit and receive PHI (personal health information) electronically, the transmission must comply with certain standards. There are code sets to identify the physician's specialty, training, and payment policies, the status of a claim, why claims have been denied or adjusted, types of health plans, benefits, patient eligibility, provider organization types, and disability types. This simplification of information exchange ultimately results in increased efficiency and available cash flow.

The HIPAA Security Rule requires covered entities to implement policies and procedures designed to prevent, detect, and contain any breaks in security. The HIPAA Officer in a physician's practice is required to monitor the security of their electronic information by conducting a risk analysis. This analysis includes following the path of each type of transmission or movement of data to look for problems. They also periodically check for security threats or gaps by reviewing audit logs and other security tracking measures.

Internet Security

If you choose correct sites and follow some general safety tips, the Internet is a safe way to obtain and transfer patient information. Here are a few key points:

- Never send any patient information over the Internet to a site that does not have a secure sockets layer (SSL). This scrambles your information as it leaves your computer and unscrambles it when it arrives at its designated address.
- Look for a lock icon on the status bar.
- Set limits on your Web browser for **cookies**. A cookie is a tiny file from a Web site left on your computer's hard drive without your permission. By examining your cookies, a Web site can learn what sites you have visited, products for which you have been searching, and files that you have downloaded. You may control your computer's cookies by setting limits on your Web browser software. Limit setters can generally be found on your toolbar under Internet options, then under either privacy or security.

 WHAT IF?

Parents ask you how to keep their child safe on the Internet. What should you say?

First and foremost, explain to the parent that direct parental observation is the best method. Encourage parents to have an open and honest discussion with their child regarding the dangers on the Internet. Computers should be kept in living rooms or family rooms. Advise parents not to let children have a computer with Internet access in his or her bedroom. Parents can require a password to be entered for Internet access. This prevents access when the parent is not present. Most Web browser programs let the parent allow access only to "safe" sites. A few sites can add filters or safety nets to a child's computer. These sites are Net Nanny (http://www.netnanny.com), Internet Guard Dog (http://www.mcafee.com/us), and CyberPatrol (http://www.cyberpatrol.com).

Viruses

Virus protection is an important security issue. A virus is a dangerous invader that enters your computer through some source and can destroy your files, software programs, and possibly even the hard drive. A worm is a specific type of virus that affects e-mail. Most computers come with virus protection software. This software will identify and stop harmful transmission. However, virus protection is not 100% guaranteed. Some ways that you can protect your computer are:

- Do not open any attachments from unknown or suspicious sites.
- Update your virus protection software regularly. Most virus protection programs offer an updating service. Virus protection updates address new worms, as well.
- Remember, new viruses are detected daily.

Downloading Information

The Internet is filled with great patient teaching resources and other information. You may decide to copy some of this material into your computer. This is **downloading**. Downloading transfers information from an outside location to your computer's hard drive. Download only files that pertain to work. Do not download screen savers, news releases, recipes, or other personal information. Do not assume that you can photocopy any material that you have downloaded and distribute it. Always ask for permission from the author. Some government and professional medical Web sites state that their material can be freely copied and used. A good example of this is the United States Department of Agriculture (USDA) Web site, which allows the food pyramids to be copied and used for teaching.

Working Offline

It is possible to access Web pages without connecting your computer to the Internet. To do this, save your commonly accessed sites on your Web browser. (If you are unsure how to do this, search your help topics for working offline). Then, to view the pages offline, click on the connection icon, select work offline, and locate your file. Remember, Web pages are regularly updated, and a page that you have saved to view offline may not be the latest version. Periodically view the online site and resave the site.

COG Electronic Mail

Electronic mail provides many benefits to the health care system. E-mail promotes good patient care, enhances communication, promotes teamwork, eliminates phone tag, and provides written documentation of messages. Since e-mail messages cannot be guaranteed to provide confidentiality, you must use reasonable measures to ensure compliance with HIPAA's Privacy Rule when handling e-mails from patients. When an e-mail is received from a patient or another sender about a patient, the message should be recorded in the patient record and then deleted from the computer. If you are using a manual or paper chart system, print the e-mail and either enter the information in the record or place the correspondence in the chart. Once the information is recorded in the chart, any paper copies should be shredded. Be sure to document any action taken or reply sent. Issue passwords for those who need access to e-mails from patients.

you need to find medical information, use a medical search or a megamedical site with links. Procedure 9-2 lists the steps necessary to search the Internet. See the listing of Web sites at the end of this chapter for some good places to start searching for medical information.

 CHECKPOINT QUESTION

6. What is a search engine?

Professional Medical Sites

At the end of the chapters in this book you see various Web addresses listed that provide you with more information on that chapter's content. These are good starting points for professional topics. But keep in mind that Web addresses change frequently. If you are unable to access a site, try eliminating the letters and symbols after a slash (/). Use the primary site address. For example, suppose you want to enter this site: http://www.fda.gov/cder/drug/consumer/buyonline/guide.htm. If you cannot access that site, try http://www.fda.gov and advance from there. Most sites will link you automatically to a new home page. Also, depending on your Web browser, you may not have to type in www. In this case, you would just type in fda.gov.

The Internet can help you communicate with patients who speak a foreign language. Some Web sites translate phrases and words. Box 9-1 lists sites that physicians are most likely to use. All medical specialties have their own special site. Hospitals have their own sites also.

BOX 9-1

SITES PHYSICIANS USE

Physicians and other health care professionals are likely to use these sites:

Journal of the American Medical Association
  http://jama.ama-assn.org
New England Journal of Medicine
  http://www.nejm.org
The Lancet
  http://www.thelancet.com
Annals of Internal Medicine
  http://www.annals.org
American Medical Association
  http://www.ama-assn.org
The Joint Commission
  http://www.jointcommission.org
Centers for Disease Control and Prevention
  http://www.cdc.gov
Clinical trials
  http://www.clinicaltrials.gov

When you start working as a medical assistant, learn the Web addresses of the specialty of your physician. For example, if you work for a neurologist, you will frequently use http://www.aan.com (American Academy of Neurology).

These sites will help you translate between English and Spanish:

- AltaVista—http://www.altavista.com (click on translate)
- Free English to Spanish translations—http://www.freetranslation.com

The Centers for Disease Control and Prevention site is also available in Spanish. You can give the following address to patients who want to view the site in Spanish: http://www.cdc.gov/spanish.

Literary Searches

According to the American Medical Association, approximately 80% of practicing physicians regularly surf the Internet for medical research information. Most research information is found through a **literary search**. A literary search involves finding journal articles that present new facts or data about a given topic. Physicians who specialize in a given area and have conducted a controlled research study write these articles. Various databases can be used to do a literary search:

- OVID will search for articles as far back as 1966. It contains access to more than 4,000 professional journals. Its address is http://gateway.ovid.com.
- PubMed will search for journal articles back to 1966 from the National Library of Medicine.
- CINAHL contains journal articles published since 1982. It has primarily journals for nurses and other allied health care professionals.

Most literary search databases require an annual subscription fee. Once you arrive at the site, you can start to search for the information. First, enter your key words. To narrow the search, you can request journal articles from all countries or limit it to the United States. You can also limit the search by selecting a time line, such as the past 6 months. Once you have done your search, a list of articles will be displayed, and you can highlight the ones you wish to see. You will be asked whether you want to see the whole article or only the abstract. An abstract is a summary of the article. It is always a good idea to print only the abstracts and allow the physician to decide which full articles he or she will want to see. Fees for downloading the complete journal article vary. Abstracts can generally be downloaded free. Your local hospital librarian is often available to assist you with literary searches and may be able to get the article for free. Some libraries will do searches for physicians on staff at no charge. Use this service if it is available.

CHECKPOINT QUESTION

7. How is a literary search different from a search on an Internet Web site?

Health-Related Calculators

The Web has numerous calculators that can be used for various health care topics:

- Due date calculator—http://www.babycenter.com/pregnancy-due-date-calculator
- Ovulation calculator—http://www.babycenter.com/ovulation-calculator
- Target heart rate—http://www.webmd.com/hw-popup/target-heart-rate-20512
- Body mass index (or BMI)—http://www.cdc.gov/healthyweight/assessing/bmi/index.html

Insurance-Related Sites

The insurance world can seem like an endless maze of papers and regulations. The Internet can help you sort through and clarify some information. Your first stop should be the patient's insurance company. Its Web address is usually listed on the back of the patient's insurance card. Bookmark these sites. Chapter 13 will get into more details on this issue. Following are a few sites that can also help you and your patients:

- For information on buying health insurance online: http://www.ehealthinsurance.com.
- The Medicare site (http://www.medicare.gov) discusses the basics of Medicare programs, eligibility, enrollment, drug assistance programs, and many frequently asked questions. This site will link you to various other options. You will also find links to report Medicare fraud and abuse.
- Patients who express concern about their health records being red-flagged because of an illness (HIV, cancer) can check a database that alerts insurance companies to "red-flagged" patients. This site is http://www.mib.com. There is a fee for using this site.

Patient Teaching Issues Regarding the Internet

Some of your patients will be very skilled at using the Internet. As discussed in Chapter 4, they can find enormous amounts of information regarding their disease, treatment options, and medications. The guidelines discussed in the Patient Education Box pertain to patients who surf the Internet. You cannot stop or limit the information that patients will search and find. Keep in mind that patients often turn to the Internet when they feel confused or hopeless about their disease or anger about the medical profession. If a patient communicates any such feelings, alert the physician.

Teach patients to acquire reliable medical information and advise them of the dangers on the Web. Some physician offices print brochures with recommended Web addresses. This is a very good education tool for patients. Some areas you should be aware of are discussed in the following sections.

Buying Medications Online

As the cost of prescription medications soar, patients look for options. It is possible to buy prescription medications over the Internet. A good Internet pharmacy will provide information on what the medication is used for, possible side effects, dosage recommendation, and safety concerns. If patients want to purchase prescriptions online, advise them to use only sites that are certified by the Verified Internet Pharmacy Practice Site (VIPPS). This certification comes from the National Association of Boards of Pharmacy and indicates that the site has been checked and is monitored for safety and quality care. Advise patients to purchase only medications that have been prescribed by the physician. For consumer safety tips, advise patients to use http://www.fda.gov/Drugs/default.htm.

CHECKPOINT QUESTION

8. If you find misleading or erroneous information on a product Web site, who can you notify?

Financial Assistance for Medications

In 2006, after many years of debate, the federal government provided drug coverage for Medicare beneficiaries. Part D Medicare provides seniors and people with disabilities with a comprehensive prescription drug benefit under the Medicare program. If a patient's coverage does not include a certain prescribed medication and a patient cannot pay for their medications, they can find many financial resources on the Web. First, you should advise patients to search the drug company's homepage, for example, http://www.pfizer.com/home. Patients on Medicare will find assistance on http://www.medicare.gov/prescription/home.asp. Another good site is http://www.needymeds.org. Physicians can access http://www.rxhope.com/home.aspx to find local financial resources for patients.

Medical Records

Patients may choose to create their own "medical records" and store personal health information on sites. Patients who travel frequently may opt for this. Microsoft and Google are two companies who offer such a service. Patients can store information about their medications, immunizations, laboratory tests, surgeries, and so on. Remind patients that this information is not secure and could be accessed by unauthorized people.

A more secure way to keep this information is to download medical record forms, complete the printed copy, and store them safely.

Medical Record Forms

The American Health Information and Management Association provides forms online for patients to record their health histories. These are available at http://www.ahima.org. The American College of Emergency Physicians has an emergency consent form (www.acep.org) that parents can sign giving permission for another person to consent to their child to be treated in case of an emergency. This is valuable for parents who travel on business and have their child stay with a relative or friend. Advance directives and legal forms for medical power of attorney are also available online. Patients should be advised to seek legal counsel and speak to the physician before completing these forms. The federal government has cards available online for patients to complete and carry with them regarding their wishes to be an organ and tissue donor at this Web site: http://www.organdonor.gov.

Injury Prevention

Injuries are a leading cause of death for children. The American Academy of Pediatrics (http://www.aap.org) has reference materials that can help parents with safety tips. The federal government sites (http://www.cdc.gov and http://www.nih.gov) also have good information that you can direct parents to search. The National Safe Kids foundation is another excellent resource (http://www.safekids.org). Questions regarding product recalls can be found at http://www.cpsc.gov.

COG Intranet

An **intranet** is a private network of computers that share data. Intranets, sometimes called *internal Webs*, are used in large multiphysician practices. An intranet is more secure than the Internet. The only people with access to an intranet homepage are people with an affiliation to the practice. Access may be limited to those within the offices or may allow for access from home computer systems. The benefits of an intranet are enhanced communication, quick access to needed information, increased productivity, and enhanced security. Common examples of data found on an intranet are:

- Policy and procedure manuals
- Marketing information
- Minutes from meetings and upcoming agendas
- Staff schedules
- Local hospital announcements or information
- Commonly used forms
- Internal newsletters
- Internal job postings
- Phone lists

- Video conference support
- Links to specialty sites

 CHECKPOINT QUESTION

9. What are the benefits of an intranet?

COG Medical Software Applications

The types of medical applications and their possibilities are endless. Every day, thousands of new software packages are released into the market. Upgrades and new versions of existing packages are also released daily. Each type of software program will have good benefits and will lack some features. The type of software that you will use will vary among different physician offices. The selection of software is based on the size of the practice, number of physicians, specialty, and the affiliated hospital's software. If the hospital software is compatible, interchanging information is relatively easy. Physician and office manager preferences play a role in the software selection. Other factors include how many users can use software at one time, can the software be used with multiple windows open, how often does the company plan to update it, and is the software HIPAA compliant with regard to security and code sets.

Never buy or install a new software program or update an existing version without permission from either the office manager or the physician.

Learning to use a particular software program and navigate quickly and efficiently through its features takes time. Most programs come with a tutorial program. On-site training is often included in the purchase price of major software applications. Training options will be discussed later in the chapter.

Medical software applications can be divided into two main groups: clinical and administrative. Clinical software packages help the physician or health care professional provide the best possible medical care to patients. Administrative software packages focus on tasks to keep the office flowing efficiently and financially strong. The next sections introduce you to what types of software capabilities are available and most commonly used. Keep in mind that new technologies are emerging every day.

Clinical Applications

As discussed in Chapter 8, clinical software is designed to help the physician, nurse, medical assistant, or other health care professional provide the most efficient, safest, and most reliable health care available. Here are some examples of the benefits that clinical software programs can bring into the physician's office:

1. Create a **virtual** patient chart. A virtual chart is a paperless chart in which all documentation is stored

on the computer. Some offices create dual charts (virtual and paper), and other offices will keep one or the other.

The advantages to a virtual charting system are that it saves filing space, increases access to patients' charts for all staff members, eliminates hunting for misplaced charts, and keeps the charts better organized and neater. Since the charting is done through keyboarding, the notes are always readable.

2. Clinical software can maintain an up-to-date list of clinical tasks organized by employee's name. For example, suppose you just discharged a patient and made a note on his chart that you need to check his laboratory tests tomorrow. The task manager would automatically assign this task to your list of duties for tomorrow. Or a physician may discharge a patient and want you to call that patient in the morning for a follow-up. The physician could assign this task to your list. This promotes organization and decreases the potential for tasks to get overlooked or forgotten.

3. The software available for prescription management and drug information is tremendous. A good program that focuses on pharmaceutical information will decrease medication errors, increase patient satisfaction, and provide better patient care, and it can be financially beneficial to the patient and to the practice. At minimum, the software should enable the physician to find the patient's name in a database, virtually write the prescription, and download it directly to the patient's pharmacy. This allows the pharmacist to fill the prescription before the patient arrives. Thus, the patient gets the medication much faster. More important, since most prescription filling errors are due to physicians' poor handwriting, this potentially lethal error is prevented. Most medication software packages red flag the physician if the prescription is contraindicated for the patient. Medications can be contraindicated because of a particular disease (e.g., asthma or diabetes), interaction with other medications the patient is taking, or an allergy. For example, assume the physician has written a prescription for Bactrim, which contains a sulfonamide. The software would find in the patient's medical record that the patient is allergic to sulfonamides. The computer would alert the physician, and the physician would select a different medication. Software also allows the physician to save the patient money. Each insurance company and hospital has a formulary of medications that it reimburses. If the physician orders a medication that is on the patient's insurance formulary, the patient saves money. If the physician selects a medication outside the formulary, the insurance company

may refuse to pay some or all of the cost of the medication.

4. Computer programs can insert laboratory reports directly into the patient's records. This is more time efficient than faxing or manually recording the results. It also eliminates transcription errors. Most software will alert the physician when a new laboratory report has been received. Laboratory reports of serious or life-threatening findings will still be telephoned to the office.

5. Perhaps one of the greatest technologies is the importing of the actual imaging study into a patient's chart. Some software allows the physician to see the radiograph or computed tomograph from the office. Without this program, the physician gets a typed written report, such as "chest radiograph shows left lower lobe infiltrate." With this technology, the physician can see the radiograph itself and thus make better clinical decisions.

6. Plastic surgeons use a wide variety of image reconstruction programs in their office. This software allows the physician to insert a picture of the patient and contrast it with the expected outcomes of the surgery. This helps patients both to decide whether the surgery is warranted and to develop realistic expectations of the surgery.

7. Many physicians' offices have a special defibrillator called an automated external defibrillator (AED). Once the AED is used on a patient, the information from the machine must be downloaded to the patient's chart for legal documentation. After use, the AED is attached to a desktop computer, and the AED sends the report into the computer and then into the patient's record. If the patient's chart is not on computer, the data can be printed on paper and placed in a conventional chart.

8. Some programs can help you with telephone triage. Triage is sorting patients. The software allows you to select a caller's topic and displays a list of relevant questions. The software also provides you some instructions for the patient. For example, assume you have a caller with abdominal pain. You type the key words "abdominal pain," and a list of questions appears. These programs log the calls with the date, time, and instructions, which provides legal protection for you.

 CHECKPOINT QUESTION

10. What is a virtual chart?

Administrative Applications

There are hundreds of administrative software packages available for physician offices. Most systems have a combination of features. Some examples of benefits administrative software can bring to the physician's office follow:

1. Appointment making and tracking are more efficient with a computer program than with a book format. As discussed in Chapter 6, good appointment software will allow you to enter appointments quickly and make changes more easily. It should allow for an unlimited comment area near the patient's name. The comment area allows you to add special notes, such as "patient is requesting a pregnancy test." Appointment software can keep a waiting list of patients who are looking for appointments or wanting to move their appointment date and time to the first available time. Appointment software can also automatically print notices to remind patients of the need to make appointments. For example, the program can be set to alert patients who have an annual Pap smear to be sent a letter each year reminding them when it is time for the next one. Appointment software can be integrated with other physicians' offices to allow you to have access to their appointment books. This allows you to see when the next available appointment is. For example, assume your physician makes a referral for Mr. Kearns to see a dermatologist. You would be able to view the schedule of the dermatologist and see when he could get an appointment and then later see if he went for his appointment. Software programs allow appointments to be made only when certain equipment is available. For example, the patient needs a biopsy that is done with a particular laser machine. The machine is available only on Tuesdays, so the program would automatically set the appointment for the patient on a Tuesday.

2. Software can allow you or the office manager to track patient flows. This can be helpful to adjust staff scheduling needs, with more help at the busiest hours or days and less staff on slower days. It can alert managers to productivity of staff members. For example, one physician may average 45 minutes per patient, while another may average 30 minutes. This allows you to schedule appointments at various intervals and thus promotes patient flow. It can track the time patients wait in the waiting room or examination room. Examining such information allows the staff to change the office flow to decrease waiting times or to indicate the need for additional staff. It can also highlight the days when patients are most likely to cancel their appointments. Patient demographics can be obtained, used for marketing, and allow the office to apply for special funding based on these demographics.

3. Software programs are needed to send insurance claims electronically. You will be able to send claims and track their progress. This allows for faster reimbursement to the practice and can identify problems of reimbursement earlier. The programs that you will use should have access to numerous plans and can be updated frequently and easily.

4. Software programs can allow integration with insurance companies and other businesses to allow for automatic quick payment and posting. This saves time and is less complicated to use than traditional accounting books.

5. Physicians' offices should have software that allows for credit card authorization. A variety of card types should be available (Visa, MasterCard, American Express).

6. Insurance software can allow you to check for patient eligibility. Most programs have enough room for the addresses and phone numbers of the primary, secondary, and tertiary providers. Case manager names should be added when available. Software can also allow for preadmission certifications to be completed and electronically submitted. Preadmission or preauthorization allows you and the patient to verify that the insurance company will cover the procedure or admission. Some software programs come with codes (ICD-9, CPT, HCPCS) and anesthesia codes preinstalled.

7. Again, programs must aim to comply with HIPAA's Privacy Rule; these programs allow you to document your adherence to these rules and regulations.

8. Other programs alert you to send collection letters. These programs have a variety of template collection letters. Always double-check the information before sending a collection letter. More information on how to collect past due accounts is discussed in Chapter 13.

9. A variety of financial software programs track accounts receivable and accounts payable. You may need to adjust the billing cycles to meet the needs of the office in which you are working. Software programs can also automate the tickler system.

10. Automated payroll software can automatically calculate tax deductions and other deductions. You will be able to arrange for direct deposit of employee checks through these software programs.

11. You will find transcription systems in most physicians' offices. These programs help you transcribe various medical reports quickly and effectively.

12. A medical office cannot run effectively without a word processing system. These systems help you write letters and other types of documentation.

13. An important part of any administrative software is the section that handles the personnel records. Contracts, disciplinary reports, performance evaluations, and so on can all be stored in a virtual personnel record.

CHECKPOINT QUESTION

11. What items may be included in a virtual personnel record?

COG Adopting Electronic Health Records Technology

Starting in 2010, the Department of Health and Human Services (HHS) requires eligible providers and hospitals to use products that have been certified in order to receive funding under the American Recovery and Reinvestment Act (ARRA). Any chosen product must meet the standards established by the Certification Commission for Health Information Technology (CCHIT). CCHIT is an independent, nonprofit organization that certifies ambulatory electronic health record (EHR) products as well as other health care information technology products. In 2006, CCHIT was named a "Recognized Certification Body" by the U.S. Department of Health and Human Services. (For more information and a list of certified products, visit http://www.cchit.org.)

Issues concerning health care reform are discussed further in Chapter 10.

Changing from a paper-based office environment to one using advanced technology takes time, money, careful decision making, and staff education, among other factors. One of the first steps in the process involves choosing a vendor. Again, the Medicare and Medicaid Incentive programs require that vendors be certified, and their products must meet stringent criteria. Below are some examples of criteria to consider (in addition to CCHIT certification) when purchasing EHR products:

- The vendor's reputation and history (check references or speak with current customers)
- The vendor's understanding of how your medical office plans to use EHR
- The product's use of customizable technology
- Easy access to product support
- Regular product maintenance and updates
- Ability to automate office workflow
- Ease of training and implementation
- Ability to send and receive electronic data to and from other health care entities, such as laboratories or hospitals
- Security of patient information

Making the Transition

Besides computer workstations, printers, and Internet access, the amount and kind of equipment required for EHR depends on the medical office's needs and budget. Other commonly used devices may include laptops and tablet personal computers (PCs), which allow greater physician mobility and require less space in exam rooms than desktop PCs. Whatever equipment setup is ultimately chosen, it should not physically impede the physician–patient relationship. For example, avoid set-ups in which the physician must turn his or her back to patients when inputting information, which might make the physician appear detached or uninterested.

Changeover to EHR usually occurs in stages. To avoid problems, the medical office should not eliminate paper charts until the EHR system is consistently working as intended. Integration of paper charts and other records can be accomplished in various ways, depending on office goals and the amount of data to be input. Some facilities keep hybrid records; personnel scan and index medical records into the system and then store paper copies in the office for a few months before destroying them. Other facilities transfer old paper records to microfiche or CD-ROM for storage and then destroy the paper sources. Off-site medical record storage facilities can house the records until time of disposal or indefinitely, whatever the physician wants. Keep in mind that implementing EHR will not eliminate the need to maintain paper documents right away. It can take months or years to fully complete the transition.

To work productively with EHR, medical assistants need training and practice. Graduating from an accredited medical assisting program, which includes training in coding, billing, and computer skills, ensures baseline preparation. Adequate education about the specific EHR system used by the medical office is also required. Medical assistants and other office staff usually undergo 1 to 2 days of initial training; after that, daily practice with EHR in the medical office allows users to get comfortable with the system. Workflow will be set by the facility according to their policies and procedures for EHR. One key point to remember is that, when implementing new technology, everyone must be willing to change. Staff may need to adjust some processes so that EHR can work effectively for the office.

COG Purchasing a Computer

Purchasing a new office computer system or updating an existing one is a very important business decision. All key members of the staff should be consulted prior to such a purchase and should be actively involved in selecting the hardware and software. Here are some general guidelines to follow when shopping for a computer and software:

- Determine your specific needs. For example, do you need both clinical and administrative applications?
- Visit physicians' offices and clinics to see what other medical office staff are using. Ask questions: How user friendly are the programs? How long did it take to educate the staff? What does the staff like and dislike about the programs?

- Try out many software packages. Most have demonstrator disks that can be used to evaluate the system.
- Interview and compare different computer vendors.

Find out:

1. If the company and its products are certified by the federal government
2. How long they have been in service
3. How many service representatives they have and whether they are available 24 hours a day
4. Specifics of the system
5. Specifics of any service and warranty contracts they provide
6. What training they provide and at what additional cost
7. How to transfer data into the new system
8. How much the system costs
9. Whether the software can be customized and at what cost
10. What is their response time for service or technical support calls
11. Whether their programs are HIPAA compliant

Independent computer consultants can be hired to evaluate your particular office and make specific recommendations. This option is often more expensive initially but can save money in the long run.

COG Training Options

To achieve the optimal benefit from any computer or software package, you must be trained in its use. There are a number of ways that this can be accomplished:

- The company from which the computer was purchased may provide personnel to train you and other staff members.
- A user manual will come with your system. You can refer to it when you have problems.
- Help screens installed with every software package allow the user to self-teach. The disadvantage of this method is that it is often time consuming.
- Most software packages come with a tutorial. This is an on-screen short course on the use of the software.
- Most computer manufacturers and software programs will have a service called a help desk, which provides technical support. It is usually accessed by calling a toll-free number and is manned by computer professionals who can answer your questions concerning the system.

A combination of these methods is the best approach to learning about your computer and software.

COG Cell Phones and Texting

In the past, medical office personnel depended on telephone answering services to communicate with

physicians. The use of cellular telephones has made wireless communication an optimal way to contact providers. You can send a text message to providers right in the office or when they are out of the office. Again, you must always keep in mind that confidentiality is an issue. Consider the following guidelines when creating a text message:

1. Refrain from using identifying information such as patients' names or medical record numbers.
2. Keep communications businesslike. For example, avoid abbreviations such as "lol" (laugh out loud).
3. Keep communications brief and to the point. For example, "please call office ASAP" or "you are needed in ICU."

With the advances in technology and more federal regulations, possiblities for electronic communication are bound to emerge and change. A good rule of thumb is to keep all communications professional and always remember to protect your patient's privacy.

AFF Computer Ethics

The computer is a must in all physicians' offices. Its capabilities are endless. It can, however, lead to invasion of patients' privacy and unethical behavior. Some key points to keep in mind are:

- Never give out your login password. New employees must be issued their own passwords.
- Never leave a screen open with patient information and walk away from the computer. Exit the file.
- Only key people need access to sensitive patient information. Some programs, such as those with laboratory results, should have individual passwords.
- Physicians can often access patient data (e.g., radiology and laboratory reports) from the hospital computers. The hospital gives the physician a special code. It is not appropriate for the physician to share this with staff members. Never use another person's password to get patient information unless instructed to do so by a supervisor. You should be given your own code by the administrator of the program.
- Do not use the office Internet access for anything other than work-related tasks. It is inappropriate to surf the Internet for personal reasons while at work.
- E-mails should be read only by the person to whom they were sent. To avoid conflicts, the physician should have his or her own e-mail account, and the practice should have a generic e-mail address. It is never appropriate for you to receive personal e-mail messages on the office's e-mail address. It is also inappropriate to access your personal e-mail while at work.
- Sensitive patient data should not be sent via e-mail from one office to the other unless it is clearly known that the recipient of the e-mail is the only one with

access to it. It is a common practice to send patient information to the consulting physician. This information may include cancer diagnosis, HIV testing, and drug abuse reports. Extreme caution must be used.

- If you are allowed access to local laboratories to obtain laboratory results, it is to be used only on patients in your practice. It is unethical and illegal to obtain other people's reports. For example, if your son had a throat culture done at the pediatrician's office and sent to the laboratory you have access to, you should not look up his results.

- Do not take advantage of your position in the medical field. Remember, you have a legal and ethical responsibility to protect patient information.

 CHECKPOINT QUESTION

12. What is a tutorial?

español
SPANISH TERMINOLOGY

Asegurese de buscar los iconos en el sitio de web para asegurarse de su credibilidad.
> Be sure you look for the icons on a Web site to ensure its credibility.

Tenga cautela al comprar medicamentos en el internet.
> Be careful if you buy medications online.

Nuestro sistema computarizado es securo y privado.
> Our computer system is secure and private.

 MEDIA MENU

- **Student Resources on thePoint**
  - **CMA/RMA Certification Exam Review**
- **Internet Resources**

Occupational Safety and Health Administration Safety and Health Topics: Ergonomics
http://www.osha.gov/SLTC/ergonomics/index.html

Typing Injuries Frequently Asked Questions
http://www.tifaq.com

U.S. Department of Health and Human Services
http://www.healthfinder.gov

Medline Plus
http://www.nlm.nih.gov/medlineplus

HealthCentral
http://www.healthcentral.com

WebMD
http://www.webmd.com

Mayo Clinic
http://www.mayoclinic.com

FamilyDoctor
http://familydoctor.org/online/famdocen/home.html

Rare Disease Search Engine
http://www.raredisease.org (this site has a database of over 1,000 rare diseases and over 900 drugs that can be used to treat rare diseases)

PSY PROCEDURE 9-1:   Caring for and Maintaining Computer Hardware

Purpose: To prolong the life of computer hardware by following certain guidelines and performing preventative maintenance

Equipment: Computer CPU, monitor, keyboard, mouse, printer, duster, simulated warranties

Steps	Reasons
1. Place the monitor, keyboard, and printer in a cool, dry area out of direct sunlight.	Sunlight can damage casings, and heat and cold are also harmful to hardware.
2. Place the computer desk on an antistatic floor mat or carpet.	Static electricity can cause memory loss, inaccurate data collection, and other adverse reactions.
3. Clean the monitor screen with antistatic wipes.	Glass cleaner is not recommended.
4. Use dust covers for the keyboard and the monitor when they are not in use.	Dust can accumulate and cause the keyboard and mouse to stick and malfunction.
5. When moving the computer, lock the hard drive.	This will protect the CPU and disk drives.
6. Keep keyboard and mouse free of debris and liquids. Dust and/or vacuum the keyboard periodically to eliminate dust particles under the key pads.	Dust and debris can be hazardous to the keyboard and cause the keys to stick, etc. Never eat or drink when using the computer.

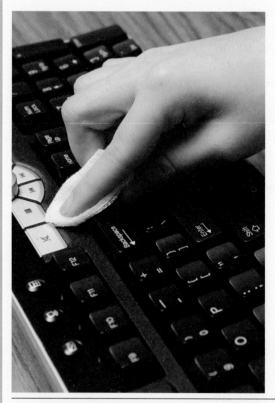

Step 6. Keep the keyboard free of dust and debris.

Steps	Reasons
7. Create a file for maintenance and warranty contracts for the computer system.	This will allow quick and easy retrieval of phone numbers, etc. if a representative is needed.
8. Handle data storage disks with special care.	Scratches, fingerprints, etc. can corrupt data.
9. **AFF** If you were the office manager, explain how you would respond to an employee who continued to spill soft drinks on her keyboard.	Prohibit eating and drinking at employee work stations. A break room should be available for eating and drinking.

PSY **PROCEDURE 9-2:** Searching on the Internet

Purpose: To quickly and effectively search the Internet, resulting in good time management
Equipment: Computer with Web browser software, modem, active Internet connection account

Steps	Purpose
1. Connect your computer to the Internet.	An Internet connection is necessary to search the Internet.
2. Locate a search engine.	A search engine is necessary to find information on the Internet.
3. Select two or three key words and type them at the appropriate place on the Web page.	Key words tell the search engine what to look for.
4. View the number of search results. If no sites were found, check spelling and retype or choose new key words.	The search engine was unable to find sites that can provide the information you requested.
5. If the search produced a long list, do an advanced search and refine your key words.	Reading through numerous sites is not time efficient.
6. Select an appropriate site and open its home page.	This allows you to view the information on the Web site.
7. If you are satisfied with the site's information, either download the material or bookmark the page. If you are unsatisfied with its information, either visit a site listed on the results page or return to the search engine.	Downloading or bookmarking the information gives you access to it in the future.
8. **AFF** You sit down to use your office computer to search for information with a patient when a co-worker's Facebook page pops up. You are embarrassed at the unprofessionalism this displays in front of the patient. Explain how you would respond in this situation.	Speak to the co-worker in person about personal use of the office computers. Refer her to the computer use policy of the office. If this does not make an impact, you could tell the office manager.

Chapter Summary

- Computers are an essential piece of technology in the medical office.
- As a medical assistant, you will use the computer for both clinical and administrative tasks. Computers will help you perform your job more efficiently, timely, and professionally.
- You will take precautions to comply with HIPAA's Administrative Simplification and Privacy Rules.
- Computers promote good patient care.
- You will be able to communicate with various health care professionals by using electronic mail.

- The Internet plays a key role in medicine.
- Patients, physicians, and medical assistants use the Internet to find new medical cures and for seeking current information about various health topics.
- You will need to be able to navigate the Web quickly and safely.
- It is essential that you stay abreast of computer technology, as it changes and improves daily.

Warm Ups for Critical Thinking

1. Log on to the Internet and locate a search engine. Search for a medical topic. It can be administrative or clinical. What are your key words? How many sites are listed? Now, using the same key words, use the advanced search engine. How many sites are listed? What are the benefits of using the advanced search method?

2. Select any five Web addresses listed in this chapter, and view the homepage. What benefits do the sites offer? What information or topics were missing?

3. Review the Patient Education Box about selecting Web sites safely. Find three Web sites that use these types of phrases or words. Do you think these sites are misleading? Do you think they pose a danger to patients?

4. Your office manager asks you to serve on a committee to purchase an electronic medical record system. Formulate a list of questions that you can ask a vendor before buying a computer system.

5. List five Web addresses for a patient who has just been diagnosed with type 2 diabetes.

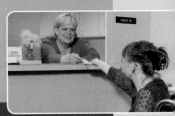

Medical Office Management, Safety, and Emergency Preparedness

Learning Outcomes

Cognitive Domain

Note: AAMA/CAAHEP 2008 Standards are italicized.

1. Spell and define the key terms
2. Describe what is meant by organizational structure
3. List seven responsibilities of the medical office manager
4. Explain the five staffing issues that a medical office manager will be responsible for handling
5. List the types of policies and procedures that should be included in a medical office's policy and procedures manual

6. List five types of promotional materials that a medical office may distribute
7. Discuss financial concerns that the medical office manager must be capable of addressing
8. Describe the duties regarding office maintenance, inventory, and service contracts
9. Discuss the need for continuing education
10. Describe liability, professional, personal injury, and third-party insurance
11. List three services provided by most medical malpractice companies
12. List six guidelines for completing incident reports

13. List four regulatory agencies that require medical offices to have quality improvement programs
14. Describe the accreditation process of The Joint Commission
15. Describe the steps to developing a quality improvement program
16. *Identify safety techniques that can be used to prevent accidents and maintain a safe work environment*
17. *Describe the importance of Material Safety Data Sheets (MSDS) in a health care setting*
18. *Identify safety signs, symbols, and labels*
19. *Describe fundamental principles for evacuation of a health care setting*
20. *Discuss fire safety issues in a health care environment*
21. *Discuss requirements for disposing of hazardous material*
22. *Identify principles of body mechanics and ergonomics*
23. *Discuss critical elements of an emergency plan for response to a natural disaster or other emergency*
24. *Identify emergency preparedness plans in your community*
25. *Discuss potential role(s) of the medical assistant in emergency preparedness*
26. *List and discuss legal and illegal interview questions*
27. *Discuss all levels of governmental legislation and regulation as they apply to medical assisting practice, including FDA and DEA regulations*
28. *Apply local, state, and federal health care legislation and regulation appropriate to the medical assisting practice setting*
29. *Describe basic elements of first aid*
30. *Identify how the Americans with Disabilities Act (ADA) applies to the medical assisting profession*

Psychomotor Domain

Note: AAMA/CAAHEP 2008 Standards are italicized.

1. Create a policy and procedures manual (Procedure 10-1)
2. *Perform an office inventory (Procedure 10-2)*
3. *Perform within scope of practice*
4. *Select appropriate barrier/personal protective equipment (PPE) for potentially infectious situations*
5. *Assist physician with patient care*
6. *Report relevant information to others succinctly and accurately*
7. *Evaluate the work environment to identify safe versus unsafe working conditions*
8. *Maintain a current list of community resources for emergency preparedness*
9. *Develop a personal (patient and employee) safety plan*
10. *Develop an environmental safety plan*
11. *Demonstrate proper use of the following equipment: eyewash, fire extinguishers, sharps disposal containers*
12. *Participate in a mock environmental exposure with documentation of steps taken*
13. *Explain the evacuation plan for a physician's office*
14. *Demonstrate methods of fire prevention in the health care setting*
15. *Complete an incident report*
16. *Incorporate the Patient's Bill of Rights into personal practice and medical office policies and procedures*
17. *Apply local, state, and federal health care legislation and regulation appropriate to the medical assisting practice setting*

Affective Domain

Note: AAMA/CAAHEP 2008 Standards are italicized.

1. *Recognize the effects of stress on all persons involved in emergency situations*
2. *Demonstrate self awareness in responding to emergency situations*
3. *Apply active listening skills*
4. *Use appropriate body language and other nonverbal skills in communicating with patients, family, and staff*
5. *Recognize the importance of local, state, and federal legislation and regulation in the practice setting*

ABHES Competencies

1. Perform routine maintenance of administrative and clinical equipment
2. Maintain inventory, equipment, and supplies
3. Maintain medical facility
4. Serve as liaison between physician and others
5. Interview effectively
6. Comprehend the current employment outlook for the medical assistant
7. Understand the importance of maintaining liability coverage once employed in the industry
8. Perform risk-management procedures
9. Comply with federal, state, and local health laws and regulations

bioterrorism	epidemic	job description	policy
body mechanics	ergonomics	mission statement	procedure
budget	expected threshold	organizational chart	quality improvement
compliance officer	incident reports	pandemic	task force

A successful and safe medical practice needs an effective medical office management process. This process must be a team effort among the physicians, nurse managers, and the office manager. A medical practice must manage risk and engage in ongoing quality improvement procedures. This chapter provides an overview of medical office management, a medical office manager's specific responsibilities, as well as a discussion of risk management and quality improvement. Emergency preparedness has become a way of life in the United States. Today's medical office personnel must be able to recognize unsafe conditions, understand fire safety issues, and guide patients and staff calmly in the event of an evacuation of the medical office.

COG Overview of Medical Office Management

Each medical office is organized in a slightly different manner, depending on the size and complexity of the setting. It has been said that change is the only constant in our lives. The health care arena is no exception. At the writing of this textbook, U.S. Congress is considering the many facets of health care reform. Although it is not certain what will transpire, we will take a look at the components of this legislation that will surely affect the management of the medical office.

Organizational Structure

The medical office's organizational structure, or chain of command, is depicted in an **organizational chart**, a flow sheet that allows the manager and employees to identify their team members and to see where they fit into the team. Figure 10-1 displays a sample organizational chart for a physician's office in which there is a partnership between two physicians. In this example, it is assumed that the physicians have an equal partnership in the practice.

CHECKPOINT QUESTION

1. What is the purpose of an organizational chart?

The Medical Office Manager

The medical office manager must be multiskilled, multitalented, and able to prioritize a variety of issues, juggle responsibilities, and communicate effectively with patients, staff, and physicians. In some settings, the medical office manager may be referred to as the business manager. Managers may be nurses, medical assistants, or administrative support personnel. Although the qualifications and educational requirements for the position vary greatly among health care organizations, a successful medical office manager must be:

- Flexible
- A positive role model for employees
- Honest and fair
- A good communicator
- A resource person for employees
- Supportive of all management decisions
- Well organized
- Able to focus on a given task
- Able to resolve conflicts
- Able to see the big picture
- A continuous learner

A medical office manager's responsibilities include varied tasks:

- Communicating with patients, physicians, and staff
- Handling staffing issues
- Writing and revising policy and procedures manuals
- Developing promotional materials
- Handling financial concerns
- Handling office maintenance
- Managing supplies and inventory
- Ensuring that the staff receives appropriate education
- Maintaining budgets
- Enforcing HIPAA regulations and other accrediting agency regulations

A medical office manager also must keep abreast of important legal issues, such as medical practice acts, employment and safety laws, patient care laws, billing and insurance regulations, and more. See Chapter 2 for more details on these topics.

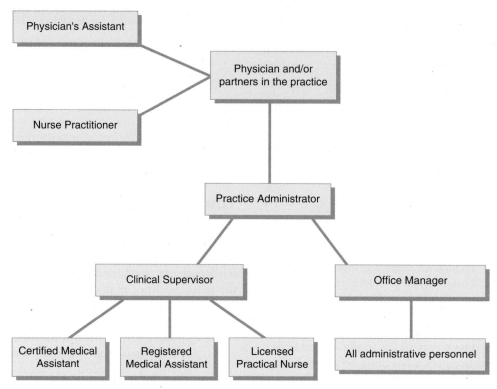

Figure 10-1 Sample organizational chart.

COG Responsibilities of the Medical Office Manager

Communication

Perhaps one of the hardest and yet most important aspects of being an effective manager is being able to communicate with fellow employees, colleagues, physicians, and patients. (The techniques for effective communication are discussed in Chapter 3.) You must be a good listener, have good interpersonal skills, and be aware of your own nonverbal language.

Communicating with Patients

Communication with patients on a management level can often be challenging. Patients come to you with a variety of complaints, such as incorrect billing, poor care, or long waits to see physicians. Of course, you must always be diplomatic. Your goal should be to correct the problem in a timely and professional manner and to alleviate any negative feelings the patient may have.

Communicating with Staff

Communication with staff members can be difficult, depending on the number of employees, number and locations of satellite centers, and the variety of shifts that are in place. There are three ways to promote communication with staff members: staff meetings, bulletin boards, and communication notebooks. It is a good idea to ask your staff for input in deciding the best way to communicate with them.

Staff Meetings

Staff meetings should be scheduled at a predictable frequency and time to allow the staff to plan (e.g., they might be held the first Monday of every month at 8 am). *Meetings should never be canceled except in a true emergency.*

Staff meetings must be well organized and should begin and end on time. Agendas should be created prior to the meeting and posted for staff review. (See Chapter 7 for information on agendas.) The agenda should be followed as closely as possible. Individual staff concerns or complaints should not be handled during a general staff meeting; the meeting should remain focused and constructive and not turn into a battleground for staff disagreements. Minutes should be taken and kept in a notebook for staff to review as needed. (See Chapter 7 for information on minutes.)

Staff meetings should be conducted in a private area out of patients' sight and hearing (Fig. 10-2). All interruptions, except for emergencies, should be avoided.

Have the telephone covered by an answering service or a prerecorded message informing callers of the time the staff will be unavailable. Lock the door, and place a sign with the time the office will reopen. Of course, you will give clear instructions to callers or visitors who have an emergency. The personnel manual should clearly state the attendance policy for staff meetings. In addition, some offices include attendance as a duty in each employee's **job description** (statement of work-related responsibilities). To improve attendance at staff

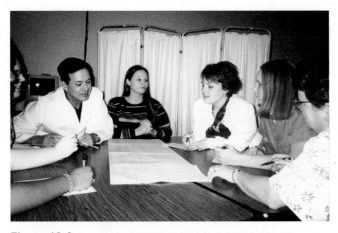

Figure 10-2 Staff meeting being conducted in a private area.

meetings, consider serving food or including an educational presentation. Involve staff as much as possible when setting the meeting agenda.

Bulletin Boards

Bulletin board postings allow employees to get a quick and easy look at new polices or procedures. To encourage staff members to read the postings, make sure the bulletin boards are attractive, well organized, and updated regularly. It is a good idea to have employees initial all messages on the bulletin board after reading them.

Communication Notebooks

A simple notebook can serve as a two-way communication tool: You can write messages to employees, and they can write back to you. Such a notebook is usually kept in the staff lounge. Again, staff members should initial any important messages after reading them. If the message is directed to you, be sure to respond as soon as possible. One medical office places a notebook with pertinent information for employees in staff restrooms and titles it "Potty Training."

Communicating Electronically

E-mail has become popular and is an easy and time-saving way to communicate with staff. Messages can be printed and kept in a binder for easy reference. E-mail messages eliminate the need for memos that must be posted or circulated. Your e-mail system will provide you with an address book that can be customized to include groups such as all employees, all clinical employees, employees and physicians, and so on.

Sometimes, the stress of daily duties prevents managers from communicating with staff members on a personal level. To be an effective manager, you should communicate not only bad news but also positive messages to your employees. You can communicate positive messages through birthday and holiday cards and employee recognition awards. Send thank you notes to the staff to compliment them when they go above and beyond the call of duty.

 CHECKPOINT QUESTION

2. What are three ways to promote communication with staff members?

Staffing Issues

Staffing issues will occupy most of your time as an office manager. These concerns include writing job descriptions, hiring new employees, evaluating present employees, taking disciplinary actions, handling terminations, and scheduling. Sometimes an office manager also becomes a coach and a counselor.

Writing Job Descriptions

Each job must have a description. The purpose of a job description is to inform the employee about the essential job duties and expectations for a given position. Job descriptions also help you in interviewing applicants and evaluating existing employees.

Each employee should receive a copy of his or her job description at the time of hiring and after any revisions to the description are made. Some medical offices have a policy requiring the employee to read and sign the job description at the time of hiring and for each annual evaluation.

Formats for writing job descriptions vary among offices. In general, the following elements are included: job title, supervisor, position summary, hours, location, employment requirements, physical requirements, duties, and the evaluation process (Fig. 10-3). The description should also include the date it was written and date of any revisions.

If possible, involve staff members in writing and revising their job descriptions. Employee participation leads to greater cooperation.

 LEGAL TIP

MAKE SURE YOUR INTERVIEW QUESTIONS ARE APPROPRIATE

Title VII of the Civil Rights Act prohibits discrimination in the workplace. To ensure that hiring practices are fair and nondiscriminatory, be careful and consistent in the types of questions asked in an interview. You may ask work-related questions like, "Are you proficient in typing?" Avoid questions that might give the appearance of discrimination. You may not ask applicants their age, race, religion, or marital status. You cannot ask about children, day care, or plans for future children.

Job Description

Title: Medical Assistant

Supervisor(s): Clinical Supervisor

Office Manager for Administrative Duties

Position summary: This is a 40-hour position that will require the employee to perform various duties including administrative, clinical, and laboratory procedures. Scheduling will be variable to meet the needs of the office.

Hours: Hours will vary to meet the needs of the office. Hours will rotate from 8:00 AM–4:30 PM and 10:00 AM–6:30 PM. You will be expected to work one Saturday per month.

Location: Our main office is located at 129 South Main Street. The satellite office is located at 56 West Road, Suite 102. This position will primarily require you to work at our main office. However, occasional days may be assigned at the satellite office.

Employment Requirements: The employee must have graduated from a medical assisting program. CMA or RMA is preferred. The employee must have a current CPR and First Aid card. One year of experience or completion of an externship is preferred.

• *Language skills:* The employee must be able to read and interpret documents and respond appropriately (verbally and/or in writing). Must be able to document in a professional manner.

• *Mathematical skills:* The employee must be able to add, subtract, multiply, and divide whole numbers and fractions.

Physical requirements: The following are physical requirements for this job: Standing: 6–8 hours/day; Sitting: 6–8 hours/day; Lifting: 50 pounds; Twisting and rotating: 45 degrees; Squatting: As needed to assist patients or to perform office tasks.

Duties: You will be expected to perform the following duties after completing the orientation process. This is a partial list; and other duties can be added as necessary.

Administrative:	
Scheduling appointments	Processing mail
Transcribing documents	Operating the telephone
Filing	Providing patient education
Completing insurance forms	

Clinical/Laboratory:	
Operating centrifuge	Obtaining vital signs
Performing phlebotomy	Administering vaccines and other medications as ordered
Performing HCT/HGB/CBC	Providing patient education
Performing pregnancy and monospot tests	Assisting the physician as directed
Obtaining visual acuities	

Evaluation process: Three evaluations will be conducted in the first year. Thirty days from start date, ninety days from start date, and then at the one-year anniversary date. Following the first year of employment, annual evaluations will be done.

I have read my job description, and I understand what is expected of me. I am able to physically perform all the required duties.

Signature of employee: _____ Date: _____

Signature of supervisor: _____ Date: _____

Signature of supervisor: _____ Date: _____

Figure 10-3 Sample job description.

Hiring and Interviewing Employees

Only after creating or reviewing an existing job description can you begin the process of interviewing and hiring a new employee. You can seek applicants through advertising in local newspaper classified sections, placement personnel at local schools that offer medical assisting programs, networking, and employment agencies.

All applicants should complete an application. State laws vary regarding the types of questions that can be asked on applications. In general, you must avoid any questions pertaining to an applicant's age, sex, race, national origin, religion, and physical or mental disabilities. If your medical facility requires a criminal background check and drug testing, the form should include this information with a place for the applicant to give necessary permission with a signature. Any employee application form should be reviewed by legal counsel prior to its use. It is always a good idea to request that the applicant bring a résumé to the interview.

Before interviewing an applicant, prepare a list of questions. Again, use caution; under law, you are not permitted to ask about some topics. Ask only questions that are job related. Ask questions like, "Tell me about a time when you disagreed with your supervisor. How did you handle it?" This type of "behavioral interviewing" will give the interviewer the most information about the candidate's job knowledge and behavior. During the interview, assess the applicant's ability to do the following:

- Perform technical skills
- Treat patients in a caring manner
- Fit into your organization
- Communicate in a professional yet friendly manner
- Remain flexible

Be consistent and fair when selecting the best candidate.

AFF ETHICAL TIP

Tough Spot

Consider this scenario: A co-worker tells you that a newly hired employee says she is a certified medical assistant (CMA), but you have a mutual friend who says this person never passed the exam. Should you share this information with anyone? *Yes*. This would constitute fraud. Unfortunately, some people are dishonest and unethical. It would be unethical for you to ignore the information. Tell the office manager who can then verify the employee's stated credentials by calling the appropriate certification registry. You can check the validity of any license or certification by contacting the licensing agency or professional organization that awards the credential. A CMA's status can be obtained by calling 1-800-ACT-AAMA. Many state medical assisting societies also have certification registries. Try going to the particular profession's Web site.

AFF WHAT IF?

You receive a call requesting a reference for an employee who was fired. What should you say?

Be careful! This situation can turn into a legal and ethical nightmare if not handled appropriately. If you give a wonderful report to the potential employer and say, "She was great; we never had any problems," you and the office may be sued by the former employee for wrongful discharge. In court, you would be asked, "If she was so wonderful, why did you fire her?" On the other hand, if you say, "She was a terrible employee, and we fired her," you can be sued for defamation of character. Because of the legal concerns in providing employment references, most organizations have a policy stating that the only information to be released is verification of employment dates and job titles. When in doubt, give no information. Ask for the caller's name and phone number, discuss the issue with the physician in charge, and then return the phone call.

Evaluating Employees

All employees must be evaluated annually. The evaluation should be a positive experience for the employee. Employee evaluations must be fair, accurate, and objective.

Some type of written evaluation should be given to the employee to read, sign, and comment on. Most forms ask employees to list their objectives and goals for the coming year. Figure 10-4 displays a sample evaluation form. Some organizations call evaluations performance appraisals.

New employees should be evaluated 1 month after their start date, again in 90 days, and then at their 1-year anniversary date. This process helps new employees gain confidence and improve weaknesses. Coaching and counseling should occur throughout the year. The employee should know what will be said during the feedback because the manager has communicated with them throughout the year. An employee should never be surprised by the feedback.

Taking Disciplinary Action

Most offices have policies regarding documentation of disciplinary action. Disciplinary actions can be verbal or written. Verbal warnings are generally done for a first-time minor occurrence (e.g., not showing up for work and not calling in). A note should go into the employee's file stating that a verbal warning was given, the date, any actions that were taken, and any comments that the employee made.

Employee Evaluation Form

Employee: *Jackie England*
Evaluation Date: *5/2/13*
Job Title: *CMA*
Ratings:

Traits	Score
Appearance	5
Communication Skills	3
Attendance	4
Quality of work	5
Reliability	4
Initiative	4
Other: *Willingness to work as a team*	5
Total Score:	30

Rating scale:
5—excellent
4—above average
3—meets job expectations
2—below job expectations
1—does not meet job expectations

Supervisor comments:
Is an excellent CMA. She is shy with patients + co-workers, but improving.

Employee goals for the next year (to be completed by employee):
I will continue to attain CEU's for recertifiction. I plan to take class on being assertive.

Employee Comments:
I love working here and appreciate having good + fair bosses.

Supervisor signature: *Diane Hall*   Date: *5/2/13*
Employee signature: *Jackie England*   Date: *5/2/13*

Figure 10-4 Sample employee evaluation form.

Written notices are used for more serious problems (e.g., breaching patient confidentiality, substance abuse) or recurrent minor ones. Employees should sign any written warning notices. These documents can be used as evidence in the event that the person is fired and brings a lawsuit for wrongful discharge. Figure 10-5 shows a sample written disciplinary action form. Determine whether the employee's credentialing agency should be notified of serious infractions.

Terminating Employees

Having to terminate (fire) an employee is never an easy or pleasant task. It is essential that policies regarding termination be followed precisely. All disciplinary actions must be clearly and objectively stated. Terminating employees for unlawful reasons or failing to follow the organization's termination policy can result in lawsuits against you and the office. When disciplining an employee, make sure to ask yourself if other employees have committed the same policy violations. Have they all been treated the same? Some reasons for termination include:

- Excessive tardiness or absenteeism
- Inappropriate dress or behavior
- Alcohol or drug use
- Endangering patients

Discipline Record

Employee Name: _Brenda Elliott_　#: _26_　Date of Warning: _5/28/13_

Warning

Date of Violation: _5/28/13_　Time: _9:15 AM_　Place: _Exam Room 1_

Description of Violation:
Brenda was assisting Dr. Baymor in surgery. She took no action when the sterile field was compromised. The possibly contaminated field was not reset. She told no one. It was questioned by the patient.

_____ Verbal Warning
_____ Written Warning
✔ Probation _30_ Days
_____ Suspension _____ Days
_____ Termination
Dana Hudson, CMA
Supervisor's Signature

Action To Be Taken:
Brenda is placed on probation for 30 days. Another occurrence will mean possible dismissal.

Date

Employee's Remarks

Do you agree with the details above:　Yes: ✔　No: _____
Comments: _I understand the seriousness of my error. It will never happen again._

Employee's Signature: _Brenda Elliott_　Date: _5/28/13_

Figure 10-5 Sample disciplinary action form.

- Lying or stealing
- Falsifying medical records or time sheets
- Breaching patient confidentiality

Scheduling

The primary goal of scheduling is to meet the needs of the office. The secondary goal is to meet the requests of your employees. You must be fair in scheduling and always follow your organization's policies for weekend and holiday or personal day requests. If possible, employees should be given time off with pay when attending seminars and meetings of their professional organization. This practice will keep morale high and encourage employees to stay current with their skills. Depending on the number of employees that you have to schedule and the complexity of the hours or shifts, you can either schedule by hand or use a computer program. If your organization is small and cohesive, you may want to assign a senior staff member to do the scheduling, or you might allow the employees to self-schedule. No matter what scheduling format is used, you are ultimately responsible for ensuring that the appropriate number and type of employees needed are scheduled.

Requests for time off should be put in writing. Depending on the size of the organization, such requests may have to be received by a given date or time. For example, the policy may read, "A request for a day off in May should be submitted by April 15. Any requests for time off filed after the cutoff date will be approved whenever possible." This eliminates repeated adjustment of the staffing schedule.

 CHECKPOINT QUESTION

3. What is the medical office manager's primary goal in scheduling?

Policy and Procedures Manuals

Every business needs written rules and regulations to ensure that its practices are within legal and ethical boundaries. Employees need written procedures to ensure consistency in the practices of the business. In the outpatient medical facility, these written policies and procedures are *required* by regulatory and accrediting agencies.

North Shore Family Practice is a group practice dedicated to providing quality care through compassion, innovation, performance and education. It is our goal to provide medical care to the community of Rochester, New York. The physicians, nurse practitioners, and all staff members are committed to working together as a team to provide the patient with the best care possible.

Figure 10-6 Sample mission statement.

5. Clinical procedures
6. Administrative procedures
7. Infection control
8. Safety measures
9. Emergency preparedness

Section 1: Mission Statement

A **mission statement** describes the goals of the practice and whom it serves. Often a mission statement provides a philosophical look at an organization. It is generally one to two paragraphs long (Fig. 10-6).

The mission statement should not only be included in the policy and procedures manual; it should also be available to patients. Often it is framed and placed in the waiting room or printed in the practice brochure.

Section 2: Organizational Structure

The organizational chart is included in this section along with policies regarding the following:

- Chain of command
- How and when to contact various members of the team
- Coverage for managers
- Physician on-call policies

Section 3: Human Resources or Personnel

This section consists of policies relating to staff responsibilities, benefits, and rules and regulations for employees. Box 10-2 lists the kinds of policies found in this section of the manual. A sample human resources policy is displayed in Figure 10-7.

It is the office manager's responsibility to coordinate the orientation and training of any new employee. A personnel manual that includes the organization's policies and outlines step-by-step procedures for each task performed in the facility becomes the new employee's information source. Even veteran employees may have to refer to the proper procedure for a task. As new procedures become available or existing procedures are changed, this is added to the procedures manual. Tips regarding policy and procedures manual are detailed in Box 10-1.

Most organizations create a policy and procedures manual that is written, maintained, and regarded as one document. A **policy** is a statement regarding the organization's rules on a given topic. A **procedure** is a series of steps required to perform a given task. Policies and procedures must be written in a clear, concise, and understandable format. Each policy or procedure is signed by the employees, indicating they have read, understand, and will adhere to the policy or procedure. Policies regarding medical office management are signed by the physician and supervisory staff.

Types of Policies and Procedures

There are many types of policies and procedures. In general, the following areas are included in a policy and procedures manual:

1. Mission statement
2. Organizational structure
3. Human resources or personnel
4. Quality improvement and risk management

Grievance procedures
Grooming, uniforms, appearance
Holiday coverage and compensation for holidays
Jury duty
Office hours
Orientation
Overtime reports
Parking
Payroll
Personal phone calls
Resignations
Sexual harassment
Sick leave and family leave
Staff meetings
Tardiness
Termination process
Time recording
Vacation days

Section 4: Quality Improvement and Risk Management

This section includes policies outlining who is in charge of **quality improvement**, the steps for developing a quality improvement plan, and explanations of incident reporting, discussed later.

Section 5: Clinical Procedures

Any task that requires intervention with a patient should be listed in this section. (Some offices separate laboratory procedures into a different section for convenience.) In addition, clinical procedures should include specific infection control guidelines for the particular procedure, patient education guidelines, and instructions for documentation. Sample documentation forms should be included in this section. It is a good idea to complete the sample form correctly so that it can serve as a model. In the medical office, these procedures may vary slightly to meet the needs of the office, physicians' requests, or manufacturers' guidelines.

Section 6: Administrative Procedures

This section includes procedures on all tasks that the administrative office staff must perform. Sample forms should also be included and updated as necessary. Examples of administrative tasks are as follows:

- Accounting and bookkeeping
- Appointment scheduling
- Collections
- Computer care and operations
- Insurance filings
- Medical records management
- Mail and postal machine operations

Benjamin William, MD
2295 Matthews Drive
Boca Raton, Florida 33432
POLICY AND PROCEDURE MANUAL

Policy title: Human Resources, Absences
Purpose: The purpose of this policy is to advise all employees of the policy for absences and to prewarn employees regarding the disciplinary steps that will be taken as a result of not complying with this policy.
Equipment/Forms necessary: No equipment or forms are required.
Explanation:

- If you are going to call in sick, you must call in two hours prior to your assigned time. Messages should be left with the answering service if the office is not open.
- If you have personal days accrued, you can use them for compensation.
- If you are going to be out sick for more than three consecutive working days, you will need to obtain a physician's note to document the illness.
- Employees are allowed six (6) absences per year without disciplinary action. Seven (7) absences will result in a verbal warning regarding attendance. Eight (8) absences will result in a written warning. Nine (9) absences will result in termination. Exceptions to disciplinary action will be reviewed on an individual basis and are at the joint discretion of the office manager and physician.

_____   _____
Susan Rogers, RMA   Benjamin William, MD
Office Manager

Date: original policy - 06/96, revised 01/00, 02/03, 02/06, 02/10, 02/13
HR: 14

Figure 10-7 Sample human resources policy.

to retain the CMA credential. The office manager may choose to keep a file for each employee with the necessary documentation. This will assist the staff in the recertification process.

As the medical office manager, you should select an educational topic for each month. In some offices, the educational topic is covered during the monthly staff meetings, whereas other offices have separate educational programs. After choosing the monthly topic, select an appropriate presenter. Suggestions for presenters include colleagues, physicians, sales representatives, local hospital staff development coordinators, and specialists. Presenters for CPR classes must be CPR instructors who are approved by a national organization. To promote attendance, create informative flyers and distribute them to all staff members. Keep attendance records for all classes given.

In addition to formal educational programs, there are other ways to keep your staff up to date. For instance, educational videos and DVDs can be rented or purchased for staff viewing; consider developing a posttest to assess for comprehension. Also, many professional magazines have continuing education articles on various topics, usually accompanied by a posttest. Finally, staff members should be sent to one or two seminars a year. Outside seminars help increase employee productivity, self-esteem, and retention.

Patient Education

All members of the health care team must constantly contribute to educating patients. As a manager, you may not provide patient education directly, but you are responsible for assisting the staff in performing this task. You can help the staff with patient education by creating booklets, developing posters, and by teaching your staff how, when, and what to teach patients and families.

Patient education brochures should be colorful and easy to read. Close attention to spelling, grammar, punctuation, and accuracy is essential. All brochures should be reviewed by a physician. Depending on your office's clientele, the brochures should be printed in various languages. Refer to Chapter 4 for more details on creating patient education brochures.

Manager Education

Managers should attend workshops and conferences and read appropriate printed materials to enhance their knowledge and skills in managing a medical office. All new managers can benefit from courses on time management, stress management, solving personnel conflicts, and budget preparation. Memberships in professional organizations can also assist the new office manager. Two such organizations are:

Medical Office Management Association
1355 South Colorado Boulevard, Suite 900
Denver, CO 80222-3331

Professional Association of Health Care Office
　Management
2929 Langley Avenue, Suite 102
Pensacola, FL 32504-7355

COG Risk Management

Risk management is an internal process geared to identifying potential problems before they cause injury to patients or employees. Potential problems are related to risk factors. A risk factor is any situation or condition that poses a safety or liability concern for a given practice. Examples of risk factors are poor lighting, clutter, unlocked medication cabinets, failure to dispose of needles properly, and faulty patient identification procedures. Such factors may lead to patient falls, medication errors, employee needlesticks, and mistakes in therapeutic intervention. Risk factors for a particular health care organization are identified through a study of patterns. As discussed later, by tracking information obtained in incident reports, risks can be identified and managed. For example, tracking of incident reports might identify particular days of the week when most negative events happen. If most events occur on Friday afternoons, perhaps staffing on Friday afternoons should be reevaluated.

Liability Insurance

Doctors today face challenges that those of a generation ago never imagined. As discussed in Chapter 2, physicians are at risk for malpractice suits and must use sound practices to decrease this risk. New medical procedures, treatments, and drugs require regular review to ensure each practice meets high standards of safety and care. Physicians need malpractice insurance to protect them from financial loss in the event of a successful lawsuit or settlement. Nurses also carry malpractice insurance, and many allied health professionals are now opting for coverage.

Many malpractice insurance companies offer services such as teaching employees to take preventative measures and to identify problems before they become threats. They also conduct risk inspections, supply self-auditing tools, and provide bulletins. Malpractice insurance Web sites have many helpful tools for office managers.

A medical office is not just subject to liability regarding patients; since it is a public place, any visitor to the office could slip and fall on a wet floor or be hurt by a picture falling from a wall. As office manager, you should assess the coverage needs of your employees and investigate the possibility of a policy that would cover any employees who need it. Insurance is a large expense but one that a medical practice must incur.

 CHECKPOINT QUESTION

6. Why do physicians need malpractice insurance?

LEGAL TIP

REPORTING OCCUPATIONAL INJURIES AND ILLNESSES

Medical and dental offices are currently exempt from maintaining an official log of reportable injuries and illnesses under the federal OSHA record-keeping rule; however, some states may require such records. You should be familiar with the laws in the state where you work and comply with any laws as necessary. All employers, including medical and dental offices, must report any work-related fatality or the hospitalization of three or more employees in a single incident to the nearest OSHA office.

Incident Reports

Incident reports, sometimes referred to as occurrence reports, are written accounts of negative patient, visitor, or staff events. Such events may be minor or life or limb threatening. The insurance company that provides the institution's liability insurance often requires incident reports.

An incident report is written or completed by the staff member involved in or at the scene of the incident. The report is reviewed by a supervisor for completion and accuracy and is then sent to a central location. Incident reports are usually given to the office manager or the physician. Depending on the type of event and organizational policy, a physician may or may not document the event on the incident report. If an unusual event happens to a patient, however, the physician should assess the patient and document the findings on the incident report. Figure 10-9 is a sample incident report.

When to Complete an Incident Report

Even in the safest settings, undesirable things can happen to patients. These events sometimes result from human error (e.g., giving the wrong medication), or they may be idiopathic. Idiopathic means that something occurred for unknown reasons and was unavoidable (e.g., an allergic reaction). Incident reports must be completed even if no injury resulted from an event. A few examples of situations requiring an incident report are:

- All medication errors
- All patient, visitor, and employee falls
- Drawing blood from a wrong patient
- Mislabeling of blood tubes or specimens
- Incorrect surgical instrument counts following surgery
- Employee needlesticks
- Workers' compensation injuries

The rule of thumb is, when in doubt, always complete an incident report.

Workplace Requirements Program for Safety and Health

SUPERVISOR'S ACCIDENT REPORT FORM

This form is to be completed by the supervisor and forwarded to the Payroll Coordinator along with a copy of the North Carolina Industrial Commission Form 19 (Workers Compensation Form) within five days of the accident. All accidents involving serious bodily injury or death must be reported to the safety and health officer immediately.

ACCIDENT DATA

1. NAME OF EMPLOYEE: or Patient
2. ADDRESS AND PHONE NO:
3. WORK DEPT. OR DIVISION: 4. SEX: ☐ MALE ☐ FEMALE   5. DATE AND TIME OF INJURY:
6. NATURE OF INJURY: 7. PART OF BODY INJURED:
8. CAUSE OF INJURY: 9. LOCATION OF ACCIDENT:
10. OCCUPATION AND ACTIVITY OF PERSON AT TIME OF ACCIDENT: 11. STATUS OF JOB OR ACTIVITY: (CHOOSE ONE)   Halted
12. NAME AND PHONE NO. OF ACCIDENT WITNESS:
13. LIST UNSAFE ACT, IF ANY:
14. LIST UNSAFE PHYSICAL OR MECHANICAL CONDITION, IF ANY:
15. UNSAFE PERSONAL FACTOR:
16. LIST HAZARD CONTROLS IN EFFECT AT TIME OF INJURY DESIGNED TO PREVENT INJURY:
17. PERSONAL PROTECTIVE EQUIPMENT BEING USED AT TIME OF ACCIDENT:
GLOVES, SAFETY GLASSES, GOGGLES, FACE SHIELD, OTHER
18. BRIEF DESCRIPTION OF ACCIDENT:
19. CORRECTIVE ACTION TAKEN OR RECOMMENDED TO DEPARTMENT SAFETY COMMITTEE:

TREATMENT DATA

20. WAS INJURED TAKEN TO (CHOOSE ONE): Hospital
21. DIAGNOSIS AND TREATMENT, IF KNOWN:
22. ESTIMATED LOST WORKDAYS: (EXCLUDING DAY OF ACCIDENT)   23. DATE OF REPORT: Month Day Year
24. REPORT PREPARED BY:
25. SIGNATURE OF SUPERVISOR:
26. SIGNATURE OF AGENCY SAFETY AND HEALTH OFFICER:

Figure 10-9 Sample incident report.

Information Included in an Incident Report

Although every agency has its own form, the following data are always included in an incident report:

- Name, address, and phone number of the injured party
- Date of birth and sex of the injured party
- Date, time, and location of the incident
- Brief description of the incident and what was done to correct it
- Any diagnostic procedures or treatments that were needed
- Patient examination findings, if applicable
- Names and addresses of witnesses, if applicable
- Signature and title of person completing form
- Physician's and supervisor's signatures as per policy

Guidelines for Completing an Incident Report

When completing an incident report, follow these guidelines:

1. State only the facts. Do not draw conclusions or summarize the event. For example, if you walk into

the reception room and find a patient on the floor, do not write, "Patient tripped and fell in reception area," because that draws a conclusion. Instead, document the incident as follows: "Patient found on the floor in the reception area. Patient states that he fell."

2. Write legibly and sign your name legibly. Be sure to include your title.

3. Complete the form in a timely fashion. In general, incident reports should be completed within 24 hours of the event.

4. Do not leave any blank spaces on the form. If a particular section of the report does not apply, write n/a (not applicable).

5. Never photocopy an incident report for your own personal record.

6. Never place the incident report in the patient's chart. Never document in the patient's chart that an incident report was completed. Only document the event in the patient's chart. (By writing in the medical record that an incident report was completed, it opens the potential for lawyers to subpoena the incident report, should there be a lawsuit.)

7. After incident reports are completed, review and track to highlight specific patterns. The resulting statistical data can be used to identify problem areas, which can be corrected through quality improvement (QI) programs.

 AFF WHAT IF?

You give the wrong medication, and the patient has a bad reaction to it. Would you be better off not documenting the medication error?

No! By not documenting the incident, you place yourself at risk. These risks can include allegations of falsifying medical records, tampering with medical records, and failing to follow reporting policies and procedures. On the incident report, do not say, "I gave the wrong medication"; just state the facts: "X medication was ordered. I gave Y medication." Then document who you told and when, what you were advised to do, and any other pertinent information. Your supervisor or the risk manager may call the medical office's insurance company to alert them to the incident. If the incident results in a malpractice lawsuit, an accurately completed incident report can prove helpful to your organization's attorney.

COG Regulatory Agencies

One of the most challenging problems for risk managers is to prevent noncompliance with regulatory agencies. As discussed earlier, numerous agencies regulate health care settings, and these rules and regulations change frequently. You can stay up to date with new changes by reading newsletters from these organizations, attending your state and local professional meetings, and frequently visiting various professional Web sites. Most states publish a monthly bulletin that reports new legislation. Every state has a Web site that will link you to legislative action. Read these regularly. Each office should have legal counsel who can assist in interpreting legal issues. It is important for a new manager to meet with the medical office's attorney to discuss legal concerns for the practice. These regulatory agencies monitor medical practices to ensure quality of care, protection of employees, and sound practices.

Centers for Medicare and Medicaid Services

The Centers for Medicare and Medicaid Services (CMS) (formerly the Health Care Financing Administration [HCFA]), a division of the U.S. Department of Health and Human Services, regulates and runs various departments and programs, including Medicare and Medicaid. This federal agency is assigned to monitor and follow two key regulations that will affect your job as a medical assistant. These two laws are the Clinical Laboratory Improvement Amendments Act (CLIA) and the Health Insurance Portability and Accountability Act (HIPAA). See Chapter 8 for information on HIPAA.

Occupational Safety and Health Administration

The Occupational Safety and Health Administration (OSHA) and the Occupational Safety and Health (OSH) Act of 1970 guarantee your right to a workplace that is free from serious hazards. The OSH Act also requires that your employer comply with occupational safety and health standards. Many states also have occupational and safety regulations that your office must follow. Unlike with those of The Joint Commission, compliance with OSHA regulations is not voluntary. Noncompliance with OSHA regulations can result in fines and closure of the health care organization. OSHA also requires that QI programs be in place to protect the health and welfare of patients and employees.

As it does with every profession, OSHA has identified safety hazards specific to medical offices. Examples are rules for blood-borne pathogen protection, use of personal protective equipment (PPE), tuberculosis prevention, management of biohazardous waste, ergonomics, and laser protection. Laser protection is needed if you are working with a physician who is operating a laser in the office. These rules and other guidelines can be found on the OSHA Web site. It also provides specific guidelines that offices must implement to ensure employee and patient safety.

The first step is to make sure that your office has an OSHA poster located in a place routinely accessed by employees, such as the breakroom or bathroom wall. This poster explains the rights of employees regarding a safe workplace and includes instructions on how to file a complaint if necessary. If you do not have this poster for your office, a free copy can be downloaded or ordered from OSHA's Web site at http://www.osha.gov. OSHA and its requirements are discussed throughout this chapter.

 CHECKPOINT QUESTION

7. What is the mission of OSHA?

The Joint Commission

The Joint Commission is a private agency that sets health care standards and evaluates an organization's implementation of these standards for health care settings. Prior to the mid 1990s, the primary focus of The Joint Commission was on evaluating hospitals and inpatient care institutions such as nursing homes. In 1996, The Joint Commission expanded its jurisdiction to outpatient and ambulatory care settings. This change was, in part, due to the shift of patient care from inpatient to outpatient services. As mentioned in Chapter 8, The Joint Commission sets standards and evaluates the care in the various health care settings. Box 10-4 lists various types of freestanding facilities for which The Joint Commission sets standards and provides accreditation.

BOX 10-4

TYPES OF FACILITIES

The Joint Commission accredits a variety of health care settings. These are some types of centers that can be accredited:

- Ambulatory care centers
- Birthing centers
- Chiropractic clinics
- Community health organizations
- Corporate health services
- County jail infirmaries
- Dental clinics
- Dialysis centers
- Endoscopy centers
- Group practices
- Imaging centers
- Independent practitioner practices
- Lithotripsy centers
- Magnetic resonance imaging centers
- Oncology centers
- Ophthalmology surgery centers
- Pain management centers
- Podiatry centers
- Physician offices
- Rehabilitative centers
- Research centers
- Sleep centers
- Student health centers
- Women's health centers

The Joint Commission surveys these centers and then assigns them an accreditation title. A survey is an on-site evaluation of the organization's facility and policies. Participation in The Joint Commission is voluntary for health care organizations; without accreditation, however, the health care organization may not be eligible to participate in particular federal- and state-funded programs, such as Medicare and Medicaid. In addition, accreditation indicates to the community that an organization has met basic practice standards, which is important for marketing its services.

The National Committee on Quality Assurance

The National Committee on Quality Assurance (NCQA) surveys and accredits 60% of all managed care organizations, which cover 85% of all insured lives in this country. To fulfill its mission "to improve the quality of health care," NCQA works with federal and state lawmakers and executive agency personnel. The NCQA Public Policy team provides information and comment letters for its government partners. NCQA also works in coalition with other involved organizations to advance policies that will improve the quality and efficiency of the health care system. At the federal level, NCQA accreditation and performance measures are valued components of health care policy. The new health care reform law has many provisions that connect to NCQA's mission and capabilities. The law builds on many of NCQA's successful activities over the past 20 years and challenges us to take more steps to work with federal and state policymakers to improve quality and value through measurement, accountability, and transparency. In 2008, NCQA established the PPC-PCMH (Physician Practice Connections) standards for offices to participate in and be recognized for by the government and insurance carriers as a PCMH (Patient-Centered Medical Home).

LEGAL TIP

THE IMPACT OF HEALTH CARE REFORM ON FUTURE OFFICE MANAGEMENT

One of the major changes in the forefront of the Health Care Reform Bill will address patient care. With the capabilities of the electronic health record, the quality of patient care will change and improve. Communication will be carried out through e-mail, and virtual office visits will be a possiblity. At the writing of this textbook, two states are testing a model for patient care called "The Patient-Centered Medical Home." A PCMH is a team-based model of care led by a personal physician who provides continuous and coordinated care throughout a patient's lifetime to maximize health outcomes. The PCMH is a health care setting that facilitates partnerships between individual patients, patients and their personal physicians, and, when appropriate, the patient's family. Source: http://www.ncqa.com.

 CHECKPOINT QUESTION

8. What are the benefits of being accredited by The Joint Commission?

COG Developing a Quality Improvement Program

The size and complexity of an organization's QI program depends on the organization's particular needs. In large facilities, numerous committees may be assigned to monitor and implement QI plans. Examples of QI plans are fall prevention, needlestick surveillance, and laboratory contamination rates. The committees will consist of staff members, including physicians. Most facilities have a specific person assigned to oversee all of these committees.

In the medical office and ambulatory care settings, QI programs tend to be more informal. Usually the office manager or senior physician is responsible for monitoring and implementing QI plans. As more outpatient centers become accredited by The Joint Commission, however, QI programs have become more structured. A few examples of quality issues that can be monitored in the physician offices are:

- Patient waiting times
- Unplanned returned patient visits for the same ailment or illness
- Misdiagnosed illnesses that are detected by another partner in the practice

- Patient or family complaints
- Timely follow-up telephone calls to patients
- Patient falls in physician's office or office building
- Mislabeled specimens sent to the laboratory
- Blood specimens that are coagulated or contaminated

Seven Steps for a Successful Program

The following seven steps are essential for creating an effective QI program:

1. *Identify the problem or potential problem.* All organizations can improve their delivery of patient care. Suggestions for improving care can come from many resources, including the following:

   - Office managers
   - Physicians (recommendations and complaints)
   - Other employees (e.g., nurses and medical assistants)
   - Patients (interviews)
   - Incident report trending (discussed earlier)

   The person responsible for QI in the medical office reviews all QI problems or potential problems and selects the one to be addressed first. Problems given top priority are those that are high risk (most likely to occur) and those that are most likely to cause injury to patients, family members, or employees.

2. *Form a task force.* A **task force** is a group of employees with different roles within the organization brought together to solve a given problem. In a medical office, the task force usually consists of a physician, nurse, medical assistant, and office manager. In large hospitals, various department managers are generally involved.

3. *Assign an expected threshold.* The task force establishes an **expected threshold** (numerical goal) for a given problem. Thresholds must be realistic and achievable. For example, if the problem is needlestick injuries, the expected threshold is a realistic number of employee needlestick injuries that the task force considers acceptable in a given period. For instance, the threshold may be one employee stick per month. It is not realistic to set the goal at zero; this may be optimal but is not achievable.

4. *Explore the problem and propose solutions.* The task force investigates the problem thoroughly to determine all potential causes and possible solutions. After various solutions are discussed, the task force decides what solution or solutions are to be implemented.

5. *Implement the solution.* The key to successful implementation of the solution is staff education. All staff members must be taught about the problem and the plan to decrease the problem. The type

of implementation will be based on the problem. For example, if the problem is patients falling at the entrance to the building, fixing the problem is likely to be complex and expensive. It may involve reengineering and construction of new walkways. If the problem is mislabeling or misspelling patients' names on laboratory specimens, the implementation will be simpler, possibly printing labels from the computer database.

6. *Establish a QI monitoring plan.* After implementation, the solution must be evaluated to determine whether it worked and, if so, how well. QI monitoring plans have three elements:
   • Source of monitoring, that is, where the numerical data will be obtained (e.g., medical record review, incident reports, laboratory reports, office logs)
   • Frequency of monitoring, that is, how often the data will be monitored and tallied (e.g., once a week, once a month)
   • Person responsible for monitoring, that is, who collects the data and presents the results in graphic form, allowing for easy comparison of data from before and after implementation of the solution

7. *Obtain feedback.* The members of the task force must review the graphs in relation to their expected threshold. Did they meet the threshold? If yes, the problem has been resolved. If the threshold was not met, the task force must determine whether the expected threshold was unrealistic or the solutions were inadequate. In either case, the problem has not been resolved; therefore, the task force must review each of the steps and make appropriate changes.

 CHECKPOINT QUESTION

9. What are the three elements of a QI monitoring plan?

COG Safety in the Medical Office

As a medical assistant, you must be aware of safety issues and practice safety measures in the medical office environment. Patients, staff, and visitors will look to you for leadership and guidance during an emergency situation. It is important for you to recognize unsafe conditions, understand fire safety issues, and guide patients and staff calmly in the event of an evacuation of the medical office. Anticipating an emergency situation and having a written plan to deal with possible emergencies is one way to assure that everyone in the office knows what to do in the event of a local or community emergency. Whether performing a routine task or assisting during an emergency, you must also practice basic personal safety through the use of proper body mechanics to minimize or avoid injury to yourself during an emergency.

Body Mechanics

Understanding and using principles of proper **body mechanics** and **ergonomics** can help you avoid both short and long term injury as you carry out your routine medical assisting duties. In the event of an emergency, practicing and using these principles will help prevent injury to you as you assist others who will be relying on you for guidance. Proper body mechanics—using the correct muscles and posture to complete a task safely and efficiently—involves following basic principles when standing, moving, lifting, or reaching. According to OSHA (http://www.osha.gov/SLTC/ergonomics/index.html), risk factors that may contribute to the injury of health care workers include:

• Force—the amount of physical effort required to perform a task (such as heavy lifting) or to maintain control of equipment or tools
• Repetition—performing the same motion or series of motions continually or frequently
• Awkward postures—assuming positions that place stress on the body, such as reaching above shoulder height, kneeling, squatting, leaning over a bed, or twisting the torso while lifting

Excessive exposure to these risk factors can result in a variety of musculoskeletal disorders in the medical assistant. Conditions that may result from poor body mechanics include low back pain, sciatica, rotator cuff injuries, epicondylitis, and carpal tunnel syndrome. Your genetic makeup, gender, age, and physical activity outside the workplace may also contribute to the development of musculoskeletal injuries. Although some injuries develop gradually over time, others may result from single events such as lifting something heavy. Following these basic principles when standing, moving, lifting, or reaching for objects may prevent injury:

1. Maintain correct body alignment.
2. Maintain a stable center of gravity.
3. Maintain the line of gravity.
4. Maintain a strong base of support.

In the clinical area, proper body mechanics is important when performing any patient care activities such as helping a patient on and off an examination table or into a chair or pushing a patient in a wheelchair. Proper body mechanics is also essential when performing administrative activities, such as lifting, carrying, or reaching for equipment and office supplies. To avoid physical strain that can lead to injury, use these proper mechanics:

• When standing: Make sure to wear comfortable shoes with good arch support to protect your feet, provide a firm foundation, and prevent slipping. When standing, keep your feet flat on the floor about 12 inches apart. Keep your back straight and stand with one foot slightly in front of the other.

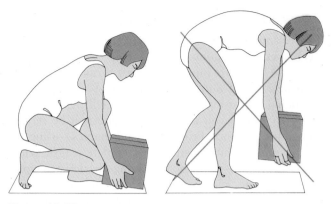

Figure 10-10 Proper and improper lifting techniques.

- When walking: Keep your back straight as you walk. If helping another person walk, you may need to place one arm around the back of the person. Keep the other arm at your side, ready to help if necessary.
- When lifting an object: Maintain a wide base for maximum stability. In a standing position, keep feet shoulder-width apart. Lower you body and keep your back straight to get close to the object. Bend from your hips and knees (never the waist), grip the object by putting your hands around it and keep it close to you (Fig. 10-10). Then, keeping your knees bent and your back straight, lift using arm and leg muscles—never your back muscles. Lift straight upward in one smooth motion. If the object is too heavy, get help.
- When pushing or pulling: If possible, push instead of pull, and use the weight of your body, especially your legs to push (or pull) an object. Your feet should be about 12 inches apart with your back straight. Lower your body to get close to the object. Bend from your hips and knees (never your waist). If the object or person is too heavy, get help.
- When reaching: If you are reaching for an object that is low, such as reaching into a bottom file drawer, squat and avoid twisting or bending. When reaching for an object that is high, reach only as high as is comfortable; otherwise, use a small step stool. Never use an office chair to stand and reach objects.

Ergonomics

Workplace ergonomics is the study of the "fit" between workers and their work environment. Short-term health problems, such as fatigue and discomfort, and long-term health problems, such as carpal tunnel syndrome and tendonitis, can often be avoided by using proper ergonomics. Equipment manufacturers, architects, and workspace planners consider ergonomics when designing devices and workstations. Consider the following techniques to reduce strain and fatigue as you work:

1. Adjust your chair:
   - Adjust your chair height so your feet are flat on the floor. Use a footrest if necessary.
   - Sit upright in the chair with your lower back and your shoulders against the backrest.
   - If the chair has armrests, your elbows and lower arms should rest lightly to avoid circulatory or nerve problems. Also, adjust armrests so that you can rest your arms at your side and relax your shoulders while working.
   - Adjust the backrest to support the natural inward curvature of your lower back. Use a rolled towel or lumbar pad for extra support.
2. Adjust your desktop:
   - Organize your desk to avoid excessive reaching.
   - If you are using a document holder, place it at the same height as the monitor and at the same distance from your eyes to reduce eye movement and strain.
3. Adjust your computer monitor:
   - Adjust the brightness and contrast to optimum comfort.
   - Position the monitor directly in front of you at arms length.
   - Position the top of the screen at eye level.
   - Tilt the monitor back 10 to 20 degrees.
   - To reduce glare, angle the monitor away from windows and direct lighting, or use a filter.
   - Make sure the monitor screen is clean.
4. Adjust your keyboard and mouse:
   - Adjust the keyboard height so that your shoulders can relax and let your arms rest at your sides (a swiveling keyboard tray can be helpful).
   - Position the keyboard close enough to prevent excessive reaching, and high enough for your forearms to be level.
   - Position the mouse beside and at the same height as the keyboard.
   - Avoid reaching for the keyboard mouse. Wrists should be in a neutral position (not excessively flexed or extended).
   - Rest your hands in your lap when not entering data, not on the mouse.
5. Adjust your lighting:
   - Close drapes or blinds and adjust lighting to reduce glare.
   - Angle the monitor away from windows.
   - Reduce overhead lighting.
   - Use indirect or shielded lighting where possible.

✓ CHECKPOINT QUESTION

10. What conditions can be prevented by using good body mechanics and principles of ergonomics?

Evaluating the Medical Office for Safety Issues

Most of us don't think about our work environment being dangerous, but every year nearly 8 out of 100 employees in hospitals, 9 out of every 100 employees in long-term care facilities, and 2 out of every 100 people who work in physician offices are injured on the job. Threats such as fires, floods, weather-related emergencies, violence, and crime are just as possible when you are at work as they are when you are at home. Other threats that can jeopardize your safety in a medical office include chemical spills, radiation leaks from x-ray machines, and needle sticks that could spread bloodborne pathogens. You could even trip over a stack of files and break your ankle! It is very important that you learn to evaluate your work environment regularly for safety issues that could affect you, other staff, visitors, and patients.

Personal and Employee Safety Plans

A personal safety plan is designed to protect you and other employees as well as your patients. The steps that OSHA requires in a personal safety plan are listed below for each category. You can use this information to develop a safety plan for your office.

1. Bloodborne pathogens
   - Have a written exposure control plan that is updated annually and explains the rationale for the equipment chosen for your office.
   - Use universal precautions and consideration of safer, engineered needles and sharps.
   - Use engineering and work-practice controls and appropriate PPE (gloves, face and eye protection, gowns).
   - Provide free hepatitis-B vaccines to employees exposed to bloodborne pathogens.
   - Provide medical follow-up in the event of an exposure incident.
   - Use labels or color-coding for items such as sharps disposal boxes and containers for regulated waste, contaminated laundry, and certain specimens.
   - Provide regular employee training on preventing pathogen exposure.
   - Properly contain and dispose all regulated waste.
2. Hazard communication
   The hazard communication standard is sometimes called the "employee right-to-know" standard. It requires that employees have access to information about hazards in the workplace. The basic requirements of this standard include:
   - A written hazard communication plan
   - A list of hazardous chemicals such as alcohol, disinfectants, anesthetic agents, sterilants, and mercury that may be stored in the office
   - A copy of the Material Safety Data Sheets (MSDS) for each chemical used or stored in the office (The MSDS describes the appropriate manner in which these items should be handled, stored, and contained in the event of an emergency [Fig. 10-11A,B].)
   - Employee training on office-based chemical hazards

3. Ionizing radiation
   If your office has an x-ray machine or other radiation-emitting equipment, there should be a list of the type of radiation used in the office. In addition, areas of potential radiation exposure should be restricted to limit employee exposure. Rooms containing radioactive material should be labeled and equipped with caution signs as needed. Employees working in these restricted areas must wear personal radiation monitors such as film badges (refer to Chapter 25).
4. Exit routes
   Your office must provide safe and accessible exits from the building in case of fire or other emergencies. Although you may want to consult with your local fire/police department and insurance company for additional information, the basic responsibilities required by OSHA include:
   - Exit routes sufficient for the number of employees in any occupied space
   - A diagram of evacuation routes posted in a visible location
5. Electrical safety
   The electrical safety standards are required to protect employees in the medical office and apply to electrical equipment and wiring in hazardous locations. If your office uses flammable gases, you may need special wiring and equipment installed. Again, you should check with your local fire department or insurance company for additional information specific to your office.

CHECKPOINT QUESTION

11. Who is protected by a personal safety plan?

Fire Safety in the Medical Office

A fire in a health care environment can be devastating. Fires not only spring up quickly, but also move quickly, destroying everything in their path. Of course, health care facilities including medical offices also have vulnerable patients who may be disabled and incapable of moving quickly to escape life-threatening smoke and flames.

Numerous agencies mandate a variety of fire-safety issues in health care facilities including local and state licensing agencies and OSHA. Although you may be aware of the fire safety issues in your home, it is also important that you be aware of fire safety issues in your work environment. These include:

- **Fire alarm and detection systems:** All health care facilities should have hard-wired, battery backup smoke detectors in every room and hallway. These are designed to detect smoke and heat and may provide information back to a communication center regarding their location.

MATERIAL SAFETY DATA SHEET

Revision #: 03

Section 1 - Product Identification & Use

Product Name:	**Advance-12A Chlorine Bleach**
Synonyms:	Liquid Swimming Pool, 12% Chlorine Bleach, Sodium Hypochlorite Solutions, Javel Water, Advance12-FP
Chemical Family:	Hypochlorite solutions
Chemical formula of Active:	NaOCl
Product Use:	Disinfectant, sanitizer, odour control, water purification, textile bleaching, commercial laundry applications.
WHMIS Classification:	Class C, Oxidizing Material Class D, Div. 2, Toxic Liquid, Skin Sensitizer Class E, Corrosive Liquid
TDG Classification:	Hypochlorite Solutions UN 1791, Class 8, packing group III
D.I.N.	02229425
REGISTRATION NO.	24922 PEST CONTROL PRODUCTS ACT
Manufacturer:	Advance Chemicals Ltd. 2023 Kingsway Ave Port Coquitlam, BC V3C 1S9 Phone: (604)945-9666, Fax: (604)945-9617
Emergency phone:	CANUTEC 24 hrs: (613) 996-6666

Section 2 - Hazardous Ingredients

Hazardous Components	%(w/w)	C.A.S. No.	LD_{50} & LC_{50}
Sodium Hypochlorite	10-12	7681-52-9	(oral, mouse)5800 mg/kg ACGIH TLV 2 mg/m^3

Section 3 - Physical Data

Physical state: liquid	Boiling point: decomposes at 40°C
Density: 1.160-1.170 g/mL	Freezing point: -6°C (5% aq. sol'n.)
pH: 12.5-13.5 @ 20°C	Vapour pressure:17.5mmHg @ 20°C
Solubility in water: 100%	Evaporation rate: no data

Odour & Appearance: The product is a clear, light green to golden yellow liquid. There is a chlorine like odour above the open liquid. The odour is due to the normal, slow but gradual decomposition process. See storage and handling conditions.

Section 4 - Fire or Explosion Hazard

Flammability: The product is not considered to be flammable.

Extinguishing media: Use an extinguishing media for surrounding the fire, or all purpose foam by manufacturer's recommended techniques for large fires. Use water to cool fire exposed containers to prevent vapour build-up and rupture. Water may also be used to flush spills away from dangerous exposures.

Hazardous Combustion Products: This product decomposes thermally above 40°C. Hazardous and toxic decomposition products may include chlorine gas, oxygen and sodium chlorate. Unvented containers will build-up internal pressure and may rupture causing a product leak. When Advance-12 is heated or comes into contact with acids, chlorine gas may be released. Vigorous reaction with oxidizable and organic materials may result in fire.

Section 5 - Reactivity Data

Stability: Under normal conditions of storage and use, this product will slowly decompose over time. The long term decomposition products are not dangerous if the product is stored in a cool, dry, well ventilated area away from direct exposure to sunlight. See also section 7, Preventative Measures.

Thermal Stability: This product will begin to decompose above 40°C. Container may rupture from excessive pressure build-up. Open cap slowly to release any pressure. Hazardous and toxic decomposition products may include chlorine gas, oxygen and sodium chlorate.

Incompatible substances: All acids, ammonium salts and aqueous ammonium hydroxide solutions, metals, oxidizers, nitrogen compounds, and methanol.

Polymerization: Will not occur.

Conditions to Avoid: High temperatures, open flame, direct sunlight (UV radiation initiates decomposition). When Advance-12 is heated, contacted with acids, contacted with oxidizers, or contacted with organic materials, a vigorous reaction may release chlorine gas and heat, resulting in a fire hazard. Allow any paper towels or rags used to wipe up spills to dry or rinse with water before discarding in an approved manner.

Section 6 - Toxicological Properties

Acute Toxicity: No data found.

Carcinogenicity: The ingredients in this product are; not classified as carcinogenic by the American Conference of Governmental Industrial Hygienists (ACGIH), or the International Agency for Research on Cancer (IARC); not regulated as carcinogens by the Occupational Health and Safety Administration (OSHA); and not listed as carcinogens by the National Toxicology Program (NTP).

Respiratory & Skin Sensitization: May cause skin sensitization and other allergenic responses. Sensitization is the process whereby a biological change occurs in the individual because of previous exposure to a substance, and as a result, the individual reacts more strongly when subsequently exposed to the product. Once sensitized, an individual can react to extremely low airborne levels, even below the TLV, or to skin contact.

Effects of Exposure:

Skin contact: Prolonged and repeated exposure often causes irritation, redness, pain, drying and cracking of the skin. Concentrated solutions may cause severe burns to the skin.

Eye contact: This product will cause irritation, redness and pain. May cause corneal damage and conjunctivitis (inflammation of the mucous membrane between the eyeball and inner eyelid).

Inhalation: This product is irritating to the nose, throat and respiratory tract.

Ingestion: This product causes severe burning and pain in the mouth, throat and abdomen. Vomiting, diarrhea and perforation of the esophagus and stomach lining may occur.

Section 7 - Preventative Measures

Recommendations listed in this section indicate the type of equipment which will provide protection against overexposure to this product. Conditions of use, adequacy of engineering or other control measures, and actual exposures will dictate the need for specific protective devices at your workplace.

Skin protection: Gloves and protective clothing made from natural rubber, neoprene or nitrile rubber should be impervious under normal conditions of use. Prior to use, user should confirm impermeability.

Eye protection: Safety glasses with side shields are recommended. Use chemical safety goggles if there is a potential for eye contact.

Other Personal Protective Equipment: Avoid contact with product by wearing chemical protective clothing and rubber boots if necessary. Eye wash fountains and safety shower facilities should be provided nearby for emergency use.

Figure 10-11A An MSDS for bleach—front page.
Source: OHSAH MSDS Database: http://msds.ohsah.bc.ca/Default.aspx

Advance-12 - MSDS Continued   Revision #: 03

Respiratory protection: No specific guidelines available. Use an NIOSH or MSHA approved air purifying respirator equipped with chlorine cartridges for concentrations up to about 8-10ppm. An air supplied or self contained breathing apparatus should be used if concentrations are exceptionally high or unknown.

Ventilation Requirements: This product should be used in a well ventilated area at all times. Local exhaust ventilation may be required and must be corrosion proof. Do not use this product in a poorly ventilated or confined area without approved respiratory protection.

Storage Requirements: Store Advance Bleach in a cool, well ventilated area. Keep away from heat, sparks and open flames. Store away from exposure to direct sunlight. Do not expose sealed containers to temperatures above 40°Celcius.

Action to take for spills & leaks: Wear chemical protective clothing, rubber gloves and suitable respiratory protection. SMALL SPILLS should be wiped up with absorbent material and disposed of in government approved waste containers. Paper towels may become extremely hot when saturated with this product and cause a secondary fire hazard. Rinse out absorbent materials used in small spill recovery with plenty of water, (see section 5, reactivity data).

LARGER SPILLS should be contained by diking with sand, soil or other absorbent, non-combustible material, then transferred into approved waste containers for proper disposal. Keep product out of sewers, storm drains, surface run-off water and soil. Harmful to aquatic life at low concentrations. Can be dangerous if allowed to enter potable water intakes. Wear appropriate respiratory protection and restrict access to non-protected personnel. Comply with all government regulations on spill reporting, and handling and disposal of waste.

The contained bleach spill can be effectively neutralized as follows;

1. Wear respiratory protection and protective clothing, gloves, glasses, etc.

2. Very slowly and cautiously, apply a dilute aqueous solution of Sodium Sulphite, or Sodium meta-Bisulphite to the spill. Mix well. This neutralizes the available chlorine content while reducing the pH to about pH 4. Check with a pH meter or test strip paper. Chlorine gas is a dangerous by-product of this reaction procedure.

3. Increase the pH of the contained spill to about pH 7 by slowly adding a dilute aqueous solution of Soda Ash or Sodium Bicarbonate. Check pH frequently.

4. The bleach spill should be neutral, with a pH of 7. Check with the appropriate local, provincial or federal agencies for proper and correct disposal methods for this product. If available, use a field test kit to check for levels of residual chlorine in the treated waste water.

Disposal methods: Dispose of contaminated product and materials used in cleaning up spills or leaks in a manner approved for this material. Consult appropriate federal, provincial and local regulatory agencies to ascertain proper disposal procedures.

Note: Empty containers can have residues, gasses and mists, and are subject to proper waste disposal as mentioned above.

Repair and Maintenance Precautions: Do not cut, grind, weld or drill in, on or near this container. Do not re-use the original container for any other product, substance, food or drink.

Section 8 - First Aid Measures

If inhaled: Remove victim to fresh air. Give artificial respiration if not breathing. Get immediate emergency medical attention.

In case of eye contact: Immediately flush eyes with clean water for at least fifteen (15) minutes, lifting the upper and lower eye lids occasionally. If irritation persists, repeat flushing and GET IMMEDIATE EMERGENCY MEDICAL ATTENTION.

In case of skin contact: Immediately flush skin with plenty of clean running water for at least fifteen (15) minutes. Remove contaminated clothing and shoes. If irritation persists, flush skin again and seek medical attention. Wash and launder clothes before re-use. If irritation persists after washing, get immediate medical attention.

In case of ingestion or swallowing: If victim is conscious and not convulsing, rinse mouth out with water, and give a glass of water to dilute stomach contents. NEVER GIVE ANYTHING BY MOUTH TO AN UNCONSCIOUS VICTIM. Immediately contact local poison control centre. Vomiting should only be induced under the direction of a physician or poison control official. If spontaneous vomiting occurs, have patient lean forward with head down to avoid breathing in the vomitus. Rinse mouth out and administer more water. GET IMMEDIATE EMERGENCY MEDICAL ATTENTION.

Emergency Medical Care: Treat symptomatically

Section 9 - Preparation Information

Advance Chemicals Limited expressly disclaims all expressed or implied warranties of merchantability and fitness for a particular purpose with respect to the product provided. The information contained herein is offered only as a guide to the handling of this specific product, and has been prepared in good faith by technically knowledgeable personnel. This M.S.D.S. is not intended to be all inclusive, and the manner and conditions of use may involve other and additional considerations.

Revised: 19 October 2006, 24 May 2007; 17 February 2010

Figure 10-11B An MSDS for bleach—back page.
Source: OHSAH MSDS Database: http://msds.ohsah.bc.ca/Default.aspx

- **Fire-fighting equipment:** A variety of fire extinguishers should be placed throughout the facility along with hose reels and fire blankets. All medical offices should have automated sprinkler systems and emergency escape lighting.
- **Fire drills:** Medical offices should regularly hold fire drills according to state licensing requirements. At the minimum, medical offices should hold one fire drill per year.

- **Training:** All staff should receive fire safety training including employee responsibilities, use of a fire extinguisher, types of fires, fire alarms, detecting and reporting a fire, and evacuating in the event of a fire. As in Figure 10-12, employees should be allowed to use an extinguisher *before* an emergency. Local fire departments offer training in the use of fire extinguishers.

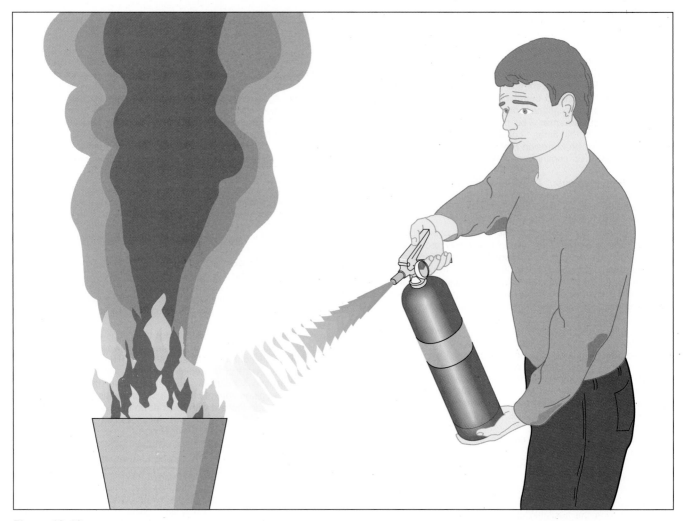

Figure 10-12 Fire extinguisher use. (LifeART image copyright © 2012 Lippincott Williams & Wilkins. All rights reserved.)

- **Hazardous Materials:** In addition to oxygen tanks, other materials in the medical office that may be hazardous include electrical equipment and medical waste.
- **Safe Exits:** All medical offices should have enough exits in enough locations to get everyone out of the building safely if necessary. Fire doors must be kept clear and unlocked, stairwells must be uncluttered and well lighted, and signs for alternative exits clearly posted in the event of a fire (Fig. 10-13). Exit signs should also be lighted in order to be seen through smoke.

Knowing the basics of fire prevention is an important aspect of your role as a professional medical assistant. To prevent fire in a medical office:

- Keep items that could fuel a fire such as paper, linen, clothing, etc., away from heat-producing devices such as lamps.

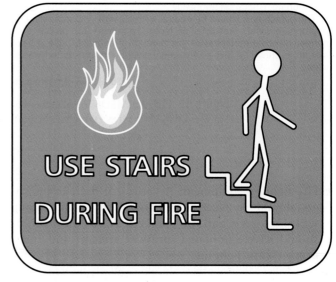

Figure 10-13 Fire safety signs should be properly posted in the medical office.

- Dispose of construction or remodeling items (oily rags, flammable liquids, sawdust, wood shavings) and other fire hazards that tend to accumulate in maintenance and storage areas.
- Ban items that emit sparks from areas that contain supplemental oxygen.
- Store cylinders or tanks that contain flammable gases or liquids away from patients and keep them capped when not in use.
- Clear hallways and stairways of trash or other items that could ignite or impede escape.

COG Emergency Preparedness

Disasters, whether arising from natural or man-made circumstances, usually strike without warning and could occur during a typical workday in the medical office. During a crisis, you should be prepared to assist not only patients and coworkers, but the community at large.

Natural disasters are outside of human control and can occur forcefully and abruptly or slowly over time. Some examples of natural disasters include:

- Drought
- Earthquake
- Epidemics
- Flood
- Hurricane
- Tornado
- Snowstorm
- Storms
- Volcanic eruption
- Tidal wave (tsunami)
- Mudslide
- Drought
- Avalanche
- Famine

Other emergencies may be caused by or controlled by humans. These include accidents involving multiple vehicles, plane crashes, or train derailments.

Emergency Medical Kit

Proper equipment and supplies should be readily available in a medical emergency. Although the office's equipment and supplies vary with the medical specialty, emergency equipment and supplies are fairly standard. This equipment should be kept in a designated location that is accessible to all staff. Standard supplies for a medical emergency kit are listed in Box 10-5. Although items used during an emergency should be replaced as soon as possible, a medical assistant or other staff member should check the contents of the emergency kit or crash cart regularly,

---

BOX 10-5

EMERGENCY MEDICAL KIT AND EQUIPMENT

The following are standard supplies that can be used to make up an emergency medical kit:

- Activated charcoal
- Adhesive strip bandages, assorted sizes
- Adhesive tape, 1- and 2-inch rolls
- Alcohol (70%)
- Alcohol wipes
- Antimicrobial skin ointment
- Chemical ice pack
- Cotton balls
- Cotton swabs
- Disposable gloves
- Elastic bandages, 2- and 3-inch widths
- Gauze pads, 2 × 2– and 4 × 4–inch widths
- Roller, self-adhesive gauze, 2- and 4-inch widths
- Safety pins, various sizes
- Scissors
- Syrup of ipecac
- Thermometer
- Triangular bandage
- Tweezers

In addition to these contents, the following equipment should be available:

- Blood pressure cuff (pediatric and adult)
- Stethoscope
- Bag-valve mask device with assorted size masks
- Flashlight or penlight
- Portable oxygen tank with regulator
- Oxygen masks
- Suction unit and catheters

Additional equipment that may be available includes:

- Various sizes of endotracheal tubes
- Laryngoscope handle and various sizes of blades
- Automatic external defibrillator
- Intravenous supplies (catheters, administration set tubing, assorted solutions)
- Emergency drugs including atropine, epinephrine, and sodium bicarbonate

---

perhaps weekly, to verify that contents are available and that no item has gone beyond the expiration date. If so, the expired items should be replaced immediately.

Emergency Action Plan

It is important for every medical office to develop a plan jointly or in consultation with the local Office of Emergency Services, Emergency Medical Services, Department of Health Services, hospital planners, and neighboring clinics.

Every medical office should have an emergency action plan, including the following:

- The local emergency rescue service telephone number (usually 911)
- Location of the nearest hospital emergency department
- Telephone number of the local or regional poison control center
- Procedures for various emergencies
- List of office personnel who are trained in CPR
- Location and list of contents of the emergency medical kit or crash cart

Whether confronted with a cardiac emergency or psychiatric crisis, medical assistants must be able to coordinate multiple ongoing events while rendering patient care. Contributing to the complexity of a medical emergency are such factors as panicky family members, the arrival of emergency personnel, and possibly language barriers. The key to being prepared is having and being familiar with a well-written plan that is functional, flexible, and easy to implement. It is important to test the plan during nonpeak hours when facilities lack optimum leadership and staff, because disasters can occur at any time. Testing should include observers to report the strengths and weaknesses of the plan and the need for training in specific areas. The plan should be modified to eliminate or minimize any vulnerability revealed during testing.

Central Operation Centers

The development of a central operation center is vital to successful disaster and emergency response operations. Although this center provides coordination of all activities, it should be located in an area that is away from the center of activities. An alternate site may also be established should the primary site become inoperable or contaminated.

The site should be equipped with adequate administrative supplies including frequently used telephone numbers, maps and marking pens, paper, floor plans of the facility (including utility shut-off valves), and locations of fire extinguishers and emergency exits. The emergency operation center should also be supplied with adequate emergency supplies including water, food, a portable radio, a first aid kit, a flashlight and batteries, and backup power.

Another important aspect of the response is to be able to adequately perform triage on a scalable basis. Preassembled patient charts should be available to quickly process a rapid influx of patients.

 WHAT IF?

What happens now?

It is difficult to think about, but the possibility of a major disaster involving an entire community is a reality. How does a medical office come back from a catastrophe? Recovery operations often take longer than the emergency itself. All health care facilities, including medical offices, must attempt to resume business after a damaging emergency. Documentation is crucial for reimbursement of damages and costs associated with response and recovery. You should assume that typical computer function may be inoperable and, therefore, backup paper billing systems should be planned for in advance of a disaster. During a recovery period, it is critical for staff members to attend to the psychosocial trauma of disaster. Staff members should be encouraged to debrief often, but this should not be forced.

 CHECKPOINT QUESTION

12. What is the purpose of a central operations center?

Epidemics and Pandemics

Each year, the virus that causes influenza causes illness in many individuals and, in some cases, death. Fortunately, a vaccine is developed every year to protect those who get the immunization against the specific virus for that year. You will come into contact with many patients who suffer from "cold-like" symptoms in the winter months, and it will be in your best interest to get this vaccine during the fall months to protect yourself.

When a disease affects numerous people within a specfic geographical area, it is known as an **epidemic**. However, when a disease affects numerous people in many areas of the world at the same time, it is known as a **pandemic**. One of the oldest examples of an epidemic that became a pandemic is the bubonic plague. According to the Centers for Disease Control and Prevention (CDC), approximately 25% of the world's population died from the plague known as "Black Death" from 1345 to 1360. This disease originated in central Asia and was carried to other countries and continents by rodents who, in turn, carried infected fleas. This disease has never been eradicated, and India reported several cases in the 1990s that resulted in heightened awareness and alerts for travelers to and from that country. Fortunately, this did not result in a global pandemic, but the ease with which people travel around the world raises concerns for all health care professionals who must plan for the possibility of an epidemic or pandemic. The CDC provides a guide for medical offices to develop a plan of action before an epidemic or pandemic occurs. This guide is called "Abbreviated Pandemic Influenza Plan Template for Primary Care Provider Offices: Guidance from Stakeholders" and can be found on the following Web site: http://www.cdc.gov/h1n1flu/guidance/pdf/abb_pandemic_influenza_plan.pdf.

PATIENT EDUCATION

BETTER SAFE THAN SORRY

Although we can protect ourselves from certain disease-causing microorganisms like the virus that causes the flu, there is always the possibility that unexpected microorganisms will cause disease in an area or, worse yet, the world. In April of 2009, the first cases of the H1N1 virus were documented in the United States, and by June of that same year, the World Health Organization (WHO) declared a global pandemic. By the fall of 2009, the worst of the pandemic of H1N1 was over for people living in the United States, partly due to the response of the CDC education efforts and the development and availability of a vaccine to immunize against this specific influenza.

We should encourage our patients to get immunized as directed by the physician each year for all types of influenza for which there are available vaccines, especially the elderly and those with chronic diseases such as asthma or chronic obstructive pulmonary disease.

Bioterrorism

Bioterriorism refers to the purposeful infliction of an agent (e.g., bacteria, virus, radiation, etc.) into a populated area with the intent to cause destruction of the environment, people, or animals living in the area. Bioterrorism is a very serious man-made threat that can trigger a large-scale emergency. The CDC classifies a biologic agent as a weapon when it is easy to disseminate, has a high potential for mortality, can cause a public panic or social disruption, and requires public health preparedness. There are many government Web sites available that provide information about various agents of bioterrorism, and they may be classified into three major categories according to the CDC:

1. Category A – These include organisms or toxins that pose the highest risk to the public and national security. Specifically, these agents have the potential to:
   - Spread easily from person to person
   - Result in high death rates
   - Cause public panic and social disruption
   - Require special action for public health preparedness
2. Category B – These agents have the potential to:
   - Spread moderately easy
   - Result in moderate illness rates and low death rates
   - Require specific enhancements of the CDC's laboratory capacity and enhanced disease monitoring
3. Category C – These agents are considered emerging threats and include pathogens that could be engineered for mass spread in the future because they are:
   - Easily available
   - Easily produced and spread
   - Potentially lethal with possible high morbidity and mortality rates

PATIENT EDUCATION

PREPARING FOR A BIOTERRORIST ATTACK

The CDC and the American Red Cross have a guide for anyone who would like more information on preparing for a bioterrorist attack (http://www.bt.cdc.gov/preparedness). Share the following informaiton with patients who are concerned and would like more information about preparing for such an attack:

- Maintain a supply of food, water, and other items for your family. Although a 3-day supply of items for each member of the family is a good start, having enough clean water and supplies for up to 2 weeks is best.
- Develop a family emergency preparedness plan. Everyone in the family should know the plan and how to respond in the event of an attack.
- Be informed and stay informed. Pay attention to the local news and follow any advice given.

Emergency Preparedness Plans in Your Community

In addition to the medical emergencies that may confront you in a medical setting, you also need to be prepared for emergencies that affect an entire community. Unfortunately, the Department of Homeland Security (DHS) reports that even people who think they are prepared for disasters often aren't as prepared as they think. In a national survey, the DHS found that 40 percent of respondents did not have household plans, 80 percent had not conducted home evacuation drills, and nearly 60 percent did not know their community's evacuation routes.

All emergencies are local. Although federal and state governments can and will step in to help in the event of a major emergency, response and recovery begins and ends with local governments. The success of those actions depends on the level of planning governments have already completed. Such plans typically reside within the public services departments, such as police, fire, and emergency services. However, you should not leave all the planning and implementation up to public service professionals. You, a member of the medical community, also have an important role to play. It is extremely important that you learn about *your* community's emergency plans and your role in those plans.

A good place to start is with your community's online Web site. Many towns and cities post their emergency preparedness plans on their Web sites. If you cannot find the plan online, call the police or fire departments or the public safety officer in your town or city. Staff there can often direct you to the right person or, even better, send you a copy of the emergency plan.

Your Role in Emergency Preparedness

The professional medical assistant can provide significant administrative and clinical contributions during an emergency. When it comes to planning, make sure that you represent the professional medical assistant on planning committees at the community, hospital, and office levels. Your role in an emergency could include the following:

- Organizing, stocking, and managing on-site medical clinics
- Performing first-aid CPR
- Serving as a liaison between the physician and others
- Interviewing patients and family members to collect pertinent personal and medical information
- Creating and maintaining medical records during and after an emergency
- Taking and recording vital signs
- Assisting physician with examinations, procedures, and treatments
- Transferring and transporting patients as needed
- Preparing and administering medications as directed by the physician

Environmental Safety Plan

If you work in a medical office that has a laboratory that uses potentially dangerous chemicals, you should have an environmental safety plan. This is a written document that outlines how your office will implement and maintain environmental safety procedures. It should include the following:

- A plan for handling and disposing of hazardous waste
- A commitment and plan to train employees on environmental safety guidelines
- Procedures to notify staff and patients in the event of an environmental emergency
- Procedures to notify fire and police of the environmental emergency
- Communication procedures
- A plan to prevent pollution in the laboratory and/or office
- Opportunities to reduce wasted resources such as energy and water
- Emergency responses to fires, spills, and similar events in the facility
- A list of safety equipment available to all personnel including fire extinguishers, safety showers, eyewash stations, spill kits, gloves, and eye protection
- A schedule of self-inspections and annual audits for the medical office
- A policy for chemical storage

 CHECKPOINT QUESTION

13. Why is it important to involve the community in disaster preparedness?

Conducting a Mock Environmental Exposure Drill

Having a written plan outlining what to do in the event of an environmental threat is a major step in being prepared. However, practicing the plan will give everyone in your office an opportunity to practice putting the plan into action. Conducting regular mock emergency drills will assure that everyone is prepared in the event a real disaster strikes. A drill can be as simple as "walking through" the evacuation of the office or as elaborate as a community-wide disaster drill. Police, fire, hospitals, etc., participate in such drills. Volunteer victims are assigned roles in the drill. The "victim" in Figure 10-14 is playing the part of a tornado surivor injured by flying debris. Box 10-6 details important parts to include when planning a mock emergency drill.

After conducting a mock emergency drill, don't forget to plan for a "postmortem" meeting, often the next day following the mock incident. This will help you identify what worked and what did not work before, during, and after the drill. The results of this analysis should be used to revise your office environmental safety plan

Effects of Stress and Emergencies

Although this chapter has described the importance of dealing with safety and emergencies in the medical office, significant consideration must be given to the

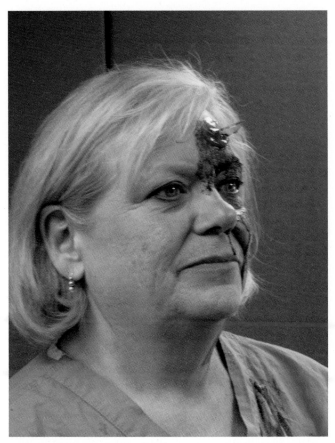

Figure 10-14 A volunteer victim in a mock disaster drill is prepared by a make-up artist to portray a tornado survivor injured by flying debris.

psychological effects of dealing with such emergencies. Often, the psychological component of a disaster is overshadowed by the acute needs of the physical casualty. Experts estimate that for every 1 physical casualty of a disaster, there are 20 psychological victims. Dealing with disasters and emergencies causes stress over a broad spectrum of individuals depending on the proximity to the disaster and the experience of the disaster on the individual. There are six categories of experience that may describe an individual exposed to a disaster:

- Primary victims: Individuals who experience maximum exposure to the disaster
- Secondary victims: Relatives and friends of the primary victims
- Third-level victims: First responders and health care personnel who participate in rescue and recovery activities
- Fourth-level victims: The community, including those who can converge, who altruistically offer help, who share the grief and loss, or are involved in some way
- Fifth-level victims: Individuals who are upset or psychologically distressed but not directly involved in the disaster
- Sixth-level victims: Those individuals indirectly or vicariously affected by the disaster

The process of coping with the disaster experience begins with feelings of disbelief, bewilderment, and difficulty concentrating. Denial is used as the primary defense. Anxiety and fear represent the next phase and are followed by varying degrees of sadness and depression.

Most victims of stress will recover using their own coping mechanisms without any residual effects. However, some individuals may be affected by acute traumatic stress or posttraumatic stress disorder (PTSD) (Box 10-7). Acute traumatic stress usually resolves within 2–4 weeks of the disaster event. PTSD may be delayed in onset up to 4 weeks and typically lasts for 4 weeks or more.

Of greatest concern is the risk that people exposed to trauma from natural or man-made disasters are at risk for the development of a major psychiatric disorder. This may include aggravation or exacerbation of any preexisting mental health condition, such as depression, generalized anxiety disorder, panic disorder, or PTSD.

BOX 10-6

MOCK EMERGENCY DRILL PLANNING

The following factors must be considered when planning a mock emergency drill:

- When and how the drill will occur
- The type of environmental exposure that will occur in the drill
- How the initial alarm will be sounded
- The type of damage and/or injuries that will result
- Individuals who should be notified of the drill
- The roles that people will play in the drill including what they should say and how they should behave
- Any special effects, clothing, or equipment required to make the drill as realistic as possible

---

BOX 10-7

CHARACTERISTICS OF ACUTE TRAUMATIC STRESS OR POSTTRAUMATIC STRESS DISORDER (PTSD)

1. Reliving the traumatic event through intrusive thoughts or images, nightmares, or flashbacks
2. Avoidance of associations of the traumatic event and feelings of numbness and detachment
3. Increased arousal as evidenced by being jumpy, nervous, or defensive much of the time
4. Difficulty sleeping and an inability to concentrate

Factors that may contribute to severe psychological reactions after an event include lack of family and social support, personal loss, adverse reactions from others, and survivor guilt. Psychological first aid for anyone suffering from a stress disorder includes:

• Immediate physical care and medical attention
• Appropriate comforting and consolation
• Protection from further threat and distress
• Facilitating some sense of being in control
• Allowing for sharing of experience, but not forcing it
• Provision of culturally appropriate ways of grieving
• Normalization of activity and routine as possible
• Facilitating links with private or community resources

Psychological response resources are also necessary for health care professionals. Disaster responders, including medical personnel, are at high risk for developing trauma-related disorders. During the disaster response, regular rest periods should be taken. Over-dedication is a risk factor for developing posttraumatic disorders.

Principles for Evacuation during an Emergency

During an emergency or natural disaster, it may be necessary to evacuate the medical office. Ideally, your facility will have an evacuation plan and will train all employees in its implementation.

It is important that you remain calm during an evacuation. How you react may determine how other employees and patients react. Encourage an orderly evacuation by walking swiftly but not running. Do not use elevators during an emergency, and, depending on the urgency of the situation, do not worry about personal belongings. You may need to close windows and lock doors as well as forward the phones or implement the answering service if there is time to do so. Again, this is something that should be determined during the planning process. Principles to consider in any evacuation plan include the following:

• Identify the person responsible for ordering the evacuation.
• Determine the facility or location that you will evacuate to. Choose a backup site, if available, just in case the planned location or facility is not available.
• Identify evacuation routes.
• Define individual staff responsibilities. Plan for the likelihood that not all staff will be available.
• Identify what critical supplies or equipment will need to be transported and who will be responsible for transporting them.
• Determine how individuals will be accounted for during and after the evacuation.
• Develop a procedure to handle patient/staff illness or death during the evacuation.
• Develop a medical office reentry plan. Who will authorize reentry after the emergency? How will the medical office be inspected to determine safety after returning?

Evacuation Plan for the Physician Office

Although it is not as involved as the scene in a hospital or nursing home, evacuating a physician office still requires planning and practice. It is important that you be familiar with the key elements of such an evacuation plan because you will, by necessity, play an important role in any emergency evacuation.

The first step is to know what constitutes an emergency requiring evacuation. This could be a fire, a chemical spill, impending weather-related emergencies, a threat of violence, or even a highly infectious patient. You should discuss the specific situations that might trigger an evacuation order in your office with your physician, office manager, and other staff and develop a policy to guide the process.

In addition to the key elements already mentioned, other items to be considered for a physician office include:

• Communicating the evacuation. This may be done verbally, through an e-mail or text message, or with an alarm. Include how patients will be notified of the evacuation before, during, and after the event.
• Determining who is responsible for giving the evacuation order. This will most likely be a physician or the office manager.
• Identifying specific staff responsiblities including who will be in charge of evacuating patients currently in the office, both those patients who are well-bodied and those who are disabled.
• Determining how patient records will be protected and/or transported.
• Identifying available transportation for the evacuation.
• Determining a meeting place for all employees once the evacuation is complete.
• Identifying exit routes from your work area. There should be at least two.
• Identifying any employees with disabilities who may require special attention during an evacuation. It should be clarified how these individuals will be assisted.
• Determining how the office will be secured during and after the evacuation.
• Identifying what, if anything, should be taken from the office and who should be responsible for seeing that the item(s) are removed and secure.
• Identifying who will communicate with emergency personnel.
• Determining if any personnel should remain behind after the primary evacuation.
• Identifying a way to account for employees during and after the evacuation.
• Identifying the person who will be responsible for notifying the public utilities (electricity, telephone, water, gas, etc.) that the building or office has been evacuated.
• Identifying and obtaining any special equipment that may be required for evacuation such as safety goggles, masks, gloves, etc.

español SPANISH TERMINOLOGY

Busco un trabajo.
I am looking for a job.

¿Tiene usted cualquier abîerto?
Do you have any openings?

¿Dónde estan las aplicaciones?
Where are the applications?

¿Soy el director.
I am the manager.

¿Vio usted lo que pasó?
Did you see what happened?

¿Cayo usted?
Did you fall?

¿Está lastimado usted?
Are you hurt?

¿Quiere usted ver un doctor?
Do you want to see a doctor?

Usted necesita obtener una radiografía.
You need an x-ray.

Tiene dolor?
Do you have pain?

Tiene dificultad para respirar?
Are you having any problem breathing?

Cuando ocurrio el accidente?
When did the accident happen?

Calmese, por favor. La ambulancia esta en camino.
Calm down, please. The ambulance is on the way.

MEDIA MENU

- **Student Resources on thePoint**
  - **CMA/RMA Certification Exam Review**
- **Internet Resources**

  Medical Group Management Association
  http://www.mgma.com

  Physicians Practice Group
  http://www.physicianspractice.com/home

  Family Leave Act/Department of Labor
  http://www.dol.gov

  Americans with Disabilities Act/U.S. Department of Justice
  http://www.ada.gov
  http://www.justice.gov

  Centers for Medicare and Medicaid Services
  http://www.cms.gov

  Clinical Laboratory Improvement Amendments Act
  http://www.cms.hhs.gov/clia

  Health Care Report Cards
  http://www.healthgrades.com

  Health Insurance Portability and Accountability Act
  http://www.cms.gov/HIPAAGenInfo

  Occupational Safety and Health Administration
  http://www.osha.gov

  National Committee on Quality Assurance
  http://www.ncqa.org

  Medscape Today from Web MD
  http://www.medscape.com/medscapetoday

  American Heart Association
  http://www.heart.org

  American Red Cross
  http://www.redcross.org

  American Safety and Health Institute
  http://www.hsi.com/

  National Safety Council
  http://www.nsc.org/Pages/Home.aspx

PSY PROCEDURE 10-1:   Create a Procedures Manual

Purpose: To communicate the proper policies and procedures to be used by all employees in a practice in order to ensure consistent, accurate, and efficient patient interaction and care
Equipment: Word processor, three-ring binder, paper, choose any procedure approved by your instructor

Steps	Reasons
1. Check the latest information from key governmental agencies, local and state health departments, and health care organizations, such as OSHA, CDC, The Joint Commission, etc., to make sure that the policies and procedures being written comply with federal and state legislation and regulations.	Serious consequences can occur if you are not conscientious about keeping abreast of changes in the medical and legal worlds. This information can be found on the Internet and in published reports.
2. Gather product information; consult government agencies, as needed. If the procedure is for new equipment, ask the sales representative for training pamphlets.	This ensures that you are using products and equipment according to the manufacturer's usage suggestions and that you are practicing within legal and ethical boundaries.
3. Title the procedure, e.g., Infection Control Procedure for Handwashing.	A logical, easily identifiable format will allow easy retrieval.
4. Number the procedure, e.g., "HR 14" means human resource section, policy 14.	All policies and procedures should be numbered to allow for easy access and identification.
5. Define the overall purpose of the procedure. This should be a sentence or two at most, explaining the intent of the procedure.	Provides the staff with a rationale for the procedure.
6. List any necessary equipment or forms. Include everything needed to complete the task. Also indicate if no special equipment or forms are necessary.	The employee will be prepared before beginning the procedure if he or she has everything needed at hand.
7. List each step with its rationale. The steps must be complete and in order. Never assume the reader knows how or when to perform a given step such as handwashing. The employee will be able to follow specific steps, ensuring patient safety.	Listing the steps in order promotes compliance and accuracy for procedure completion.
8. Provide spaces for signatures. Administrative procedures are signed by the physician and office manager. Clinical procedures usually are signed by the clinical manager and a physician. Employees must have a space to sign.	The employee's signature will verify that he or she has read and understands the procedure.
9. Record the date the procedure was written. If changes are needed, the procedure is rewritten, signed, and dated again. The previous dates also are generally listed.	By recording the date, you ensure that you are reading the most current revision. It will also help you know when a new revision should be considered.
10. **AFF** Describe how you would explain to employees why they were asked to work in a group to create a procedure manual.	It is important to work effectively with a group to accomplish the task of creating a procedure manual. Employees from different areas of the practice will bring different perspectives to the task.

PSY PROCEDURE 10-2:   Perform an Office Inventory

Purpose: To maintain a sufficient amount of supplies needed to perform daily administrative, clinical, and laboratory duties involved in patient care.
Equipment: Equipment: Inventory Form, Reorder Form

Steps	Reasons
1. Using forms supplied by your instructor, count and record the amounts of specified supplies.	Established forms will promote consistency.
2. Record amount of each item.	As always, accuracy is important.
3. Compare amount on hand with amount needed.	These amounts will be established based on usage.
4. Complete reorder form based on these numbers.	You must also consider the time it will take for the ordered supplies to arrive to avoid running out.
5. Submit reorder forms to office manager.	Although many individuals may count supplies, the duty of ordering should be placed on one or two employees, usually a supervisor.
6. Document your actions per the ordering procedure.	Proper documentation prevents duplication in ordering.
7. **AFF** Explain how you would respond to an employee who continually takes a vacation day when the office plans to take inventory.	Explain to the employee that this is an important part of having an efficient work place. Everyone must do their part as a member of the team. Being a team player is essential.

- Effective management of the medical office is essential for a health care organization to succeed in the competitive marketplace.
- A good manager must be able to perform a variety of tasks in an organized and efficient manner.
- An office manager will be communicating simultaneously with patients and staff, handling staffing issues, developing policy and procedures manuals, creating promotional materials, preparing budgets, and overseeing educational programs.
- The medical office manager must keep current on legal requirements related to office operations.
- QI programs have many benefits to health care organizations. They can identify potential problems for patients and employees.
- After identifying the problem, a task force can create solutions to resolve them.
- QI programs are also required by various agencies. Four important agencies are The Joint Commission, OSHA, CMS, and your state health department. You must stay alert to new regulations from these agencies. Patients place trust in all health care workers and health care settings. We must all work hard to provide good quality care to all patients every time they are treated.
- Dealing with a medical emergency in the office or community will require you to:
- Communicate clearly and calmly.
- Recognize the need for immediate medical intervention.
- Perform emergency procedures immediately and competently.
- Provide first aid and life support measures that can mean the difference between life and death.
- Reassure the patient and family members.
- Work with the physician and other health care team members efficiently and with confidence.

Warm Ups for Critical Thinking

1. Review the list of qualities that a manager should have. Which ones do you have? How would you acquire the others? Should any other qualities be listed?

2. Review the types of sections that are often included in policy and procedures manuals. Now assume that you are to help a physician set up a practice. How would you organize your policy and procedures manual? Create one sample sheet for each section of your manual. Be sure to include all necessary elements when you write your policies and procedures.

3. Create a list of potential patient or employee problems that could be solved with a QI program. Be sure to include some administrative, clinical, and laboratory examples. Then select three problems and develop a list of solutions for each problem.

4. Plan a mock fire drill for a medical office: assign employees to certain tasks and design a form to document the drill.

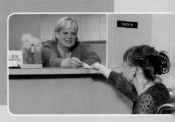

Good management of finances is essential for a medical practice to succeed. This unit introduces you to various aspects of medical office finances, beginning with a chapter on credit and collections, in which you learn the process of collecting fees. Next, you will learn bookkeeping and banking skills as well as other accounting responsibilities. Most of the income for the physician's practice is through insurance reimbursements. To be able to collect fees from insurance companies, you must understand coding. This information is covered in the last three chapters. A financially strong practice is good for the patients, the community, and you.

CHAPTER

11

Credit and Collections

Outline

Fees
Fee Schedules
Discussing Fees in Advance
Forms of Payment
Payment by Insurance Companies
Adjusting Fees

Credit
Extending Credit

Legal Considerations

Collections
Legal Considerations
Collecting a Debt
Collection Alternatives

Learning Outcomes

Cognitive Domain

Note: AAMA/CAAHEP 2008 Standards are italicized.

1. Spell and define the key terms
2. *Discuss physician's fee schedules*
3. Discuss forms of payment
4. Explain the legal considerations in extending credit
5. Discuss the legal implications of credit collection
6. *Discuss procedures for collecting outstanding accounts*
7. *Describe the impact of both the Fair Debt Collection Act and the Federal Truth in Lending Act of 1968 as they apply to collections*

8. *Describe the concept of RBRVS*
9. *Define Diagnosis-Related Groups (DRGs)*
10. *Describe the implications of HIPAA for the medical assistant in various medical settings*
11. *Discuss all levels of government legislation and regulation as they apply to medical assisting practice, including FDA and DEA regulations*

Psychomotor Domain

Note: AAMA/CAAHEP 2008 Standards are italicized.

1. Evaluate and manage a patient account (Procedure 11-1)
2. Write a collection letter (Procedure 11-2)
3. *Perform collection procedures*

Affective Domain

Note: AAMA/CAAHEP 2008 Standards are italicized.

1. *Apply ethical behaviors, including honesty and integrity in performance of medical assisting practice*
2. *Demonstrate sensitivity and professionalism in handling accounts receivable activities with clients*
3. *Demonstrate sensitivity to patient rights*
4. *Recognize the importance of local, state, and federal legislation and regulations in the practice setting*

ABHES Competencies

1. Perform billing and collection procedures
2. Use physician fee schedule

Key Terms

adjustment

aging schedule

collections

credit

executor

installment

participating providers

patient co-payment

professional courtesy

write-off

The medical practice must operate in a financially sound manner to continue to serve the patient's needs. The office depends on the fees generated by patient visits, laboratory work, and in-office procedures. Without these fees, the medical office would be unable to pay for staff, office space, and supplies. Therefore, collecting fees, whether paid by the patient, an insurer, or a third party, is essential for the medical practice to succeed. Box 11-1 shows how to determine whether your office is collecting fees satisfactorily.

COG Fees

Fee Schedules

Generally, the physician sets the fees for office visits, laboratory work, and in-office procedures based on the UCR concept: (1) U (usual) fair value of the service; (2) C (customary) competitive rates charged by other physicians; and (3) R (reasonable), that which meets the other two criteria. Fee setting also considers the resource-based relative value scale (RBRVS), by which fees are based on the relative value of a particular service and adjusted for geographical differences. (See Chapter 13 for more information about UCR fees and Chapter 15 for more information about RBRVS.) A physician's fee schedule also takes into consideration the costs of operating the office, such as rent, utilities, malpractice insurance, salaries, and so on. A list of the services and procedures offered in an office along with descriptions, procedure codes, and

---

BOX 11-1

DETERMINING A PRACTICE'S COLLECTION PERCENTAGE

Medical practices should evaluate their method of collections periodically to determine the effectiveness of their practices. A collection analysis lets you identify the strengths and weaknesses of the system.

To do a collection analysis, determine the monthly production from the first day of each month to the last day. This will be the total charges posted to all patients' accounts. Next, determine the revenues the practice received. Computer systems will automatically total payments received during a specified time. Divide revenue by production to determine the collection percentage. Analysis of the collection percentage should reveal the percentage of the collection of all outstanding debts to the practice.

Collection percentage = monthly revenue received ÷ monthly production

Most medical practices average 8% to 20% loss yearly. Experts consider a collection percentage above 80% to be reasonable. Performing a 2-year collection percentage comparison analysis will help you evaluate past collection effectiveness.

Code	Key	Mod	Par Fee	Non Par Fee	Allowed Amount
50010			$690.30	$655.79	$754.16
50010			$690.30	$655.79	$754.16
50020			$1,112.72	$1,057.08	$1,215.64
50021			$522.30	$496.19	$570.62
50040			$1,009.84	$959.35	$1,103.25
50045			$921.52	$875.44	$1,006.76
50060			$1,116.74	$1,060.90	$1,220.04
50065			$1,128.28	$1,071.87	$1,232.65
50070			$1,172.52	$1,113.89	$1,280.97
50075			$1,451.88	$1,379.29	$1,586.18
50080			$976.28	$927.47	$1,066.59
50081			$1,336.92	$1,270.07	$1,460.58
50100			$1,033.66	$981.98	$1,129.28
50120			$945.54	$898.26	$1,033.00
50125			$980.30	$931.29	$1,070.98
50130			$1,010.09	$959.59	$1,103.53
50135			$1,110.42	$1,054.90	$1,213.14
50200			$138.72	$131.78	$151.55
50205			$696.55	$661.72	$760.98
50220			$1,015.02	$964.27	$1,108.91
50225			$1,168.36	$1,109.94	$1,276.43

Figure 11-1 Sample Medicare fee schedule.

prices must be available to patients. Federal regulations require that a sign to this effect be posted in the office.

There may be several fee schedules based on the reimbursement schedules of different insurance companies. **Participating providers** are doctors who agree to participate with managed care contracts and other third-party payers in exchange for building a solid patient base. Patients covered under participating plans will have a different fee schedule from patients who are private payers (paying with no money from insurance). Each managed care plan, workers' compensation company, Medicaid carrier, and Medicare plan has a different fee schedule. See Chapter 15 for further discussion of third-party payers.

A Medicare fee schedule has three columns. A participating fee is the amount paid to physicians who participate or agree to accept a certain fee. A nonparticipating fee is the amount paid to physicians who do not have agreements with Medicare. A limiting charge is the amount a physician can charge a Medicare patient. Figure 11-1 is a sample Medicare fee schedule.

 CHECKPOINT QUESTION

1. What is meant by "participating provider?"

Discussing Fees in Advance

It is always a good policy to discuss fees with patients in advance. This ensures that patients are aware of the charges. Patients will need to know in advance whether the medical office is a participating provider with their insurance carrier. Managed care companies usually require that the patient pay a certain share of the bill, known as the **patient co-payment**, or co-pay. A good and easy way to initiate a discussion of fees is by providing an office brochure that lists not only the office's address, telephone number, and hours but also office policies regarding fees and collections, third-party payments, and how they are handled. Patients should understand that co-pays are to be paid at the time of service. Such information should be included in the office brochure. Many offices post a sign in the waiting area stating this.

Ideally, you should collect the entire amount due from a new patient on the first visit. Obviously, the less credit you extend, the lower your accounts receivable and the better the cash flow. As discussed in Chapter 5, many problems associated with collection (acquiring funds that are due) come from patients who move and leave no forwarding address or those who go from one practice to another. Be sure you get complete information including the names, numbers, and relationships of contacts able to give you information about a patient's new location. You should also get a picture identification, such as a driver's license, on a patient's first visit. (See Chapter 5, The First Contact: Telephone and Reception.)

Forms of Payment

Depending on the medical office's policies, patients can usually pay for services in several ways: cash, personal check, debit card, or credit card (e.g., Visa, MasterCard, Discover). If a new patient is paying by check, get two forms of identification.

By agreeing to accept a credit card payment, the medical office also agrees to pay the credit card company a percentage (usually 1.8%) of the total charge. Although this may seem costly, it is sometimes more cost effective to receive payment by credit card than to receive it in installments—or not at all—from the patient.

 CHECKPOINT QUESTION

2. List four forms of payments accepted by most physician offices.

Payment by Insurance Companies

By far, the largest proportions of fees are paid by insurance companies. Therefore, it is imperative that patients' insurance information be kept current. Most medical practices require that a patient submit a medical insurance card for each visit; this way, changes in insurance can quickly and easily be noted. Remember, always make a copy of both sides of the patient's insurance card and place it in the appropriate section of the chart for billing reference. Most insurance companies offer online services such as checking coverage, eligibility for procedures, co-pays, etc.

Adjusting Fees

Sometimes, **adjustments** (changes in a posted account) must be made to a standard fee, as when the medical office accepts a set insurance rate for a service that is lower than the practice's rate. You must charge the patient the regular fee for the service; when the insurance carrier sends payment, however, the explanation of benefits (EOB) will show how much you may collect for the service. The difference between the physician's normal fee and the insurance carrier's allowed fee will be adjusted in the credit adjustment column on the patient's account.

Other fee adjustments include **professional courtesy** fees, in which other health care professionals are charged a reduced rate. The physician may choose not to charge a fee at all; this too is considered a professional courtesy and should not be confused with writing off a fee. (A **write-off** is cancellation of an unpaid debt; these generally can be claimed as deductions on the practice's federal taxes.) Again, you charge the regular fee and then adjust the designated amount in the adjustment column with "professional courtesy" in the description column. Some practices offer discounts for paying in full. You would handle this as earlier described for adjustments (charge the full amount and adjust off the discount).

 CHECKPOINT QUESTION

3. What is the difference between a fee adjustment and a write-off?

COG Credit

Extending Credit

It is not always possible for patients to pay the entire bill when costs are incurred. Depending on the medical office's policy, **credit** may be extended to patients on an installment plan. Collection experts have estimated that billing one patient costs the practice about $8 per month. This total includes the time it takes to prepare the statements, the supplies needed, and so on. Extension of credit to a patient is a decision that is sometimes made solely by the physician. The practice will make the decision to extend credit in house or to arrange financing through a bank or other lending facility. If the credit is extended by the practice without the use of a third party, credit to a patient should be extended only after checking the patient's credit history (Box 11-2). Many offices outsource their credit and billing functions. There are medical billing companies that manage the practice's accounts receivable, prepare the insurance claims, offer training to the employees, and provide other related services.

BOX 11-2

WHAT IS A CREDIT SCORE?

There are three major credit reporting firms—Experian, Transunion, and Equifax. Credit reports can help you make better-informed decisions about granting credit. A credit rating or score is assigned to consumers who have credit. It is a number between 300 and 850 that evaluates your risk as a lender. This score will determine whether you extend credit and also determines interest rates if you charge interest. The Web site addresses for these companies are listed at the end of the chapter.

AFF ETHICAL TIP

Paying the Doctor with Eggs?

There was a time when patients paid for their medical care with eggs from their farm. Those days are long gone. In today's complicated financial world, it is necessary for a physician practice to behave as any other business. Although it is legal to charge patients reasonable interest rates, finance charges, and late payment fees, risk managers suggest avoiding them. Even the American Medical Association, which advises physicians on matters such as ethical principles and finances, warns that patients may be put off by their doctor charging these fees. Doctors are in the business of taking care of people, but they must pay their bills. These charges may create bad will or be seen as a conflict from a caring and helpful physician. You must use empathy and treat patients with respect—even the ones who have trouble paying.

Legal Considerations

When a medical practice extends credit to a patient, it may charge interest on the patient's unpaid balance. If this is the case, the medical office is legally required to disclose this information to the patient, along with any other fees or charges incurred by the patient's acceptance of credit. This legal documentation, called a truth-in-lending statement, must be filed in the patient's medical chart (Fig. 11-2).

Different states have different laws concerning the extension of credit. Generally, credit cannot be denied based on age, gender, race, marital status, religion, national origin, or source of income (e.g., if a patient receives public assistance). If your facility has given

Bruce C. Collin, M.D.   305 Madison Avenue
                                                                       Anderson, Indiana 46027

I agree to pay $_____ per week/month on my account balance of $_____.

Payments are due by the _____ of each _____ and will begin _____.
                                        (week/month)   (date)

Interest will/will not be charged on the outstanding balance (see Truth-in-Lending form below for rate of interest).

I agree that if payments are not made in the full amount stated above or if payments are not received on time, the entire account balance will be considered delinquent and will be due and payable immediately.

I agree to be responsible for any reasonable collection costs or attorney fees incurred in collecting a delinquent account.

_____   _____
Date   Signature

This disclosure is in compliance with the Truth-in-Lending Act.

_____   _____
Patient's Name   Address

_____   _____
Responsible Party (if other than patient)   City, State, Zip Code

1.	Cash Price (Medical and/or Surgical Fee)	$
	Less Cash Down Payment (Advance)	$
2.	Unpaid Balance of Cash Price	$
3.	Amount Financed	$
4.	FINANCE CHARGE	$
5.	Total of Payments (3 + 4)	$
6.	Deferred Payment Price (1 + 4)	$
7.	ANNUAL PERCENTAGE RATE	%

The "Total of Payments" shown above is payable to Bruce Collin, M.D. at the address shown above in _____ weekly/monthly installments of $_____, the first installment being payable on this date _____, and all subsequent installments are due on the same day of each consecutive week/month until paid in full.

_____   _____
Date   Signature

Figure 11-2 Truth-in-lending form.

credit to one patient, you typically may not refuse the same arrangement to another patient. Some states have laws limiting the amount of interest that can be charged. The practice's accountant should be able to provide the information required by the state and municipality.

 CHECKPOINT QUESTION

4. On what grounds is it illegal to deny credit?

COG Collections

When a patient has an unpaid bill or has not paid an installment per a credit agreement, those funds must be collected. **Collection** is defined as the process of acquiring funds that are owed. Collecting an unpaid debt is costly to any business. Collecting fees can also be time consuming, and collecting practices are regulated by a variety of consumer protection laws. Many medical practices outsource their billing to companies specializing in billing and debt collection.

Legal Considerations

The Fair Debt Collection Act of 1996 requires debt collectors and creditors to treat debtors fairly. It prohibits harassment, misrepresentation, threats, disseminating false information about the debtor, and engaging in unfair or illegal practices in attempting to collect a debt. Certain procedures should be followed when attempting to collect a debt. A debt collector—in this case, the medical assistant or billing clerk—must exercise reasonable restraint when contacting a patient about a bill. Attempting to collect a debt from a patient's estate requires particular diplomacy.

kept on a large sheet of paper. Figure 11-3 is a sample of a manual report. Figure 11-4 shows a computerized billing screen.

Aging of accounts is a measure of the practice's ability to collect its fees. Nearly all fees (80%) should be collected within 30 days. If the aging shows a high percentage (50%) of fees being collected 30 days or more after billing, the practice's billing and collection procedures should be reviewed. Procedure 11-1 outlines the steps in aging accounts.

 CHECKPOINT QUESTION

5. What is meant by aging of accounts?

Collecting Overdue Accounts

The three most common ways of collecting an overdue account are sending an overdue notice to the patient, telephoning the patient to let him or her know the account is overdue, and informing the patient at his or her next office visit.

Overdue Notices

With a manual system, overdue notices are fairly simple to prepare. Often, they consist of a copy of the patient's monthly billing with the words "overdue" or

---

Elkin Neurologic Center
1222 Brook Blvd
Edenton South Carolina 22617
331-561-8821

June 20, 2013

Christine Stultz
149 Fourth Street
Reedtown, SC 22617

Dear Mrs. Stultz,

This is to inform you that your account is more than 90 days past due. I know that you value your good credit rating, and I would like to speak with you as soon as possible about taking care of this obligation.

I will expect your payment of the balance of $250.00 by Friday, June 30, 2013.

I look forward to hearing from you.

Sincerely,

Tiffany Stone, CMA
Credit Manager

Figure 11-5 Sample collection letter.

"second notice" stamped in red. Alternatively, a form letter with spaces for the patient's particulars may be sent. Figure 11-5 is a sample collection letter. If a computer billing program is used, the computer often can automatically generate overdue notices. Procedure 11-2 describes how to compose a collection letter.

Telephoning the Patient

If written notices bring no response, you may have to telephone the patient to inquire about an overdue account. Always ask when payment may be forthcoming and document the reply on the patient's account. If payment is not received as promised, contact the patient again. (See Legal Tip.)

 AFF **LEGAL TIP**

BE CAREFUL WHEN LEAVING MESSAGES ON ANSWERING MACHINES

Patients are required to sign an authorization form for release of information at their first visit to a medical office. This form can be designed to give permission to leave a message on their answering machines. Because many people work during the day, you may need to leave a message for the patient to call you back. This is fine if they have given you permission. Because you cannot be sure who will retrieve the message, you must protect the patient's rights. The Health Insurance Portability and Accountability Act of 1996 Privacy Rule prohibits disclosing information that would link the patient to a particular physician or medical treatment. Your message must not include any such information. For example, it would be improper to leave a message asking for payment on a past due account. It would be within the law, however, to ask the person to call you back. You should only give your first name and telephone number. Do not state the nature of the call.

In-Office Reminders

A patient can be reminded of an overdue balance when he or she comes to the office to see the physician. To handle this situation discreetly, simply give the patient a copy of the most recent overdue notice. Once again, ask when payment may be forthcoming and follow through. Computer systems may offer the option of a message on the computer screen when the patient's overdue account is retrieved. This alerts anyone working with the patient either to discuss payment or to refer the patient to someone in the office who will explain that payment is expected. The more contact you have with the patient, the more likely he or she will pay. If payment is not mentioned, the patient may believe that you are not worried about it. Some physicians prefer not to discuss fees and accounts with patients; others will want to know when a patient's account is past due and will feel comfortable mentioning it to the patient.

 CHECKPOINT QUESTION

6. What is the proper and legal way to leave a message on a patient's answering machine or voice mail?

Collection Alternatives

Sometimes, it is more cost effective for collections to be handled outside the medical office. Three common options include collection agencies, small claims court, and credit bureaus. Collection agencies specialize in collecting debts. For either a fee or a percentage of the debt, the collection agency attempts to collect the monies due by the methods listed earlier. In addition, the collection agency can represent the medical practice in small claims court and can have the bad debt listed with credit-reporting agencies.

The medical practice can, of course, sue patients in small claims court or list patients with credit bureaus, but it is often more time and cost effective to hire an outside agency.

 CHECKPOINT QUESTION

7. What are three ways of collecting overdue accounts?

SPANISH TERMINOLOGY

Necesito cobrar el monto total de su cuenta.
I need to collect the balance on your account.

¿Puede pagar parte de su deuda?
Can you pay some of your balance?

Esta es una carta de cobro.
This is a collection letter.

Usted le debe dinero a esta oficina.
You owe this office money.

MEDIA MENU

• **Student Resources on thePoint**
  • **CMA/RMA Certification Exam Review**
• **Internet Resources**
  Collections & Credit Risk
  http://www.collectionscreditrisk.com
  Fair Debt Collection Practice/Federal Trade Commission Statutes
  http://www.ftc.gov
  National Credit Systems
  http://www.nationalcreditsystems.com
  Experian
  http://www.experian.com
  Transunion
  http://www.transunion.com
  Equifax
  http://www.equifax.com/home/en_us

PSY PROCEDURE 11-1: Evaluate and Manage a Patient's Account

Purpose: To monitor the activity on a patient's credit account in order to keep the collection ratio at a maximum rate

Equipment: Simulation including scenario; sample patient ledger card with transactions; yellow, blue, and red stickers:

Yellow for accounts 30 days past due
Blue for accounts 60 days past due
Red for accounts 90 days past due

Scenario: Stephen Hill was seen first on March 3, 2008. His total bill that day was $250.00 for a level 2 consultation. He paid $50.00 as he was leaving. He returned to the office on April 9, 2013, for a revisit. His limited office visit was $50.00. He paid nothing that day. He has no insurance. It is now May 4, 2013. Post the charges and payment on a ledger card. Make a copy of the ledger card and place the appropriate sticker.

Steps	Purpose
1. Review the patient's account history to determine the "age" of the account. If payment has not been made between 30 and 59 days from today's date, the account is 40 days past due, and so on.	Aging accounts lets you know what action to take.
2. Flag the account for appropriate action. Place a yellow flag (sticker) on accounts that are 30 days old. Place a blue flag on accounts that are 60 days old. Place a red flag on accounts that are 90 days old.	Color coding the ledger cards lets everyone know the status of the account. In a computerized accounting system, the status of the account is determined automatically.
3. Set aside accounts that have had no payment in 91 days or longer.	You will write collection letters to these patients (see Procedure 11-2).
4. Make copies of the ledger cards.	These copies will serve as the patient's monthly statement.
5. Sort the copies by category: 30, 60, or 90 days.	Keeping each type together will make the next step quicker and easier.
6. Write or stamp the copies with the appropriate message, for example, "30 days past due" or, "Your account is 30 days past due, please remit."	The messages you placed on the accounts will hopefully generate payment. The messages will be designed to become stronger as the account ages. In these cases, the patient may need more than a gentle nudge.
7. "Mail" the statements to the patients.	
8. Follow through with the collection process by continually reviewing past due accounts.	Following up on collection attempts and promises is the most important part of the process. Patients need to know that there will be continuous and consistent attempts to receive payment. They will be more apt to pay.
9. **AFF** When you call a patient with a seriously past due account, he informs you that he has not paid because his wife passed away and he can hardly get through the day. Explain how you would respond.	Express your sympathy and the sympathy of the entire office. Be calm and gentle in your speech. Explain to the patient that arrangements must be made to pay the account. Give him a specific date and amount to pay. Send him a self-addressed, stamped envelope.

PSY PROCEDURE 11-2:   Composing a Collection Letter

Purpose: To obtain payment from a patient whose account is more than 90 days old
Equipment: Ledger cards generated in Procedure 11-1, word processor, stationery with letterhead

Steps	Purpose
1. Review the patients' accounts and sort the accounts by age.	Sorting the accounts will make the task quicker and easier.
2. Design a rough draft of a form letter that can be used for collections.	A rough draft gives you the opportunity to review and edit your letter.
3. In the first paragraph, tell the patient why you are writing.	Let the patient know that you are attempting to collect a debt.
4. Inform the patient of the action you expect. Example: "To avoid further action, please pay $50.00 on this account by Friday, May 1, 2013."	Being specific will let the patient know exactly what you expect and enable you to follow up more efficiently.
5. Proofread the rough draft for errors, clarity, and accuracy, and then retype.	Errors in a letter may translate to the patient as inattention to detail and, therefore, to your collection followthrough.
6. Take the collection letter to a supervisor or physician for approval.	Since you are serving as an agent of the facility, you should be sure the contents of the letter are appropriate.
7. Fill in the appropriate amounts and dates on each letter. Ask for at least half of the account balance within a 2-week period.	Each letter will have a different amount based on the account activity.
8. Print, sign, and mail the letter.	
9. **AFF** You are helping a co-worker get her collections letters in the mail. You notice several errors in the letters. Explain how you would respond.	Show her the errors and joke about your spelling capabilities. Offer to proofread for her in the future.

Chapter Summary

- The financial status of a medical office is based on the ability of the staff to collect the physician's fees.
- Fee collection must be done in a professional manner and in accordance with state and federal laws. Technology affords the medical office the ability to streamline procedures, and collection practices are more efficient with computer systems.

- Aging accounts and communicating with patients in a fair and professional manner ensures a constant cash flow and success in managing the finances of the outpatient medical practice.
- Keeping the delicate balance between taking care of people and running a business can be a challenge.

Warm Ups for Critical Thinking

1. Write a script for leaving a message on a patient's answering machine asking them to return your call.
2. A patient has an overdue account balance. She is coming in for a visit today. What would you say to her?
3. A patient tells you that he does not believe he owes the amount on his statement. He says his insurance will pay. You have received a statement from his insurance indicating that he owes the balance on the account. What do you say to him?
4. Create a collection letter that you would send to a patient's executor or patient's estate.
5. A patient promises to come by and bring you $100.00 on Friday. The payment is now 5 days late. What will you say when you call the patient?

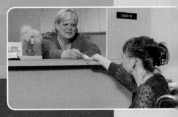

CHAPTER 12

Accounting Responsibilities

Outline

Learning Outcomes

Cognitive Domain

Note: AAMA/CAAHEP 2008 Standards are italicized.

1. Spell and define the key terms
2. Explain the concept of the pegboard bookkeeping system
3. Describe the components of the pegboard system
4. Identify and discuss the special features of the pegboard daysheet
5. Describe the functions of a computer accounting system
6. List the uses and components of computer accounting reports
7. Explain banking services, including types of accounts and fees
8. Describe the accounting cycle
9. Describe the components of a record keeping system
10. Explain the process of ordering supplies and paying invoices
11. *Explain basic booking computations*
12. *Differentiate between bookkeeping and accounting*
13. *Describe banking procedures*
14. *Discuss precautions for accepting checks*
15. *Compare types of endorsements*
16. *Differentiate between accounts payable and accounts receivable*
17. *Compare manual and computerized bookkeeping systems used in ambulatory health care*
18. *Describe common periodic financial reports*
19. *Explain billing and payment options*
20. *Identify procedure for preparing patient accounts*
21. *Discuss types of adjustments that may be made to a patient's account*

Psychomotor Domain

Note: AAMA/CAAHEP 2008 Standards are italicized.

1. *Prepare a bank deposit (Procedure 12-9)*
2. *Perform accounts receivable procedures, including:*
   a. *Post entries on a daysheet (Procedures 12-1, 12-2)*

each transaction one by one. Add the previous balance to the fee or subtract the payment from the previous balance to check whether the new balance listed is correct. If the posted charges are correct, total each column again. Do not erase or white-out errors; draw a line through the erroneous entry and enter the transaction on a new line. When you re-enter a transaction on the daysheet, use the ledger card again.

The daysheet is important because it keeps track of accounts receivable. The accounts receivable total changes every time a charge, payment, or adjustment is made to an account. You should perform a trial balance at the end of each month. Add the totals of each ledger card with an outstanding balance. The total should match the running total kept on the daysheet. This practice ensures the accuracy of your financial records.

Completed daysheets are filed chronologically in a ledger (a book of accounts) with the most recent daysheet on top. Completed daysheets are important legal documents and must be kept for at least 7 years for tax purposes. They should be stored in a safe, dark area to avoid loss or fading.

CHECKPOINT QUESTION

2. What are five sections of a pegboard daysheet?

Ledger Cards

The ledger card is a financial record for each patient. Most ledger cards include areas for the responsible person's name, address, telephone number, and insurance information. Figure 12-2 is a sample ledger card. Patient information appears on the top of the ledger card; the bottom portion is used to record the patient's financial activities.

DATE	DESCRIPTION	CHARGES	CREDITS PYMNTS.	ADJ.	BALANCE
	BALANCE FORWARD ➤				20 00
5/2/13	OV	50 00			70 00
2/10/13	BC/BS ck (5/2)		60 00	10 00	—⊘—
5/25/13	OV, Lab	120 00			120 00

FORM MR 10   PLEASE PAY LAST AMOUNT IN BALANCE COLUMN ➤

Figure 12-2 Sample ledger card.

A photocopy of an individual's ledger card is sent as a bill. If you use a copy of the ledger card for billing, make sure that no information other than the billing name and address is visible through the window of the envelope. Allowing other information to be visible is a breach of privacy.

The ledger card is a legal document and should be kept for the same length of time as the patient's medical record. Ledger cards are filed alphabetically in a ledger tray. A medical practice may require more than one ledger tray. Ledger cards with outstanding balances are kept separate from paid ledger cards; this makes it easier to photocopy the monthly bills or find a ledger card when a patient calls about an outstanding bill. If the office uses only one ledger tray, the ledger cards with outstanding balances are filed alphabetically in the front of the ledger tray, with the paid ledger cards filed alphabetically in the back.

Encounter Forms and Charge Slips

The **encounter form** and the charge slip are preprinted patient statements that list codes for basic office charges and have sections for the patient's current balance and next appointment. Most encounter forms and charge slips have three-part copies:

1. The first copy is kept by the facility for auditing purposes (all are numbered).
2. The second copy is given to the patient for insurance filing (if the patient files the insurance claims).
3. The third copy, which has a carbon line at the top to match your ledgers and daysheets, is given to the patient as a receipt of services.

Charge slips are smaller versions of an encounter form and are designed to be used in conjunction with ledger cards. They often have different-colored no-carbon-required (NCR) copies. Figure 12-3 shows a computer-generated encounter form and a charge slip used in a manual system. You can see the same information found in a computerized system in the screen shot in Figure 12-4.

CHECKPOINT QUESTION

3. What is an encounter form?

Posting a Charge

The charge column of the daysheet is for original charges incurred for services received by the patient from the physician or staff on a specific date. Examples include office visits, electrocardiograms, blood work, hospital visits, consultations, and fees for returned checks. As discussed previously, charges in a medical office are based on a fee schedule or list of charges determined by the usual, customary, and reasonable charges of similar providers in similar localities who practice under similar circumstances. Procedure 12-1 outlines the steps for posting a charge.

Patient Name: _____

Patient ID #:_____ DOB: _____ Sex: _____

PCP: _____

SSN: _____ Financial Class:_____

Phone:_____ (home)_____ (work)

Medical Record #: _____ Date of Service: _____

Benefit Pkg: _____ Copay $_____

Encounter #: _____

Service Provider: _____

Appt. Status: ☐ Scheduled ☐ Same Day ☐ Walk-in

Check-in Time: _____ Check-out Time: _____

Escorted to Exam Room: _____ Time Patient Seen: _____

Appointment Time: _____

Is Patient Being Seen in Relation to:
☐ Motor Vehicle Accident ☐ Workman's Compensation

Appointment Failure Reason:
☐ Patient Cancel ☐ No Show ☐ Walk Out ☐ PHA Cancel

TYPE OF VISIT

✓	CODE	DESCRIPTION	FEE	✓	CODE	DESCRIPTION	FEE	✓	CODE	DESCRIPTION	FEE	✓	CODE	DESCRIPTION	FEE
		OFFICE VISITS-EST.				**OFFICE VISITS-NEW CONT.**				**PREVENTATIVE, NEW**				**COUNSELING**	
	99211	Minimal			99204	Compreh.			99385	E&M 18-39			99401	15 Min.	
	99212	Focused			99205	Comp. & Complex			99386	E&M 40-64			99402	30 Min.	
	99213	Expanded				**NURSE VISIT**			99387	E&M 65 & over			99403	45 Min.	
	99214	Detailed			99211	Minimal				**CONSULTATION**			99404	60 Min.	
	99215	Compreh.				**PREVENTATIVE, EST.**			99241	Focused					
		OFFICE VISITS-NEW			99395	E&M 18-39			99242	Pre-Op Consult					
	99201	Focused			99396	E&M 40-64			99244	2nd Opinion					
	99202	Expanded			99397	E&M 65 & over									
	99203	Detailed													

PROCEDURES

✓	CODE	DESCRIPTION	FEE	✓	CODE	DESCRIPTION	FEE	✓	CODE	DESCRIPTION	FEE	✓	CODE	DESCRIPTION	FEE
	88170	Aspiration - Cyst			11200	Skin Tag Removal				**IMMUNIZATIONS/INJECTIONS**				**IMMUNIZATIONS/INJECTIONS CONT.**	
	20600	Aspiration - Joint (Small)			20550	Trigger point/Tendon Inj.			G0009	Administration Fee - Pneumovax			J2203	Triamcinolone Inj.	
	20605	Aspiration - Joint (Interm.)							G0010	Administration Fee - Hepatitis B			J3420	Vitamin B$_{12}$	
	20610	Aspiration - Joint (Large)				**SPECIALTY SERVICES**			95115	Allergy Injection Single				**IN-HOUSE LABORATORY**	
	16020	Burn Dressing			99070	Ace Bandage			95117	Allergy Injection Multiple			89050	Cell Count, except blood	
	69210	Ear Irrigation			E0110	Crutches			90788	Antibiotic IM			89060	Crystalanalysis	
	10120	Foreign Body Removal, Skin			29130	Finger Splint			J2910	Aurothioglucose			82948	Glucose	
	10060	I&D Abscess, simple			29125	Wrist Splint			G0008	Flu Vaccine			85013	HCT	
	90780	IV Infusion Therapy			99080	Form Completion			J1600	Gold Injection			85018	Hemoglobin Screen	
	12001	Laceration Repair, Simple				**TESTING/SCREENING**			90731	Hepatitis B			81025	Pregnancy	
	13160	Laceration Repair, Extens.			95004	Allergy - Skin Test			90741	Immune Globulin			81002	Urinalysis, Dipstick	
	64450	Medial Nerve Infiltration			92557	Audiometry			90724	Influenza			81000	Urinalysis, Full	
	17110	Molluscum/Wart Rmvl			93000	EKG			J9217	Lupron 3.75 mg			G0001	Venipuncture	
	94640	Nebulizer			92506	Hearing Screen			J9217	Lupron 7.5 mg				**OTHER PROCEDURES**	
	82270	Stool for Blood (Hemocult)			86580	PPD			J9250	Methotrexate 2-5 mg					
	12001	Suturing, Superficial			94010	Pulmonary Function			90732	Pneumovax					
	13100	Suturing, Complex			94760	Pulse Oximetry, Single			90718	Td					
	11050	Skin Les./Wart Cautery			45330	Sigmoidoscopy, Flexible			90782	Therapeutic SQ or IM					

P = PRIMARY   S = SECONDARY   S1-S9 = NUMBERED SECONDARY

DIAGNOSIS

✓	CODE	DESCRIPTION	✓	CODE	DESCRIPTION	✓	CODE	DESCRIPTION
	789.0	Abdominal Pain		780.6	Fever		462	Pharyngitis (sore throat)
	879.8	Abrasion/Laceration		704.8	Folliculitis		486	Pneumonia
	995.3	Allergic Reaction		535.5	Gastritis		V70.3	Pre-Marital Testing
	477.9	Allergic Rhinitis		558.9	Gastroenteritis		V72.81	Pre-op Cardiac Exam
	285.9	Anemia		274.9	Gout		V72.83	Pre-op Exam, Other
	413.9	Angina		V72.3	Gyn Exam		601.0	Prostatits
	300.00	Anxiety		784.0	Headache		600	Prostatism
	716.90	Arthritis		389.9	Hearing Loss		782.1	Rash
	427.9	Arrhythmia		536.8	Heartburn/Indigestion		569.3	Rectal Bleeding
	493.90	Asthma		573.3	Hepatitis		530.81	Reflux
	611.72	Breast Lump		455.6	Hemorrhoids		V81.2	Screening for Cardiac Condition
	490	Bronchitis		553.9	Hernia		780.3	Seizure Disorder
	727.3	Bursitis		401.9	Hypertension (NOS)		473.9	Sinusitis
	354.0	Carpal Tunnel Syndrome		272.4	Hyperlipidemia		848.9	Strain/Sprain
	682.9	Cellulitis		242.00	Hyperthyroidism		438	Stroke
	786.50	Chest Pain		251.2	Hypoglycemia		305.90	Substance Abuse
	575.1	Cholecystitis		380.4	Impacted Cerumen		099.9	STD
	372.3	Conjunctivitis		780.52	Insomnia		727.00	Tenosynovitis, Tendonitis
	496	COPD		564.1	Irritable Bowel Syndrome		451.9	Thrombophlebitis
	414.9	Coronary Artery Disease		719.40	Joint Pain		246.9	Thyroid Disease
	290.9	Dementia		592.0	Kidney Stones		435.9	TIA
	311	Depression		464.0	Laryngitis		463	Tonsillitis
	692.9	Dermatitis		724.2	Low Back Pain		011.90	Tuberculosis
	250.01	Diabetes, IDDM		710.0	Lupus		465.9	Upper Respiratory Infection
	250.00	Diabetes, NIDDM		V70.0	Medical Exam/Physical		599.0	Urinary Tract Infection
	558.9	Diarrhea		346.9	Migraine		V04.8	Vaccination, Flu
	562.10	Diverticular Disease		278.0	Obesity		V03.9	Vaccination, Pneumovax
	780.4	Dizziness		382.9	Otitis Media		616.10	Vaginitis
	995.2	Drug Reaction		614.9	Pelvic Inflammatory Disease		424.9	Valvular Heart Disease
	782.3	Edema		533.9	Peptic Ulcer Disease		079.9	Viral Syndrome
	780.7	Fatigue/Tiredness/Malaise		443.9	Perpheral Vascular Disease			

Comments:

PREVIOUS BALANCE	$
TODAY'S CHARGES	$
PAYMENT	$
BALANCE	$

RETURN APPOINTMENT:
_____ Days _____ Weeks _____ Months
APPT. LENGTH: _____ PROVIDER: _____

APPT. REASON:

PROVIDER SIGNATURE:

Adult

Philadelphia
Health Associates
Tax ID #23-2350500
PHA Group # PH75923

☐ 3550 Market Street
Philadelphia, PA 19104
(215) 823-8660

☐ The Bourse Building
111 S. Independence Mall
East • 7th Floor
Philadelphia, PA 19106
(215) 625-9100

OTHER DIAGNOSIS

✓	CODE	DESCRIPTION	✓	CODE	DESCRIPTION

PHA-019 (6/95)

Figure 12-3 Sample encounter form and charge slip.

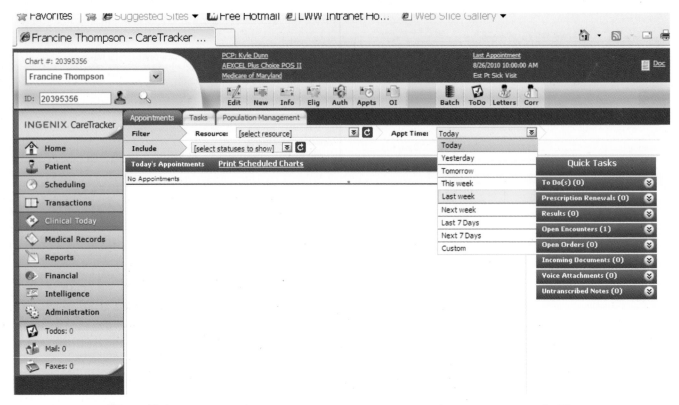

Figure 12-4 Computerized patient encounter screen. Courtesy of Ingenix® CareTracker™.

Posting a Payment

Payments received by the practice may include insurance checks received in the mail, money orders, credit card payments, or cash received from patients. Procedure 12-2 outlines the steps for posting payments and adjustments.

Processing a Credit Balance

Sometimes an account is overpaid, either by the patient or the insurance company. Such an overpayment is termed a credit (money owed to the patient or insurance carrier). This will show on the patient's ledger card as the last balance, with brackets (e.g., [25]) indicating a credit (Procedure 12-3). Brackets indicate the opposite of the column's usual meaning. For example, the balance column normally shows patients' debits, or amounts patients owe to the doctor. Brackets around an amount indicate the opposite, namely, that the doctor owes the patient money.

Processing Refunds

Credits are handled in one of two ways: (1) the credit stays on the account and is subtracted from the charges on the patient's next visit, or (2) the patient is mailed a refund for the amount of the overpayment. How an overpayment is handled depends on office policy and the amount of the overpayment. Generally, overpayments under $5 are left on account as a credit, whereas overpayments over $5 are refunded. Procedure 12-4 indicates how to process refunds.

Posting a Credit Adjustment

The adjustments section is used to indicate nonstandard office fees and to credit an account for uncollectible monies. Below are three specific situations that require a credit adjustment.

Example 1. The physician wishes to give a registered nurse a 25% professional discount on charges incurred for an office visit. You enter the fee from the fee schedule in the charge column, show in the description column an office visit with a professional discount of 25%, and put the 25% in the adjustment column. Assume an office visit is $40. You put $40 in the charge column and $10 (25% of $40) in the adjustment column. The patient owes your facility $30 for this visit.

Example 2. Most medical offices participate with certain insurance groups, which means the physician has signed an agreement with the insurance carrier to accept the fee for services set by that carrier instead of the physician's normal fee. Again, you must charge the same fee for the procedure. When payment is received, however, the explanation of benefits from that carrier will show the agreed-on amount for that procedure. You will post the payment in the normal way, but you must write off the difference between the physician's standard fee for this procedure and the agreed-on amount. Assume the doctor charged $40 for an office visit and the insurance carrier's agreed-on amount was $35. You would post $40 in the payment column and $5 in the adjustment column to arrive at the agreed-on amount.

Example 3. Most facilities require that you write off the balance of an account when you turn it over to a collection agency to keep better control of the accounts receivable. Therefore, if the patient's balance is $1200, you would show "collection agency" in the description column of the ledger and put the $1200 in the adjustment column, which would bring the balance to 0. Procedures 12-5 and 12-6 list the steps for posting an adjustment and collection agency payment.

Posting a Debit Adjustment

Generally, a credit adjustment reduces the patient's account balance, whereas a debit adjustment adds to the patient's account balance. Below are three specific situations that require a debit adjustment.

Example 1. You receive a nonsufficient funds (NSF) check from the bank today. The check was given to you by a payment made earlier in the month and posted as such to his account (see What If? box). The previous payment is no longer valid. Therefore, you must eliminate that payment because the patient now owes it again. Because this is not an original charge, you may not use the charge column for this entry. To post this debit adjustment to the patient's account, you will show NSF in the description column and the amount of the NSF check in the adjustment column with brackets. Procedure 12-7 describes the steps for processing NSF checks.

Example 2. Assume that you have turned over an account to a collection agency and the patient comes in later to pay the amount owed. You must first put the money back on the account, or you will create a credit balance. Place the ledger card on the daysheet, and in the description column, write "reverse collection." Again, this is not an original or new charge, so you do not use the charge column. Show the amount in the adjustment column in brackets because you are adding the amount to the patient's balance. You may now show the payment in the payment column.

Example 3. Your office requires that you refund all money over $5 to the patient or insurance carrier. You must also post this to eliminate the credit balance on the account. Place the ledger card on the daysheet, and in the description column, write "refund to patient" (or insurance carrier). To eliminate a credit balance, you must debit the account. You put the amount of the refund in the adjustment column in brackets, indicating that it is a debit, not a credit adjustment. Procedure 12-4 describes the steps in processing refunds.

CHECKPOINT QUESTION

4. How does a credit adjustment differ from a debit adjustment?

Posting to Cash-Paid-Out Section of Daysheet

Some insurance carriers adjust for money overpaid to your facility by holding that amount out of money they are paying your facility for other patients. Although you are posting the correct amounts in the payment column for each patient, the check amount from the insurance carrier is short the refund or kept-out money. You write this in the cash-paid-out section of the daysheet, explaining, "insurance refund on account of [patient's name]." It is also a good idea to make a copy of the explanation of benefits and staple it to the back of your daysheet for future reference. Procedure 12-8 describes how to balance a daysheet.

 AFF PATIENT EDUCATION

PHYSICIAN CHARGES: WHAT HAPPENS TO THE DIFFERENCE?

The concept of writing off the difference in the amount the physician charges and the amount a third-party payer pays is often misunderstood by patients. Many patients think that this means the physician has overcharged them. You can help clear up confusion by saying something like this: "The doctor charges $50.00 for a level 1 exam. When we file a claim with your insurance company, they only 'allow' $40.00 for that particular exam. The doctor has made an agreement with your insurance company to accept less in exchange for being your choice of physician."

Let's say a patient's coverage requires her to pay 20% of the bill. Insurance will pay their portion of what they allowed, which would be 80% of $40.00 or $32.00. The patient pays $8.00. This would leave a balance of $10.00, which is the difference in what was charged and what was allowed. This $10.00 is adjusted off of the account. This amount is written off only when the doctor is a participating provider with the insurance company. If you break it down, most patients will understand and appreciate the lesson.

Computerized Accounting

Most medical office accounting software available today is easy to use and requires a minimum of computer skills. Computer programs fulfill many of the same functions as a pegboard system but do so much faster. Instead of recording entries on a daysheet, you key entries into a computer. You can print out invoices and receipts for patients and insurance companies. Since most practices have computer stations in several locations, the patient's account can be quickly and easily retrieved in all areas of the office, enabling everyone involved in the patient's

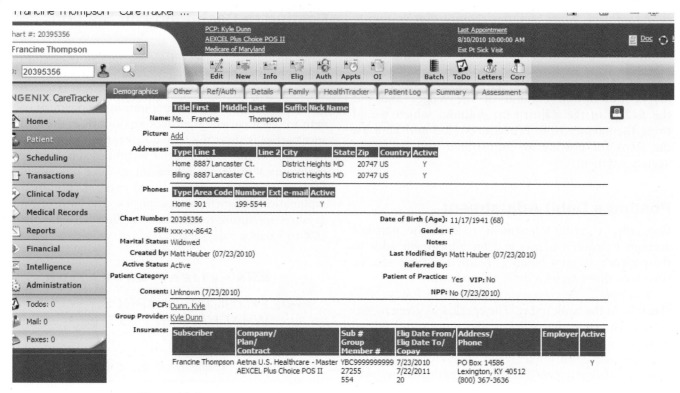

Figure 12-5 Patient account screen shot. Courtesy of Ingenix® CareTracker™.

care to access information about third-party coverage, co-payments required, and so on.

Computer bookkeeping programs have a variety of advantages over pegboard bookkeeping. Computer programs work as expanded calculators and perform the arithmetic functions, such as balancing individual accounts and the day's totals. Many bookkeeping programs also can write checks. Some programs manage electronic banking between the office and bank. The office may have computerized many functions, including bookkeeping, making appointments, and generating other office reports, such as forms for insurance reimbursement. It is essential that data stored on the computer be backed up in a reliable way in case the computer crashes. Figure 12-5 shows a screenshot of the equivalent of the patient's ledger card.

Posting to Computer Accounts

If you understand the fundamentals of accounting and how to post entries manually, you will be able to use a computer system with ease. When you post charges into the computer database, in most systems, you use a local or access code to indicate a certain procedure or service. For example, you may enter 211 to post a level 2 office visit for a new patient. When the information prints on the claim form, the CPT (Current Procedural Terminology) code 99212 will appear (see Chapter 15). Figure 12-6 is a screen shot showing a charge posted to a patient's computerized account.

To post payments, first retrieve the patient's account. The software will take you through the process. You enter the source and amount of the payment, the allowed amount for the service, and any necessary adjustments. As in a manual system, this information is provided on the insurance carrier's explanation of benefits (EOB). Calculations are automatic and error free. Figure 12-7 shows a screen shot for posting an insurance payment in a computerized system.

Computer Accounting Reports

Depending on the software package, you can easily generate daily, monthly, and yearly reports on transactions of an individual physician in a group practice. Daily and weekly reports provide the same information found on the bottom of a daysheet in a manual accounting system. At any given time, you can request a report that displays the practice's period-to-date and year-to-date financial status.

Computer systems record the daily activities described earlier for the manual system, and bookkeeping software enables you to create a closing report that prints a list of the day's financial activities. You may run a trial daily report or a final daily report. In a trial report, the information keyed in that day is printed for review. You correct any errors before running a final report. As on the daysheet, you categorize receipts as cash, check, and so on. A check register report can print the amount of the daily deposit and a list of checks for the day.

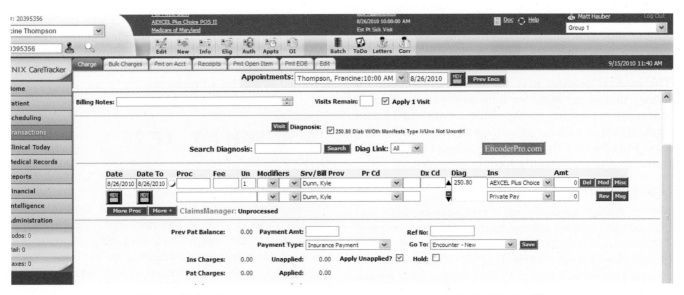

Figure 12-6 Charge posting screen shot. Courtesy of Ingenix® CareTracker™.

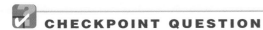

CHECKPOINT QUESTION

5. What is a local or access code?

COG Banks and Their Services

Types of Accounts

Besides physical location, several factors are important when choosing a bank for the office business account. These factors include the monthly service fees, overdraft protection programs (protection against bouncing checks), interest-bearing accounts, and returned check fees.

Checking Accounts

A checking account allows you to write checks for funds that are deposited in the account. Each day, you will deposit to a checking account the money collected in the office. At the time a new checking account is opened, checks are ordered with a check order form. The administrative medical assistant must maintain the checkbook and ensure that checks are reordered as needed.

Banks offer a variety of options for checking accounts. Variables include monthly service charges, maximum amounts of checks written, minimum balance requirements, and so on. Interest-bearing checking accounts pay interest if the balance is kept above a certain amount. Most banks set the minimum checking account balance at $500 to $2500. The bank pays this interest in exchange for the use of your money for loans and other transactions. If you drop below the minimum balance, however, you will not earn interest. Most banks also charge a monthly service fee and a fee for each check written for the period the balance was below the limit. Some banks waive the monthly

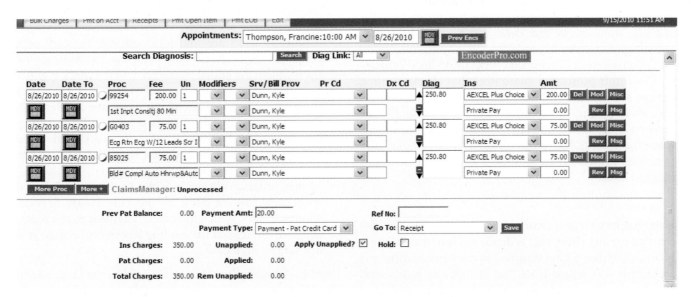

Figure 12-7 Insurance payment posting screen shot. Courtesy of Ingenix® CareTracker™.

service fee if the office agrees to maintain a minimum balance in another account, such as a savings account.

Savings Accounts

The medical practice may use a savings account for money that is put aside for long-term plans or money that is not needed for writing checks. A savings account pays interest at a higher percentage rate than a checking account, allowing the money to grow. Funds can be transferred to the checking account as needed.

Money Market Accounts

Money market accounts are a combination of a savings account and an interest-bearing checking account. The minimum balance is usually much higher than that of a checking account (as much as $2,500), but the interest rate also is much higher. These accounts offer limited check-writing privileges, including an initial deposit of $2,000 and minimum balance of $500 per check.

Bank Fees

Banks charge fees for services. In an effort to get new business, banks offer special services and plans for small business, including the medical office.

Monthly Service Fees

Bank policies concerning monthly fees or service charges vary widely. A **service charge** is a fee charged monthly for using an account. The charge can be a fixed amount or may be an individual charge for each check written on the account. As discussed, some banks do not levy a service charge if a specific minimum balance is maintained for the account.

Overdraft Fees and Protection

According to NYtimes.com, in 2010, banks generated $20 billion in overdraft fees. As of July 1, 2010, the Federal Reserve requires that banks obtain a customer's consent before they can charge overdraft fees for automatic teller machine transactions and debit purchases. Banks now encourage customers to opt in for the protection to avoid the embarrassment of returned checks or declined cards.

Overdraft protection guarantees that checks written against the account will be paid even when there is not enough money in the account at the time. Usually, the bank pays the checks and retrieves the money owed to it when the account balance is restored. Many banks offer overdraft protection as a "loan," and the customer is charged a fee.

Returned Check Fee

Some banks charge a **returned check fee**, which is a fee charged for any check that is deposited into the checking account but that is later returned to the bank because the account it was issued from had insufficient funds with which to pay the check. Such a check is often referred to

as a bounced check. Most facilities charge this amount to the patient. Because this is an original charge, the bad check fee is listed in the charge column of the patient ledger and daysheet, with the amount of the check being recorded as a debit adjustment.

WHAT IF?

What if a patient's check is returned for nonsufficient funds?

As a courtesy, you may call the patient and explain that the check has been returned for nonsufficient funds. Many times, the patient will instruct you to send the check back through the bank. You will need to make a separate deposit slip from the daily deposit of money taken in that day.

If this is not an option, then the patient should come into the office and pay the amount of the check plus any fees your office charges for a returned check. The returned check would then be given back to the patient since he or she has now paid cash for the amount. It is a good practice to flag the patient's account and even to demand cash only for future payments. Some businesses use a check service that electronically approves a check. There is a fee for this service.

Types of Checks

Most medical offices use the standard business check, but when certain circumstances require, there are other types available:

- Certified checks are stamped and signed by the bank to verify that the amount of the check is being held in the account for payment. The check is written from the customer's account.
- Cashier's checks are sold to a customer for cash or a personal check. The check is written by the bank, giving the recipient the added guarantee that the check is good.
- Traveler's checks are a convenient and safe way to carry cash when traveling. They are available in denominations of $10, $20, and $50, and if lost, they can be replaced. Traveler's checks are signed when bought and are countersigned (signed again) in the presence of the payee.
- Money orders, although not checks, can be purchased with cash from a bank or the U.S. Postal Service. Money orders, which guarantee payment to the recipient, are often used for mailing payments because it is not safe to mail cash.

Box 12-1 highlights other terms used in the language of banking.

COG Banking Responsibilities

Writing Checks for Accounts Payable

Another financial responsibility of the medical assistant may be to handle accounts payable, or pay the bills. The accounts payable in a medical office usually include rent, utilities, taxes, salaries, vendors of supplies and services, patient refunds, and petty cash reimbursement. The accounts are usually paid by check. Banks require signature cards for each person authorized to sign checks. In most cases, this is limited to the physician or physicians. Some medical offices require two signatures, especially if the check is over a certain amount. Computer systems allow you to enter information in the proper field and print checks. Software systems also keep track of every transaction

using a check. When using a manual system, type or write legibly. Use the current date and write the amount of the payment in both figures and words and the name of the payee. Complete the memo line for reference. Record the date, check number, amount of the check, and payee on the check registry. Post this transaction to the appropriate account in the general ledger or apply it to the proper category in a computer system by entering the type of payment on the proper screen. Recording transactions in the proper account or category is important when preparing the office taxes. Subtract each amount from the check register balance.

Receiving Checks and Making Deposits

When checks are received in the office, they are first endorsed. To endorse a check requires writing (or rubber stamping) on the back of the check the name and number of the account into which it will be deposited (Fig. 12-8). This way, if the payments are lost or stolen, no one else can cash them. It also ensures that the bank deposits the payments to the correct account. An endorsement stamp can be purchased from your bank or an office supply store.

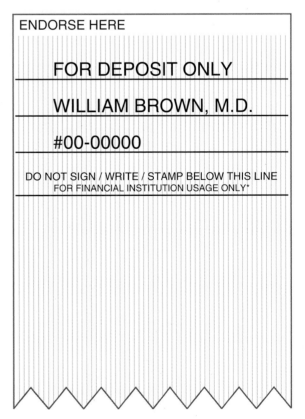

ENDORSE HERE

FOR DEPOSIT ONLY

WILLIAM BROWN, M.D.

#00-00000

DO NOT SIGN / WRITE / STAMP BELOW THIS LINE
FOR FINANCIAL INSTITUTION USAGE ONLY*

Figure 12-8 An endorsed check.

After all payments are posted, total all of the checks and all cash received that day. This total should match the totals of the payments column on your daysheet. Detach the deposit sheet from the daysheet and stamp the back with the endorsement check stamp. If a computer program is used, print out a deposit slip. Wrap the deposit slip around the checks and complete a bank deposit slip for the account to which the deposit is made. The deposit can be hand delivered or mailed to the bank.

A hand-delivered deposit may be taken to a teller, who will issue a deposit receipt, or dropped in a depository. If the deposit is mailed, make sure sufficient postage has been affixed to the envelope. Never include cash payments in a deposit that is mailed or placed in a depository. Cash deposits should always be hand delivered, and a teller's receipt should always be obtained. Procedure 12-9 describes how to make a bank deposit.

Reconciling Bank Statements

All banks mail monthly statements to account holders on which are listed all transactions since the last closing date. This bank statement must be reconciled, or compared for accuracy, with your records each month.

The statement consists of a list of all checks written and their amounts, all deposits made and their amounts, any electronic transactions, and any service charges. Verify that all checks and deposits are listed correctly. Make a check mark on the checkbook stub of each check that has been paid by the bank. On the back of the statement is a worksheet that explains how to balance the account (Fig. 12-9). Following the steps listed on the worksheet makes balancing the account fairly easy. The steps for reconciling a bank statement are listed in Procedure 12-10.

1. Subtract any fees or charges that appear on this statement from your checkbook balance.
2. Add any interest paid on your checking account to your checkbook balance.
3. List the checks you have written that have not been paid (these checks did not yet appear on your bank statement). You can also include in this list any withdrawals you have made since the ending date of the banking statement that do not appear on the statement.

Check Number	Amount
6217	32.94
6218	50.00
6219	119.24
Total	202.18

4. If you have entered deposits or other additions to your checkbook that do not appear on the statement, list them here:

Date	Amount
12-8-13	592.00
Total	592.00

5. Enter the ending balance from your statement here: 9542.91
Add the total deposits from Step 4:   + 592.00
Subtract the total from Step 3:   − 202.18
Total (this should equal your checkbook balance):   9932.73

If these balances do not equal your checkbook balance:
• Check the addition and subtraction in your checkbook
• Check the amount of each transaction in your checkbook with the amount shown on your statement
• Check to see that all transactions from your previous statement have been accounted for
• Call your bank manager for assistance

Figure 12-9 Completed reconciling worksheet.

CHECKPOINT QUESTION

6. What information is found on a bank statement?

COG Petty Cash

A petty cash account is a cash fund kept in the office specifically for small purchases, such as buying postage stamps or office supplies. The value of the petty cash account should always remain the same. A petty cash fund is always a designated sum of money. When money is taken from the fund, a voucher (Fig. 12-10) or receipt is placed in the fund to verify the purchase. The remaining cash and the sum of the vouchers should always equal the designated sum; for example, a petty cash fund of $40 with $13 in actual cash should have receipts that amount to $27.

Petty cash funds should be kept separate from patient cash payments. All cash should be kept in a securely locked area. One person should be designated to maintain the petty cash fund and issue vouchers. A voucher with an attached receipt should always be placed in the petty cash box, both to provide proof of the purchase and to keep the account balanced. The petty cash fund normally is replenished once a month. To replenish the fund, cash a check in the amount of the total of the vouchers. The money is placed in the fund, and the vouchers are removed and filed (Procedure 12-11).

Some offices keep a petty cash expense record. This record is similar to a checkbook that keeps track of the account balance as checks are written, such as personal checkbook. This expense record also categorizes purchases so that they can be included with the monthly office expenses. Purchases such as stamps and office and medical supplies can be deducted as office expenses and added to the accounts payable expense record.

AFF ETHICAL TIP

Honesty is the Best Policy

Physician-employers put their trust in their employees every day. In the clinical area, they trust that their assistants will be conscientious and careful. In the administrative area, they trust that employees will be completely honest and trustworthy. Borrowing $5.00 out of petty cash for lunch is not acceptable. When handling money for the facility, follow established procedures to the letter. "Cross every 't'" and "dot every 'i'" so there will be no reason to doubt you. Fortunately, most physicians and their medical assistants enjoy a mutual respect and loyalty. By following the rules, you will prove to your employer that you are worthy of his or her trust.

CHECKPOINT QUESTION

7. List six guidelines for managing petty cash.

COG Overview of Accounting

Accounting is the compilation of a business's financial records. It is necessary for assessment of the practice's financial history and current financial stakes, which serves as the basis for sound financial management. The medical office, like other businesses, requires strict adherence to sound record-keeping practices. Records must be maintained in an orderly fashion so you can retrieve financial information at any time and to present an organized picture of the business's finances. A system of checks and balances is an integral part of record management. Generally, the check-and-balance status of accounts is examined monthly by comparing the total of all accounts with outstanding balances against the running total taken from the daily logs of all financial transactions. The practice's accountant will also closely

PETTY CASH RECEIPT		
	12/1	20 13
Supplies:	14.	32
Postage:	1.	17
Travel Expenses:		
Other: fish food	4.	00
Approved 12/1/13 L. Davis, CMA	TOTAL	19.49
Received Above Amount		
19.49		HP, CMA

Figure 12-10 Completed petty cash receipt.

scrutinize these records at scheduled intervals for tax-reporting purposes.

Although manual accounting systems are still used, computer accounting is available as part of most medical software packages, and the many advantages include efficient tracking and analysis of critical information, improved productivity, and smarter business decisions. General ledger, payables, receivables, inventory, purchasing, cash flow, bank reconciliation, collections, fixed assets, and many other applications integrate with each other so you can manage the office's core processes efficiently and effectively.

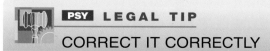

PSY LEGAL TIP

CORRECT IT CORRECTLY

It is illegal to falsify any financial documents. Accurate record keeping is essential. The Internal Revenue Service will examine the practice's financial records. You may be held liable for errors or omissions to these documents. White-out is a great product, but should not be used in a medical office. There are documented cases of suspected fraud when financial records were corrected with white-out. Corrections to ledger cards, daysheets, petty cash records, etc. are made just as they are in the medical record. Draw a single line through the wrong number, and place the correct one above or below. You should be able to see the item being corrected. If the space is too small for this, cross out the entire transaction and start a new one. Initial the correction.

Accounting Cycle

The finances of medical practices operate in one of two 12-month intervals or durations. The office **accounting cycle** follows either a fiscal year (a consecutive 12-month period starting with a specified date) or a calendar year (January through December). The yearly interval used depends on the way the practice's accountant has structured the business. For example, the medical practice can exist as a sole proprietorship or as a professional corporation.

The federal **Internal Revenue Service (IRS)** examines a business's income statements for the amount of profit and owed tax four times a year by quarterly estimated tax returns. The practice's annual tax return is a summary of the quarterly returns and reports the final year-end profit or loss (income minus expenses equals profit or loss) for the fiscal or calendar reporting period. If financial records are scrupulously maintained all year, preparation of the annual income tax return should

merely be a summation of existing accounting facts. Well-maintained office records not only facilitate IRS returns but also provide data that define the practice's business picture.

There are many reasons for a physician along with an accountant to review financial data on a regular basis. Financial records reflect growing expenditures and growth in the business. Conclusions drawn from financial data can affect future financial decisions. For example, analysis of the practice's accounts receivable can predict the amount of salary increases. Tax records must be available in case of an IRS inquiry or **audit** (review of accounts). Records such as receipts should be retained for 7 years, but records such as bank statements, canceled checks, and IRS tax returns should be kept for the duration of the business.

COG **Record-Keeping Components**

The practice's financial records should include a running record of income, accounts receivable, and total expenditures, including **payroll** (employee salaries), cash on hand, and **liabilities** (amounts the practice owes). Expenditures can be broken down into categories (Box 12-2). This is important because it enables the record keeper to track the practice's expenses and provide the physician

BOX 12-2

CATEGORIES OF EXPENDITURES

- Office supplies: items used by the facility's employees, such as paper, pencils, daysheets, and ledger cards
- Medical supplies: items used for patients, such as examination gowns, electrocardiograph paper, syringes, and tongue depressors
- Drugs: drug purchases, such as injectables; some facilities keep a separate column for these purchases, and others put this amount in the medical supplies category
- Payroll: gross amount paid to employees
- Taxes: taxes paid, such as the Federal Insurance Contributions Act tax, Medicare, federal withholding, state withholding (listed separately)
- Rent: amount paid to rent the facility
- Utilities: gas, electric, telephone
- Maintenance: routine care of the facility, such as cleaning personnel
- Travel: physician's car lease payment, gas mileage if paid to employees, and so on
- Personal: any money used personally by the physician

and accountant with a cohesive picture of the practice's expenses at tax time.

Categories can be accommodated by several types of bookkeeping systems; a simple business checkbook does not allow this. Pegboard systems allow the bookkeeper to write the check once over the **check register** (a place to record checks) or the ledger sheet and then have multiple pages with columns to distribute an expense into categories, including a back sheet for payroll. These columns are totaled and balanced at the completion of each check register sheet and can be subtotaled monthly, quarterly, and annually (discussed later in the chapter). Keeping a monthly accounts payable disbursement sheet lets the administrative medical assistant easily compare past years' expenses for the same part of the year.

Software packages offer the most sophisticated way to maintain financial records, not just for the categorization of expenses but also for the rapid formation of financial reports. Automating accounts payable does, however, require a personal computer (PC), software, and the training to use it.

There are advantages and disadvantages to both computer systems and paper records. Each practice should make this decision based on its particular volume and needs. Either system (pegboard or computer) can provide the practice and its accountant with the ability to pay and track expenses and to furnish the financial data necessary to create reports.

Multiple **summation reports**, such as the payroll report, itemized category report, account balances, and the **profit-and-loss statement**, must be prepared for the practice's accountant. If financial data are entered diligently into the bookkeeping system, preparing monthly, quarterly, or yearly reports should not be a daunting task. Income tax accounting cycles are divided into quarters: January through March, April through June, July through September, and October through December. Payroll reports show the amount of taxes being withheld and made monthly, quarterly, or annually. Normally, the practice's accountant will send you necessary reports and have you mail the checks.

Accounts Payable

Ordering Goods and Services

There are many economical ways to purchase office supplies or equipment. For instance, purchasing cooperatives (co-ops) offer bulk rate discounts by allowing physicians to order in a pool with other purchasers. Vendors may offer discounts for buying in volume or for paying promptly. Large warehouse-type merchandisers and companies with discount catalogs also offer competitive prices. Researching and cost-comparing office products and medical supplies can be time consuming,

but it is worth the effort, especially for items used frequently. Compare past invoices with prices in new catalogs.

Besides cost, other considerations come to bear when purchasing office supplies. For example, office supply companies often provide free delivery, but office warehouse chains may charge a fee or require a minimum order for free delivery. Quality also plays a role. Supplies should be of standard quality as well as economical. It is common to use several office supply vendors according to quality or pricing of specific goods.

Office supplies or equipment can be ordered in a number of ways. Once an account is set up, offices can place orders by telephone, fax, mail, or e-mail. These orders can be paid monthly by check or by credit card. It is preferable to pay for supplies by check or credit card rather than by cash, but when cash purchases are necessary, retain a detailed receipt for tax purposes. Credit card purchases can be made online, over the telephone, or by mail, but for security reasons credit card account numbers should not be faxed.

When placing orders for supplies, give the office's account number to the vendor or write it on the order form. It is a good idea to use a **purchase order** that lists the supplies ordered and their order numbers, so that order numbers for frequently ordered items can be pulled from the previous purchase order; this saves time with subsequent orders. Be sure to record the charges for your order and verify them against the bill later. It is also handy to keep a list of all vendors, telephone numbers, and account numbers. Procedure 12-12 lists the steps for ordering supplies.

 CHECKPOINT QUESTION

8. When purchasing office supplies, what factors besides price should you consider?

Receiving Supplies

When goods are delivered to the office, a receipt or **packing slip** listing the enclosed items should always accompany the order. The office staff member who receives the supplies must check the packing slip against the actual contents to ensure that all supplies are in the shipment. The person should initial the packing slip, which shows that all goods were received. When it is time to issue checks for payables, the assistant can then pay the **invoice** or bill. These receipts or packing slips should be placed in a bills pending file, so that they may be compared to the bill when it arrives. If the bill has already been paid by check or credit card, the invoice should be placed in the appropriate account's paid file; there should be such a file for each fiscal or calendar year.

PSY WHAT IF?

What if all of the supplies ordered from a particular vendor are not in the shipment?

Check the packing slip to see that the item was actually sent (Fig. 12-11). The form should indicate whether the item or items are being shipped separately, out of stock, or discontinued. If the item is listed on the form as having been shipped, you will need to call the supplier. The supplier will need an order number from the packing slip. The missing item may have just been left out. Be sure to document the date, findings of the call, and name of the person you spoke with. Place a reminder on your calendar to follow up if the item is not there when promised. Do not pay for something you do not get.

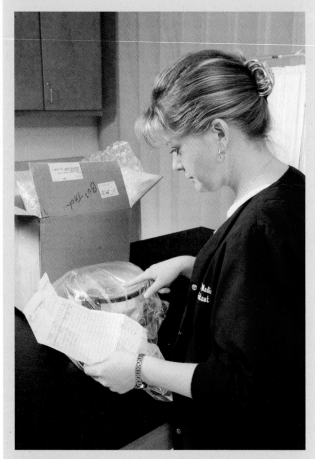

Figure 12-11 The medical assistant should be sure supplies are received and checked carefully.

Paying Invoices

Invoices for supplies and other types of bills payable by the practice should be kept together in a bills pending file to avoid loss or misplacement of a bill. Bills can be paid daily, weekly, biweekly, or monthly.

Manual Payment

Manual payment of bills requires a checkbook and checks (Procedure 12-13). The practice's accountant may recommend use of a log or record book into which is entered information about each check, such as payroll taxes or the breakdown of expenses for a monthly credit card bill. The large checks and checkbooks available from banks and business printers offer more space for writing memos or itemizing a check. Each check, once written, is detached from a **check stub**, which remains in the checkbook. If you make a mistake while writing a check, void the check and stub and staple the voided check to the stub. Never make corrections on the facility's checks. Check stubs should be filed with other fiscal or calendar year records and kept for the life of the practice.

The information recorded on the check stub includes the check number, the date the check was issued, the payee (the party to whom the check was written), and the full amount of the check. Notes should be written on both the memo section of the check and on the check stub. For example, when entering the purchase of a new beeper, the note might read, "payee: Office Communications" or "new beeper for Dr. Smith." The check is then attached to the bill or invoice and signed by an authorized individual.

Memos or notations on check stubs can be referenced later if a question arises concerning payment by a particular check. A log or record book enables the bookkeeper to make entries for each expense, categorize expenses, and maintain detailed payroll records. Unlike one-write (pegboard) or computer systems, multiple entries must be made by hand to track office bill paying. This can seem laborious when compared to other bookkeeping systems, but it may be ideal for smaller practices.

Pegboard Payment

The same pegboard system that is used for accounts receivable may be used for bill paying; it has several advantages over the ordinary manual method of paying bills. Instead of using a daysheet, a **check register** page is used to record the checks that have been written. The check is then aligned on the pegboard over the register page and is filled out as with any other check (Fig. 12-12). Pegboard checks have a carbon or transfer strip, and on this strip is written the date, the payee, the check number, and the amount. The information written on the strip is recorded automatically on the check register. These check-writing systems are referred to as one-write systems for this reason. The check can be addressed directly beneath the payee line and mailed in

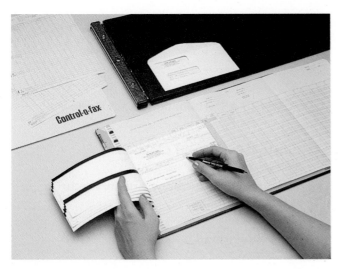

Figure 12-12 Sample pegboard check and check register. (Courtesy of Control-o-fax, Waterloo, IA.)

a window envelope, which saves the time it would take to address an envelope.

The pegboard check register has approximately 20 columns that can be used to categorize expenses, such as rent, insurance, office supplies, utilities, service contracts, postage, and any other applicable categories. All entries on the check register are totaled when the register is completed; these totals are carried forward to the new register page. Each fiscal or calendar year begins with a new first page (page 1), and the last check register page will have totals for the entire year. The check register provides a system of checks and balances even before the bank statement arrives because the check register must be balanced, as with a bank statement.

The check register also allows entries for bank deposits, and the back page of the register is used for payroll record keeping. As with pegboard accounts receivable, completed pegboard check registers are filed in a separate binder in chronological order, with the most recent register on top.

Computer Payment

A computer accounts payable system has all the advantages that a pegboard system offers: access at a glance to check registers, itemized categories and their totals, payroll records, and entries for bank deposits. To use such a system, you must have a PC, accounts payable program software, printer, and bank checks that are compatible with the software and printer. The initial expense with a computer system is much higher than that of manual or pegboard systems. Office personnel will need computer training to use the program. Also, since it runs on electricity, a computer may not work during power failures. A good computer accounting program will, however, provide functions for both accounts receivable and accounts payable. Financial

data should be recorded in three forms: on the computer's hard drive, on a magnetic tape or CD, and in printout form (hard copy).

Although entering data in the computer may be time consuming at first, this becomes less of a concern with practice. Furthermore, financial reports can be compiled and printed in a fraction of the time required with manual or pegboard systems. The computer program can also perform the record-keeping arithmetic; as a result, mathematical errors are practically nonexistent.

Paying bills by computer requires using the software to open the check-writing file. Checks are presented on the computer screen in the same way that a paper check would normally appear, and the information that is required to appear on the check is entered on the computer keyboard. The information is stored, and the check is printed out; the computer program automatically subtracts the amount of the check from the account's balance. The bookkeeper can print one check at a time or a batch of checks together.

The computer can "memorize" checks so that the information on them can be recalled and reprinted without re-entering it; this is especially helpful with payroll checks. A good accounting program also allows for bill and backup reminders. Of course, it is essential to back up financial data in case of computer problems.

 CHECKPOINT QUESTION

9. Whether using a manual, pegboard, or computer accounts payable system, two steps must always occur when ordering and receiving supplies. What are they?

COG Preparation of Reports

The bookkeeper must also prepare reports for the practice's accountant or the IRS based on financial data stored in the office's bookkeeping system. For this reason, care should always be taken when recording financial data.

The manual system, when assisted by the use of a log or record book, should be able to provide monthly, quarterly, and annual summaries for income, expenditures, and payroll. It is advisable to have subtotals and totals for these periods for tax payment purposes.

The pegboard system is also practical for providing summaries of income, expenses, and payroll and can be totaled monthly, quarterly, and yearly. Each day-sheet, check register, and payroll journal is individually totaled, with all balances forwarded to the next page. These records are stored in binders and kept for future reference.

A computer system of accounting offers all of the previously mentioned reports along with other more complicated reports that generally require more advanced accounting skills. The great advantage with a report generated by a computer is that the computer will perform all of the mathematical calculations for the time frame requested.

COG Assisting with Audits

An audit may be informal (in-house) and used to assist the practice's accountant with tax preparation, or it may be a formal audit by the IRS. If meticulous attention to record keeping has been paid throughout the year, the preparation time needed for such an audit should be minimal. It is important to save all bank statements, copies of annual and quarterly tax returns, and receipts for expenditures. Canceled checks and payroll records should be readily available.

Manual and pegboard systems can provide spending category and payroll summaries in addition to examination of the actual entries for the period being audited. A computer accounting system can provide all of this plus reports such as profit-and-loss statements, which normally would be compiled by an accountant.

español SPANISH TERMINOLOGY

Tenemos que cobrar los impuestos de su sueldo.
Taxes must be taken out of your paycheck.

Usted necesita completar estas formas.
You need to complete these forms.

Gracias para su pago.
Thank you for your payment.

Gracias por su cheque.
Thank you for your check.

Este es su recibo.
This is your receipt.

Este es el total.
This is your balance.

Esto es su crédito.
This is your credit.

No pague esta factura.
Do not pay this bill.

Su cheque ha sido devuelto por fondos insuficientes.
Your check was returned for insufficient funds.

Su cuenta ahora está a cargo una agencia de cobros.
Your account has been sent to a collection agency.

MEDIA MENU

- **Student Resources on thePoint**
  - **CMA/RMA Certification Exam Review**
- **Internet Resources**

  Superbill Forms and Creations
  http://www.physicianshelp.com

  Comptroller of Currency Administrator of National Banks
  http://www.occ.treas.gov

  The Accounting Library
  http://www.accountinglibrary.com

  Quickbooks Online
  http://payroll.intuit.com/index.jsp
  http://www.quickbooks.intuit.com

  Microsoft Business Solutions
  http://www.microsoft.com/en-us/dynamics/default.aspx

  Internal Revenue Services
  http://www.irs.gov

PSY PROCEDURE 12-1:   Post Charges on a Daysheet

Purpose: To keep a daily and running account of all charges to patients in the medical practice
Equipment: Pen, pegboard, calculator, daysheet, encounter forms, ledger cards, previous day's balance, list of patients and charges, fee schedule
Computer and medical office software: Follow the software requirements for posting credits to patient accounts

Steps	Purpose
1. Place a new daysheet on the pegboard and record the totals from the previous daysheet.	A new sheet should be used each day. Transferring the totals from the day before enables you to keep a running total.
2. Align the patient's ledger card with the first available line on the daysheet.	Each line should be used. It is easy to accidentally overlap entries.
3. Place receipt to align with the appropriate line on the ledger card.	Proper alignment makes neat and legible entries.
4. Record the number of the receipt in the appropriate column.	This enables you to cross reference and provides two forms of tracking.
5. Write the patient's name on the receipt.	This is the section that will appear in the name section.
6. Record any existing balance the patient owes in the previous balance column of the daysheet.	This total must be added to any charges because this amount is already owed.
7. Record a brief description of the charge in the description line.	This will tell you and the patient what the charges were for.

Statement					
DATE	DESCRIPTION	CHARGES	CREDITS PYMNTS.	ADJ.	BALANCE
	BALANCE FORWARD →				
	OV, Lab				

Step 7. Write a description in the proper line of the daysheet.

8. Record the total charges in the charge column. Press hard so that marks go through to the ledger card and the daysheet.	Totaling the charges for a visit saves room on the ledger cards and the daysheets.
9. Add the total charges to the previous balance and record this number in the current balance column.	The current balance is what is already owed plus the new charges.
10. Return the ledger card to appropriate storage.	Cards should be returned promptly for quick and easy retrieval.

PSY PROCEDURE 12-2: Post Payments on a Daysheet

Purpose: To keep a daily and running account of all payments made to accounts in the medical practice
Equipment: Pen, pegboard, calculator, daysheet, encounter forms, ledger cards, previous day's balance, list of patients and charges, fee schedule
Computer and medical office software: Follow the software requirements for posting credits to patient accounts

Steps	Purpose
1. Place a new daysheet on the pegboard and record the totals from the previous daysheet.	A new sheet should be used each day. Transferring the totals from the day before enables you to keep a running total.
2. Align the patient's ledger card with the first available line on the daysheet.	Proper alignment makes neat and legible entries.
3. Place receipt to align with the appropriate line on the ledger card.	Each line should be used. It is easy to accidentally overlap entries.
4. Record the number of the receipt in the appropriate column.	This enables you to cross reference and provides two forms of tracking.
5. Write the patient's name on the receipt.	This is the section that will appear in the name section.
6. Record any existing balance the patient owes in the previous balance column of the daysheet.	This total must be added to any charges because this amount is already owed.
7. Record the date of service being paid for, source, and type of the payment in the description line.	Such information makes tracking the payment easier and gives vital information that can be easily retrieved.
8. Record appropriate adjustments in adjustment column.	In many cases, it is illegal not to write off certain adjustments.
9. Record the total payment in the payment column. Press hard so that marks go through to the ledger card and the daysheet.	Because you are using a write-it-once system, your marks must go through three thicknesses.
10. Subtract the payment and adjustments from outstanding/previous balance, and record the current balance.	Subtracting these amounts will give you the the current amount owed.
11. Return the ledger card to appropriate storage.	Cards should be returned promptly for quick and easy retrieval.

PSY PROCEDURE 12-3: Process a Credit Balance

Purpose: To determine and record monies that have been paid on an account beyond what is owed
Equipment: Pen, pegboard, calculator, daysheet, ledger card
Computer and medical office software: Follow the software requirements for processing a credit balance in patient accounts

Steps	Purpose
1. Determine the reason for the credit balance and be sure it is recorded in the explanation column of the ledger card.	An explanation will help you discuss the account with the patient.
2. Place brackets around the balance indicating that it is a negative number.	Brackets indicate the opposite of the usual action of a certain column. For example, when totaling the daysheet, a number in brackets would be subtracted instead of added.

Statement					
DATE	DESCRIPTION	CHARGES	CREDITS PYMNTS.	ADJ.	BALANCE
	BALANCE FORWARD →				
			<47 00>		

Step 2. Place brackets around number.

Steps	Purpose
3. Write a refund check by following the steps in Procedure 12-4.	A credit indicates that a patient's account has been overpaid.

PSY PROCEDURE 12-4: Process Refunds

Purpose: To return money to the proper person or company when more money has been paid on an account than is owed
Equipment: Pen, pegboard, calculator, daysheet, ledger card, checkbook, check register, word processor letterhead, envelope, postage, copy machine, patient's chart, refund file

Steps	Reasons
1. Determine who gets the refund—the patient or the insurance company.	The explanation of benefits will list the patient's responsibility.
2. Pull patient's ledger card and place on current daysheet aligned with the first available line.	Proper alignment makes neat and legible entries.
3. Post the amount of the refund in the adjustment column in brackets, indicating it is a debit, not a credit, adjustment.	The brackets will instruct you to perform the opposite action of the column.
4. Write "Refund to Patient" or "Refund to _____" (name of insurance company) in the description column.	This information will be needed to discuss the account with the patient.
5. Write a check for the credit amount made out to the appropriate party (see Procedure 12-13).	Refunds should be made in a timely fashion. It is unethical to keep money that does not belong to the practice.

(continued)

PSY PROCEDURE 12-4: **Process Refunds** *(continued)*

Steps	Reasons
6. Record the amount and name of payee in the check register.	This follows proper procedure for writing a check.
7. Mail check with letter of explanation to patient or insurance company.	Place any identifying numbers in the letter to help match the refund to the proper person. Again, this should be done as soon as possible after writing the check.
8. Place copy of check and copy of letter in the patient's record or in refund file.	You must keep complete and accurate records of all transactions.
9. Return the patient's ledger card to its storage area.	Cards should be returned promptly for quick and easy retrieval.

PSY PROCEDURE 12-5: **Post Adjustments to a Daysheet**

Purpose: To keep a daily and running account of all adjustments made to patients' accounts in the medical practice
Equipment: Pen, pegboard, calculator, daysheet, encounter forms, ledger cards, previous day's balance, list of patients and charges, fee schedule
Computer and medical office software: Follow the software requirements for posting credits to patient accounts

Steps	Reasons
1. Pull the patient's ledger card and place on current daysheet aligned with the first available line.	Proper alignment makes neat and legible entries.
2. Post the amount to be written off in the adjustment column. Press hard so that marks go through to the ledger card and the daysheet.	Because you are using a write-it-once system, your marks must go through three thicknesses.
3. Subtract the adjustment from the outstanding/previous balance, and record in the current balance column.	Subtracting these amounts will give you the current amount owed.
4. Return the ledger card to appropriate storage.	Cards should be returned promptly for quick and easy retrieval.

PSY PROCEDURE 12-6:   Post Collection Agency Payments

Purpose: To apply payments made to collection agencies to patients' accounts, adjusting any amount paid to the collection agency.
Equipment: Pen, pegboard, calculator, daysheet, patient's ledger card

Steps	Reasons
1. Review check stub or report from the collection agency explaining the amounts to be applied to the accounts.	There may be more than one patient's account paid in a single check. You must determine the amount for each individual account.
2. Pull the patients' ledger cards.	Pulling all cards that are needed will minimize interruptions.
3. Post the amount to be applied in the payment column for each patient.	This amount should be subtracted from the outstanding amount for a particular date of service.
4. Write "payment from collection agency" in the explanation column.	This makes tracking the amount owed easier.
5. Adjust off the amount representing the percentage of the payment charged by the collection agency.	Subtracting the amount paid to the collection agency clears out the outstanding balance.

PSY PROCEDURE 12-7:   Process NSF Checks

Purpose: To document, record, notify patients, charge back amount "paid," assess fees and retrieve funds when the medical practice has a check returned due to nonsufficient funds (NSF)
Equipment: Pen, pegboard, calculator, daysheet, patient's ledger card

Steps	Purpose
1. Pull patient's ledger card and place on current aligned with the first available line.	Proper alignment makes neat and legible daysheet entries.
2. Write the amount of the check in the payment column in brackets indicating it is a debit, not a credit, adjustment.	Brackets tell you to do the opposite action of that expected in a particular column. Normally, the adjustment column is subtracted from the outstanding balance. Brackets instruct you to add the amount instead.
3. Write "Check Returned for Nonsufficient Funds" in the description column.	An explanation will make it easier to track transactions and determine specific reasons.
4. Post a returned check charge with an appropriate explanation in the charge column.	If the office charges a returned check fee, it should be posted here. This amount is designed to discourage returned checks and to cover administrative costs.
5. Write "Bank Fee for Returned Check" in the description column.	If the bank charges the practice with a fee, then you will pass this charge along to the patient.
6. Call the patient to advise him or her of the returned check and the fee.	The patient should be notified immediately in order to rectify the situation.
7. Construct a proper letter of explanation and a copy of the ledger card and mail to patient.	Even though the patient is notified by phone, details should also be recorded in writing.

(continued)

PSY PROCEDURE 12-7:   Process NSF Checks *(continued)*

Steps	Purpose
8. Place a copy of the letter and the check in the patient's file.	A copy of the letter placed in the patient's chart proves the communication with the patient actually happened.
9. Make arrangements for the patient to pay cash to cover the check and fees.	Requiring cash will eliminate the possibility of another returned check.
10. Flag the patient's account as a credit risk for future transactions.	It is helpful to know of possible future problems with payment of an account.
11. Return the patient's ledger card to its storage area.	Cards should be returned promptly for quick and easy retrieval.
12. **AFF** You see a patient whose check was returned for nonsufficient funds out at a soccer game. He whispers to you to keep quiet about the bad check. Explain how you would respond.	Assure him that you do not discuss patients outside of the office.

PSY PROCEDURE 12-8:   Balance a Daysheet

Purpose: To ensure an accurate daily total of charges, payments, and adjustments to patients' accounts in the medical practice
Equipment: Daysheet with totals brought forward, calculator, pen

Steps	Purpose
1. Be sure the totals from the previous daysheet are recorded in the column for previous totals.	You must have these previous totals in order to keep a running balance of the accounts receivable.
2. Total the charge column and place that number in the proper blank.	
3. Total the payment column and place that number in the proper blank.	
4. Total the adjustment column and place that number in the proper blank.	
5. Total the current balance column and place that number in the proper blank.	
6. Total the previous balance column and place that number in the proper blank.	
7. Take the grand total of the previous balances, add the grand total of the charges, and subtract the grand totals of the payments and adjustments. This number must equal the grand total of the current balance.	This will prove that the daysheet is balanced and there are no errors.
8. If the numbers do not match, calculate your totals again, and continue looking for errors until the numbers match.	The daysheet must be accurate before moving onto a new daysheet.
9. Record the totals of the columns in the proper space on the next daysheet.	You will be prepared for balancing the new daysheet.

PSY PROCEDURE 12-9: Complete a Bank Deposit Slip and Make a Deposit

Purpose: To place money collected in the medical practice into a safe and secure bank account
Equipment: Calculator with tape, currency, coins, checks for deposit, deposit slip, endorsement stamp, deposit envelope

Steps	Purpose
1. Separate the cash from the checks.	These will be recorded separately on the deposit slip.
2. Arrange bills face up and sorted with the largest denomination on top.	Most bill counters in banks are loaded in this manner. Sorting the bills is also a courtesy to the bank.
3. Record the total in the cash block on the deposit slip.	
4. Endorse the back of each check with "For Deposit Only."	This is one safety practice to reduce the possibility of fraud and/or forgery.
5. Record the amount of each check beside an identifying number on the deposit slip.	This helps ensure the identity and accuracy of each check.
6. Total and record the amounts of checks in the line on the deposit slip labeled "total of checks."	This amount will be added to the amount of cash.
7. Subtotal and record the amount of cash and checks for the total deposit.	Add the amount of cash and the amount of checks.
8. Record the total amount of the deposit in the office checkbook register.	This step will keep the checkbook balance accurate and current.
9. Make a copy of both sides of the deposit slip or office records.	Keeping records helps you prove any errors for future discrepancies.
10. Place the cash, checks, and completed deposit slip in an envelope or bank bag for transporting to the bank for deposit.	Deposits should be made as soon as possible to prevent loss or theft. If using a night deposit box, pay close attention to your surroundings and stay safe.

PSY PROCEDURE 12-10: Reconcile a Bank Statement

Purpose: To ensure the accuracy and sound financial practices of the bank accounts of the medical practice
Equipment: Bank statement, reconciliation worksheet, calculator, pen

Steps	Purpose
1. Compare the opening balance on the new statement with the closing balance on the previous statement.	You must know where your last bank statement ends and where the current one begins.
2. List the bank balance in the appropriate space on the reconciliation worksheet.	Since there is no standard format for a reconciliation statement, be sure you are using the proper blank.

(continued)

PSY PROCEDURE 12-10: **Reconcile a Bank Statement (continued)**

Steps	Purpose
3. Compare the check entries on the statement with the entries in the check register. Place a check mark beside each check listed as paid on the statement.	This will help you identify the outstanding checks.

Withdrawals / Debits

DATE	AMOUNT	DESCRIPTION		REFERENCE #
02-12	38.90	Food Lion	✓	436674796
02-12	500.00	Melton Custodial Servic	✓	426580282
02-13	1200.00	Lewis Realty	✓	446480157
02-13	22.00	John Little	✓	456974902
02-14	150.00	HS Brown, Florist	✓	466748392

Step 3. Place check marks next to checks listed as paid.

Steps	Purpose
4. List the amounts of the checks without checkmarks (outstanding checks).	These have not cleared the bank.
5. Total outstanding checks.	
6. Subtract from the checkbook balance items such as withdrawals, automatic payments, or service charges that appear on the statement but not in the checkbook.	These transactions are reflected in the bank statement but not in the checkbook.
7. Add to the bank statement balance any deposits not shown on the bank statement.	This gives you the proper current balance in the account.
8. Make sure that the balance in the checkbook and the bank statement agree.	This will ensure the accuracy of the current balance in the account.

PSY PROCEDURE 12-11: **Maintain a Petty Cash Account**

Purpose: To keep a small amount of cash on hand to cover expenses such as postage due, reimbursement for emergency supplies, etc.
Equipment: Daysheet and an exercise from the workbook about establishing and maintaining a petty cash fund

Steps	Reasons
1. Count the money remaining in the box.	This amount will remain in the box.

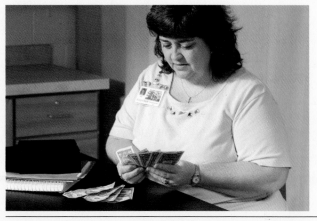

Step 1. Count the cash from the box.

Steps	Reasons
2. Total the amounts of all vouchers in the petty cash box to determine the amount of expenditures.	This total will represent the amount of money used.

PSY PROCEDURE 12-11: **Maintain a Petty Cash Account (continued)**

Steps	Reasons
3. Subtract the amount of receipts from the original amount in petty cash.	This should equal the amount of cash remaining in the box.
4. When the cash has been balanced against the receipts, write a check only for the amount that was used.	You will keep the same amount of petty cash unless instructed otherwise.
5. Record totals on the memo line of the check stub.	This is proper procedure for writing a check.
6. Sort and record all vouchers to the appropriate practice accounts.	The next step in the accounting is to post the amounts to the individual accounts of the practice.
7. File the list of vouchers and receipts attached.	Records of all business transactions must be kept.
8. Place cash in petty cash fund.	Added to the amount already in the box, this will replenish the petty cash box.
9. **AFF** A co-worker asks to borrow money from petty cash for bus fair home. She promises to pay it back tomorrow. Explain how you would respond.	Absolutely refuse her request. Perhaps you could find another way to help her.

PSY PROCEDURE 12-12: **Order Supplies**

Purpose: To maintain the materials and supplies needed to operate a medical practice efficiently
Equipment: 5 × 7 index cards, file box with divider cards, computer with Internet (optional), medical supply catalogues

Steps	Purpose
1. Create a list of supplies to be ordered. Knowing what supplies you are ordering will help you know what catalogs will be needed. Making a list of all the needed items will help you organize the ordering process.	Employees will report supply needs as they occur.
2. Create an index card for each supply on the list by placing the name of the supply in the top left corner and including name and contact information of vendor(s) and product identification number.	This establishes a record of the supplies used in the facility.
3. File the index cards in the file box with divider cards alphabetically or by product type.	This allows for quick access and makes reordering easier.
4. Record the current price of the item and how the item is supplied. Make a note of any price breaks on larger quantities, etc.	The price should be written in pencil because this allows you to change the price as needed. You will save money by taking advantage of special discounts for larger quantities.
5. Record the reorder point. This is the point where you reorder an item.	When supplies on hand reach half of the amount you need, you will know to reorder.

PSY PROCEDURE 12-13: Write a Check

Purpose: To disperse money to individuals or companies from the medical practice by preparing checks from a checking account

Equipment: Simulated page of checks from checkbook, scenario giving amount of check, check register

Steps	Purpose

1. Fill out the check register with the following information:
  a. check number
  b. date
  c. payee information
  d. amount
  e. previous balance
  f. new balance
	This is all crucial information and must be recorded accurately.

2. Enter the date on the check.	Dates are also crucial to a bookkeeping system.
3. Enter the payee on the check.	Without a payee, the check is nonnegotiable.
4. Enter the amount of the check using numerals.	This is the amount paid by the bank. It will be compared to the written amount below, ensuring that the amount has not been tampered with.
5. Write out the amount of the check beginning as far left as possible and making a straight line to fill in space between dollars and cents.	This practice creates a double check system that helps to verify the authenticity of the check.
6. Record cents as a fraction with 100 as the denominator.	According to banking guidelines, this is the customary way to write a check.
7. Obtain appropriate signature(s).	Many offices require more than one signature to help reduce the possibility of employee theft.

Step 7. A properly completed check.

8. Proofread for accuracy.	Accuracy is important in everything a medical assistant does.

Chapter Summary

- Accounting is a complex process involving many legal issues. As a medical assistant, you must keep neat and well-organized accounting records.
- Whether a medical practice uses a manual bookkeeping system, such as the pegboard system, or a computer system, you may be responsible for keeping records of accounts payable, accounts receivable, and petty cash.
- You may also be responsible for banking functions, such as receiving checks, making deposits, and reconciling monthly bank statements. To carry out these responsibilities effectively, you must record all transactions accurately and promptly.
- Computers have made the daily bookkeeping practices much easier, but you must understand the principles of accounting applied in the manual system if you are to use the computer system.
- Using the appropriate banking services will allow the day-to-day financial operations to be efficient, accurate, and secure.
- Managing the supplies and equipment in a practice, ordering goods and services efficiently and economically, and paying invoices are important duties of a medical assistant.
- With the computer being used for many administrative medical office functions, it is imperative that you keep abreast of changes and new opportunities to make this process more efficient and up-to-date.

Warm Ups for Critical Thinking

1. Your daysheet deposit slip and your posting proofs do not agree. How do you find the error?
2. Your office is considering going from a pegboard system to a computer bookkeeping system. What features should you look for in the software?
3. Explain the advantages of using computerized accounting systems.
4. When might a manual bookkeeping system using a pegboard be used?
5. A vendor continually mixes up your orders, and the physician asks you to look for a new vendor. How do you decide which one to recommend? What factors influence your choice of one office supply vendor over another?
6. The physician asks you, the office manager, how much money is owed to him. How do you gather the information needed to answer his question?

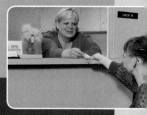

Outline

Health Benefits Plans
Group Health Benefits
Health Care Savings Accounts
Individual Health Benefits
Government-Sponsored
(Public) Health Benefits
Managed Care
Health Maintenance
Organizations

Preferred Provider
Organizations
Physician Hospital
Organizations
Other Managed Care Programs
Workers' Compensation
Filing Claims
Electronic Claims Submission
Explanation of Benefits

Reimbursement
Diagnostic Related Groups
Resource-Based Relative Value
Scale
Policies in the Practice

Learning Outcomes

Cognitive Domain

Note: AAMA/CAAHEP 2008 Standards are italicized.

1. Spell and define the key terms
2. *Identify types of insurance plans*
3. Discuss workers' compensation as it applies to patients
4. *Identify models of managed care*
5. *Describe procedures for implementing both managed care and insurance plans*
6. *Discuss utilization review principles*
7. *Discuss referral process for patients in a managed care program*
8. *Describe how guidelines are used in processing an insurance claim*
9. *Compare processes for filing insurance claims both manually and electronically*
10. *Describe guidelines for third-party claims*
11. *Discuss types of physician fee schedules*

12. *Describe the concept of RBRVS*
13. *Define Diagnosis Related Groups (DRGs)*
14. Name two legal issues affecting claims submissions

Psychomotor Domain

Note: AAMA/CAAHEP 2008 Standards are italicized.

1. Complete a CMS-1500 claim form (Procedure 13-1)
2. *Apply both managed care policies and procedures*
3. *Apply third-party guidelines*
4. *Complete insurance claim forms*
5. *Obtain precertification, including documentation*
6. *Verify eligibility for managed care services*

Affective Domain

Note: AAMA/CAAHEP 2008 Standards are italicized.

1. *Demonstrate assertive communication with managed care and/or insurance providers*
2. *Demonstrate sensitivity in communicating with both providers and patients*
3. *Communicate in language the patient can understand regarding managed care and insurance plans*

4. *Apply ethical behaviors, including honesty/integrity in performance of medical assisting practice*

ABHES Competencies

1. Prepare and submit insurance claims
2. Serve as liaison between physician and others
3. Comply with federal, state, and local health laws and regulations

Key Terms

assignment of benefits	crossover claim	health care savings account (HSA)	plan maximum
balance billing	deductible	health insurance	preexisting condition
birthday rule	dependent	independent practice association (IPA)	preferred provider organization (PPO)
capitation	diagnosis-related groups (DRGs)	insured	resource-based-relative-value scale (RBRVS)
carrier	eligibility	managed care	
claims	employee	Medicaid	third-party administrator (TPA)
claims administrator	explanation of benefits (EOB)	Medicare	usual, customary, and reasonable (UCR)
coinsurance	fee-for-service	peer review organization	utilization review (UR)
coordination of benefits	fee schedule	physician hospital organization (PHO)	
co-payments	group member		

In the United States, **health insurance** is funded by a combination of employer and employee contributions and tax-funded coverage. In addition to the numerous Blue Cross and Blue Shield plans, health benefits also are provided by other insurance companies, self-funded group plans, and government plans such as Medicare and Medicaid. The benefits vary with each plan and from state to state. Approximately 80% of Americans are enrolled in health benefits plans of one sort or another. Consequently, most of the patients you will encounter in the physician's office have some type of health insurance. With so many different companies and plans, it would be impossible for you to know each patient's insurance plan requirements, but as a medical assistant, you will need to know where and how to obtain such information so that you can complete and file claim forms appropriately. You must keep abreast of changes as you are notified. You will also need to learn the special terminology associated with health insurance claims. In addition, you may need to instruct patients about insurance matters.

COG Health Benefits Plans

Group Health Benefits

Group health benefits are sponsored by an organization, such as an employer, a union, or an association. A person covered by group health benefits is either an **employee** or a **group member**, who by virtue of employment or membership in an organization may participate in and receive benefits from a health plan. Coverage in health plans differs greatly, so you need to know the **eligibility** of the patient for services being provided by your office. For example, birth control is frequently not covered unless there is medical necessity.

Benefits may be either **insured** or self-funded. Commonly, health benefits are referred to as insurance. It is, however, important to distinguish between the actual benefits and the vehicle used to fund and provide them.

With insured benefits, the employer, employee, or both pay a monthly premium to an insurance company. The insurance company, in turn, is obligated to pay for any eligible health benefits. Self-funded benefits on the surface appear the same as insured benefits. They are paid for in the same manner as group health benefits, but instead of the employer paying the insurance company to invest the money to cover payments, they invest it themselves. They pay an insurance company or other agency to process **claims** and make payments on their behalf. Any payment for medical services that are not paid by the patient or physician is said to be paid by a *third-party payer*. In this case, the payer is an agent for the self-funded plan and is, therefore, known as a **third-party administrator (TPA)**. Many employers now choose to self-fund their group benefit plans rather than insure them.

You will need to be aware of these funding differences as they relate to state and federal regulations. For instance, insured benefit plans are subject to state regulations. Many states mandate that certain types of benefits be included in any insurance plan. These mandated benefits vary from state to state but often include such medical services as childhood immunizations, routine diagnostic care, and treatment for substance abuse.

For a group benefit plan to cover (pay for) eligible expenses, the patient must meet several criteria, called eligibility requirements. These are defined in the policy or plan document and may include a minimum number of hours worked per week and a waiting period from the date of employment before benefits become effective.

The eligibility of a **dependent** (spouse, children) is based on the employee's eligibility. Certain eligibility limitations apply to dependent children. For example, children are usually eligible until they are 18 or 21 years old. The age limitation is usually extended if the child is disabled or a full-time student. Eligibility usually requires that children be the unmarried natural or adopted children of the employee, unmarried stepchildren, or children for whom the employee has legal guardianship.

To confirm a patient's eligibility, check the back of the patient's identification (ID) card (Fig. 13-1) for a Web address or phone number to contact the **claims administrator** for the health benefits plan.

Group and individual health benefits describe contractual agreements and how the policies are paid. Both groups and individuals can choose from many different types of plans, such as traditional, HMO (health maintenance organization), and PPO (preferred provider organization). These types are further discussed later in this chapter.

Health Care Savings Accounts

Health care savings accounts (HSAs) are often offered as an employee benefit. Employees save money through payroll deduction to accounts that can only be used for medical care. Money is put into a health savings account before it is taxed and can be withdrawn instantly for qualified medical expenses as needed; any dollars remaining can be carried over to be spent in future years or invested to accumulate savings for health needs after retirement. HSAs are not designed to replace a regular health insurance policy but work in conjunction with a high-health insurance policy, which costs less. In effect, an employee would pay for medical care, using his or her tax-free HSA dollars, until he or she spends up to the deductible. A **deductible** is the predetermined amount the policy holder must incur before the insurance begins paying. Once the deductible is met, the health insurance pays for most or all of the employee's medical expenses for the rest of the year. Employees choose their own doctors and level of care. HSAs are gaining popularity, and experts say they are here to stay.

CHECKPOINT QUESTION

1. Under what circumstances is a dependent eligible for coverage by a parent's insurance policy?

Individual Health Benefits

Individual health benefits policies are purchased by an individual from an insurance company. The individual

---

UnitedHealthcare®
myuhc.com
PAID Prescriptions, L.L.C.
Rx Bin 610014 UHEALTH
REBECCA B. KEIFER
Member # 123-45-6789

UnitedHealthcare
Options PPO

Group # 555555
COPAY: Office Visit $10 ER $50
SPECIALIST OV $15

ABC Company

Electronic Claims Payer ID 87726

MTH

Call toll-free 866-351-6830 for Member Services

This card does not prove membership nor guarantee coverage.
For verification of benefits, please call Member Services.

IMPORTANT MEMBER INFORMATION
For authorization of health care services specific to your plan, you must call the number on the front of this card prior to the service to receive the highest level of benefits (see your benefit description for details). In emergencies, call Member Services within 48 hours.

Claim Address: PO BOX 740800, Atlanta, GA 30374-0800

United HealthCare Insurance Company

Issued: 01/04/14

Figure 13-1 Patient identification card.

pays premiums directly to the insurance company, and the insurance company pays either the doctor or the hospital directly if they are a participating provider or reimburses the individual for eligible medical expenses.

For patients with individual health benefits, the criteria for completing and filing claims are the same as for patients with group health benefits. Individual health policies commonly have less generous coverage, however, than group health plans have. An individual policy may also have a rider that limits or eliminates benefits for certain illnesses or injuries based on the determination of the underwriter at the time the policy was issued. The Health Insurance Portability and Accountability Act of 1996 (HIPAA) includes a provision to protect employees changing jobs from being denied benefits for preexisting conditions (see Appendix A). There can, however, be a waiting period for coverage of pre-existing conditions.

With the cost of health care skyrocketing and more insurance companies limiting what they will cover, many people have more than one health care insurance policy. It is extremely important that you know which insurance you bill first (primary) and which to bill the remainder of the charges (secondary).

Government-Sponsored (Public) Health Benefits

Government-sponsored benefit programs are funded and regulated by the federal government or individual states. Government programs have been developed over the years to assist persons who do not otherwise have health benefits, such as the elderly, the indigent, and others unable to obtain benefits. Government programs include Medicare, Medicaid, TRICARE/CHAMPVA, and workers' compensation.

Medicare

In 1965, the Social Security Act established **Medicare** to provide health insurance for the elderly. Elderly persons were defined as Social Security recipients age 65 or older. In 1972, amendments to the Social Security Act expanded Medicare coverage to two additional high-risk groups: disabled persons who have been receiving Social Security benefits for 24 months and persons suffering from end-stage renal disease.

Medicare Part A covers hospital expenses and is provided at no additional charge to persons eligible for Social Security benefits. Medicare Part B pays for physician fees, both inpatient and outpatient, diagnostic testing, certain immunizations (influenza and pneumonia), and specific screening tests (PSA, mammograms, Pap smears, bone density testing, colorectal screening). Part B Medicare is optional, and the participant is charged a monthly fee. The fee is deducted from the monthly Social Security benefits.

Persons signing up for or receiving Social Security benefits are automatically enrolled in both Part A and Part B Medicare when they reach age 65 years. If they do not wish to participate in Part B, they must decline it. Both Part A and Part B of Medicare have deductibles and co-payments, and as with most health insurance policies, these generally increase yearly.

A patient with Medicare coverage who is actively employed and covered by the employer's plan will have secondary Medicare benefits. A retired person age 65 or older who has health insurance in addition to Medicare will have primary Medicare benefits. Physicians are required to submit claims to Medicare on behalf of Medicare patients. These claims must be filed within 1 year of the time the service is incurred. (See section on filing claims for more information.)

After the deductible has been met, Medicare Part B reimburses the physician 80% of the Medicare-approved charges. The patient is responsible for the remaining 20% of the Medicare-approved fee. Under certain circumstances, if paying the 20% causes undue financial hardship, the physician may not charge the remaining 20%. The Centers for Medicare and Medicaid Services (CMS) can provide forms with the requirements, and the forms should always be used. In addition to Medicare, the Social Security Act of 1965 established Medicaid, a program of health care coverage for the poor. If patients are financially unable to pay the 20%, they may be eligible for Medicaid. This is referred to as a **crossover claim** because the patient is eligible under both Medicare and Medicaid, and the claim crosses over automatically from one coverage to the other. In this situation, Medicare is primary, and Medicaid is secondary. Medicare will accept original claims (no copies) filed on CMS-1500 universal claim forms only.

The CMS, which was known as the *Health Care Financing Administration (HCFA)* prior to July 1, 2001, is a government agency that oversees the financial aspects of health care in the United States (Box 13-1). The CMS has adopted a revised Current Procedural Terminology (CPT) coding system that must be used for Medicare claims. Medicare B claims use the standard CPT codes. For equipment, supplies, and services not listed in the CPT code, the CMS has established the Healthcare Common Procedure Coding System (HCPCS) codes (see Chapter 15).

It is important to ask the patient about supplemental or secondary coverage. This policy, which patients may purchase on their own, usually covers the deductible and charges not covered by Medicare. In this case, filing a second claim is necessary.

✔ CHECKPOINT QUESTION

2. What is the difference between parts A and B of Medicare coverage?

WHAT IS THE CMS?

The CMS is the federal agency that administers Medicare, Medicaid, and the State Children's Health Insurance Program (SCHIP). About 100 million people—1 in 3—now have government coverage through Medicaid, Medicare, or military or federal employee health plans. More than 10 million others are eligible for Medicaid but have not signed up. The CMS also performs quality-focused activities, including regulation of laboratory testing, development of coverage policies, and quality-of-care improvement. The CMS maintains oversight of the survey and certification of nursing homes and continuing care providers, including home health agencies and intermediate-care facilities for the mentally retarded. It makes available to beneficiaries, providers, researchers, and state surveyors information about these activities and nursing home quality.

To ensure public and expert involvement in running their programs, the CMS maintains a number of chartered advisory committees. These committees, whose meetings are open to the public, provide advice or make recommendations on a variety of issues relating to CMS's responsibilities and activities.

Medicaid

Medicaid provides health benefits to low-income or indigent persons of all ages. Often, eligibility for Medicaid is based on a patient's eligibility for other state programs, such as welfare assistance. Medicaid is governed by both federal and state statutes and rules and then implemented on a state and local level. Although the federal government stipulates the minimum health care coverage, states can provide coverage beyond the minimum. Therefore, Medicaid eligibility and benefits vary from state to state. At a minimum, Medicaid provides 100% coverage for the following:

- Inpatient hospital care
- Outpatient treatment and services
- Diagnostic services
- Family planning
- Skilled nursing facilities
- Diagnostic screenings for children

Many states use a managed care type of Medicaid coverage in which recipients make a co-payment based on their income and are assigned a primary care physician as a "gatekeeper."

Since circumstances that make recipients eligible for coverage change from month to month (i.e.,

employment), Medicaid patients receive a new ID card each month. Make a photocopy of the card for the patient's file on the first visit of each month. Most states have online eligibility and authorization verification capabilities. Because reimbursement is considerably less than other insurances, not all physicians accept Medicaid patients, nor are they required to do so. If Medicaid patients are accepted, you need to be familiar with Medicaid as administered in your state.

CHECKPOINT QUESTION

3. List six types of medical expenses that are covered at 100% by Medicaid.

AFF WHAT IF?

What if a patient comes in to see the physician but does not have her Medicaid card?

Most states offer Medicaid providers the ability to verify eligibility on any given date of service online. By searching for the Department of Human Services on the Web in almost any city, you can be directed to this feature. This is especially helpful since Medicaid eligibility is managed on a monthly basis, and sometimes patients will not receive their cards before the first day of a new month. Before this capability existed, many times patients were sent away if they did not have their cards with them. As long as you have an ID number or Social Security number, you can verify eligibility instantly.

TRICARE/CHAMPVA

TRICARE is administered by the U.S. Department of Defense and provides medical coverage for dependents of active service personnel, dependents of service personnel who died during active duty, and retired service personnel. When Congress realized that CHAMPUS costs could be controlled with managed care, they mandated that HMOs and PPOs (discussed later in this chapter) be added to the coverage. This three-part system is now called TRICARE. This system requires that participants be assigned a primary care manager (PCM). The PCM is named on the beneficiary's card.

If a patient lives within 40 miles of a uniformed services hospital and that facility is unable to handle the needs of patients covered by TRICARE, a statement of unavailability is required for treatment by a physician's office or civilian hospital. Patients who live more than 40 miles from a uniformed services hospital do not need this statement to be treated in a physician's office or civilian hospital and for the physician or hospital to be reimbursed.

The Civilian Health and Medical Program of the Veterans Administration (CHAMPVA) covers dependents of veterans who have total and permanent service-connected disabilities. CHAMPVA is administered by the area Veterans Administration hospital. Once admitted to the CHAMPVA program, patients select their own physician; this allows them the same benefits as private insurance.

COG Managed Care

Health care costs in the United States have grown at about twice the general rate of inflation. As a result, the United States now spends more for health care services than any other industrialized nation, both as a percentage of gross national product and per person. In the United States, most people obtain health coverage through their employer. The exceptions are Medicare for the elderly, TRICARE for retired military personnel and their dependents, Medicaid for low-income Americans, and those who buy their own health insurance.

The rapid rate of health care inflation encouraged employers to begin offering **managed care** programs, which are typically less costly than traditional insurance coverage systems. Managed care programs vary greatly, but all involve a different relationship between the insurer, health care provider, and covered individual from that of traditional insurance programs. To understand this difference, we first discuss the traditional insurance system.

In traditional insurance systems, the covered patient may seek care from any provider. Normally, the patient and physician decide what care is needed. Then, services are rendered, and the insurer pays a portion of the provider's bills (after deductibles and coinsurance). The insurer has no relationship with the provider.

In managed care systems, however, the insurer has a contractual relationship with the provider. The contract usually establishes what prices will be charged for each service and the conditions under which a service would be covered. Most managed care programs contain the following elements:

- *Precertification of hospital admissions* (often also called *utilization management [UM]* or **utilization review [UR]**). A patient can be admitted to a hospital for certain conditions only if that admission has been certified (approved) by the insurer. The goal of this requirement is to ensure that a patient's care is provided in the most cost-effective setting. For example, many surgical procedures that used to require an inpatient hospital stay can now be performed in an outpatient setting if proper education and support are available to the patient. Conflict between a UR guideline and the physician's requirements for the patient can be appealed

to an impartial **peer review organization** composed of physicians and specialists who will review the case and make the final recommendation.

- *Approved referrals.* As discussed in Chapter 6, in many managed care plans, a specialty physician can provide services to a managed care patient only on referral from the patient's primary care physician. The purpose is to ensure that the services provided by the specialist are medically necessary and, again, provided in the most cost-effective setting. Payment of a claim depends on the completion of the appropriate form.

- *Network.* A network consists of providers (physicians, hospitals, pharmacies, and other providers and suppliers) who have signed contracts with the insurer or **health maintenance organization (HMO)** to provide services to covered persons in individual, group, or public health plans. A patient is normally required to use network providers to receive full coverage. The financial penalties (lost coverage) are often very high if a patient does not use these providers.

- *Assignment of benefits.* By contract, the network provider cannot bill the patient for any amounts not paid by the insurer (no **balance billing**) except for co-payments, coinsurance, and deductibles. If payment for a service provided by a network physician or hospital is denied by the insurer because it was not properly authorized, the provider cannot bill the patient for these services unless the contract does not contain a hold-harmless clause for the patient. This puts teeth in the control features of the managed care program.

Most physicians have contracts with more than one managed care program, and each of these programs has its own requirements and reimbursement schedules. So that the physician can provide the patient with needed health care services, while ensuring that the physician is paid for his or her services, it is necessary to consider the requirements of each patient's program. UM or precertification requirements are extremely important. Check the patient's ID card for details (see Fig. 13-1). UM requirements may apply to inpatient services or to a variety of outpatient and doctor office services.

Until you are very familiar with the requirements of each of your patient's managed care programs, you should call the number on the ID card before a patient is admitted to a hospital (on a nonemergency basis), referred to another physician, or scheduled for specific laboratory, radiologic, or other tests or evaluations. For inpatient admissions, the UM firm may ask for the diagnosis, the procedure or procedures to be performed, and other related information before approving the admission. Once the procedure is approved, the UM firm may only approve a specified length of stay in the hospital. Failure to comply with the precertification requirements results in a financial penalty for the patient and possibly also for the physician and the hospital.

It is important to be familiar with physicians within the network. The physician, hospital, laboratory, or other provider you normally refer a patient to may not be in the patient's managed care network. By calling the UM number to check, you can avoid penalties and improve the satisfaction of the patient with your services. Many times, these requirements can be met electronically as companies improve their technology.

 CHECKPOINT QUESTION

4. What are the four key elements of a managed care program?

Health Maintenance Organizations

It is easiest to understand how an HMO functions if we contrast it with a traditional health insurance program. In the traditional insurance system, the relationship between the covered individual and the insurer or self-insurer is purely financial. In return for receiving a paid monthly premium, the insurer promises to reimburse (indemnify) the individual if he or she incurs certain types of covered medical expense. There are often limits to coverage (exclusions and limitations), and normally, the coverage has a deductible (amount below which services are not reimbursable) and **coinsurance** (the patient pays a percentage of the medical expense after the deductible is satisfied). For example, the patient pays the first $200 (deductible) in physician charges each year starting January 1; then insurance pays 80% of covered charges, and the patient must pay the other 20%.

The covered individual seeks medical services and thereby incurs an expense. The individual, not the insurer, must pay for this expense. If the medical treatment is covered as defined in the insurance policy, the insurer will reimburse the patient a portion of the amount incurred after deductibles and coinsurance.

In contrast to traditional insurance companies, an HMO promises to provide covered services rather than pay for them. In this respect, the HMO acts as both an insurer and a provider of service. HMO policies are written differently from insurance policies. The HMO policy lists the medical services that the member is entitled to receive and the physicians and hospitals that will provide these services. The HMO has a contract with both the patient and provider. It must provide covered services to the member either directly from its own physician staff and hospitals or indirectly from physicians and hospitals contracted to provide the services promised to the member. The HMO, rather than the patient, is responsible for the costs of medical services, and providers bill the HMO rather than the patient when a reimbursable service is rendered to an HMO member.

This is one reason HMOs do not normally use deductibles and coinsurance, which are standard features of health insurance programs. A patient does not receive a provider's bill, so deductibles and coinsurance cannot apply. Instead, HMOs use predetermined **co-payments** (e.g., $10 per physician office visit) to reduce premium prices.

HMOs come in many forms. An HMO contracts with employers to cover their employees. The medical group and hospitals contract with the health plan to provide the services required in the health plan's contract with employers. Rather than paying for these services on a **fee-for-service** basis, a company pays the physicians per employee. Consistent with its history, the health plan does not pay the medical group a fee for each service provided. Instead, it pays each party based on the number of members enrolled in the health plan. This is often called **capitation** because there is one payment per member. Capitation payments are also used by other types of HMOs.

As group model HMOs developed (they were called prepaid group practices until 1973 federal legislation changed their names), nongroup physicians organized into an entity called an **independent practice association (IPA)**. The early IPA HMOs were often sponsored by a local medical society and were developed to allow independent physicians to compete with prepaid group practices.

IPA HMOs contract with employers in the same manner as group model HMOs, and their members receive covered services from IPA physicians. The HMO's contracts with physicians are different, however, because these physicians are not organized into a single multi-specialty group practice. IPA physicians are paid in a number of ways. Some are paid on a capitation basis, and some may be paid on a fee-for-service basis using a **fee schedule** established by the HMO. Often, a portion of any reimbursement is withheld by the HMO and paid only if the HMO's total medical expense is within budget; this encourages the physician to be cost conscious in caring for patients.

In some of these HMOs, the IPA is a separate corporation, often owned by physicians. With this structure (still called an IPA HMO), the IPA contracts with physicians, and the HMO contracts with the IPA instead of directly with each physician.

Over the years, HMOs have continued to evolve, and many are now a mixture of these discussed models. As a medical assistant, you must know what type of relationship the practice has with an HMO before you can determine how the practice is reimbursed. Most HMOs require claims to be submitted even if payment is capitation rather than fee-for-service. Many HMOs also require the collection and transmission of other patient information, which is not required in the traditional insurance industry. Of course, this information is provided with the patient's permission.

CHECKPOINT QUESTION

5. How does an HMO differ from a traditional health insurance program?

 PATIENT EDUCATION

HELP PATIENTS UNDERSTAND THEIR OBLIGATION

As discussed in Chapter 2, the contract between a physician and his patient implies that the *patient* will pay the physician for his services, not the patient's insurance company. When a physician participates with an insurance company, he may be required to file a patient's claims, but this is not the case with all third-party payers. Although patients have the ultimate responsibility of paying the physician, they tend to think that a physician should wait for their insurance to pay. A physician who does not choose to participate with a particular third-party payer is not obligated to extend credit to a patient. Of course, most practices choose to offer filing the patient's claim as a courtesy. Because of the nature of a physician's work, most physicians are willing to make reasonable credit arrangements, but patients should understand that their physician is not legally obligated to file their claims or extend credit.

Understanding the claims filing process will give patients the opportunity to take a more active role in their physician's reimbursement. Direct patients to their insurance company's Web site, keep abreast of changes, and be willing to discuss these matters openly. Help patients understand their obligations to the physician and their insurance company's obligations to them. This approach will not only benefit the patients, but will also improve your collection ratio.

Preferred Provider Organizations

Whereas HMOs promise to provide services and have a financial risk in their relationships with subscribers, a **preferred provider organization (PPO)** is a type of health benefit program whose purpose is simply to contract with providers and then lease this network of contracted providers to health care plans. The PPO network is not risk bearing; it does not have any financial involvement in the health plan. PPOs are typically developed by hospitals and physicians as a vehicle to attract patients, although some are developed and managed by insurance **carriers**.

PPOs contract with participating providers, including hospitals and physicians. These contracts allow the PPO to contract with insurers and other purchasers of health care services on behalf of the participating providers, who typically accept less than their normal charges and agree to follow the UM and other administrative protocols as specified by the PPO.

Typically, a health plan with a PPO offers benefits at two levels, commonly referred to as in network and out of network. Unlike in an HMO, patients may visit any provider they wish for services. If the provider is in network (a participating provider), the levels of benefit for the patient are greater than if the patient receives services from an out-of-network (nonparticipating) provider.

A typical health plan with a PPO may look like the breakdown shown in Figure 13-2.

As you can see from the example, each time the patient sees an in-network provider, he or she receives significantly better benefits. A primary difference between an HMO and PPO, therefore, is that patients can see any physician of their choice and receive benefits; they simply have an incentive in the form of higher benefits when they see an in-network provider.

As part of your responsibilities, you should identify the PPOs with which the physician has contracted and determine the administrative requirements set forth by each PPO in the contract. To understand the necessary administrative procedures agreed to by the physician, review all managed care contracts carefully. Also be aware that most PPOs have a provider relations representative who works with the contracted providers (physicians) to answer questions and clarify procedures. The PPO is typically operated by a group of hospitals or physicians or by an insurance company or independent organization. Physicians agree to participate in PPOs to serve their existing patients who now have PPO plans and sometimes to gain additional patients who seek the services of a PPO physician.

Participating physicians have agreed to perform certain administrative services for PPO patients. Commonly, the physician's office must accept assignment of benefits and provide claims filing services for the patient. The physician agrees to accept the reimbursement by the claims administrator as payment in full and agrees not to bill the patient for any difference between the physician's usual charge and the PPO-negotiated charge for

Example of a Health Plan with a PPO		
Benefit	In-network	Out-of-network
Deductible	$100	$300
Coinsurance	90%	70%
Routine care	$200 per calendar year	-0-
Mental health	80%	50%
Office visit	$10 co-pay; no deductible	70%

Figure 13-2 A health plan with a PPO.

PLEASE
DO NOT
STAPLE
IN THIS
AREA

CARRIER

	PICA	**HEALTH INSURANCE CLAIM FORM**	PICA	

1. MEDICARE	MEDICAID	CHAMPUS	CHAMPVA	GROUP HEALTH PLAN	FECA BLK LUNG	OTHER	1a. INSURED'S I.D. NUMBER	(FOR PROGRAM IN ITEM 1)
(Medicare #)	(Medicaid #)	(Sponsor's SSN)	(VA File #)	(SSN or ID)	(SSN)	(ID)		

2. PATIENT'S NAME (Last Name, First Name, Middle Initial)

3. PATIENT'S BIRTH DATE MM | DD | YY   SEX   M   F

4. INSURED'S NAME (Last Name, First Name, Middle Initial)

5. PATIENT'S ADDRESS (No., Street)

6. PATIENT RELATIONSHIP TO INSURED   Self   Spouse   Child   Other

7. INSURED'S ADDRESS (No., Street)

CITY   STATE

8. PATIENT STATUS   Single   Married   Other

CITY   STATE

ZIP CODE   TELEPHONE (Include Area Code) ( )

Employed   Full-Time Student   Part-Time Student

ZIP CODE   TELEPHONE (INCLUDE AREA CODE) ( )

9. OTHER INSURED'S NAME (Last Name, First Name, Middle Initial)

10. IS PATIENT'S CONDITION RELATED TO:

11. INSURED'S POLICY GROUP OR FECA NUMBER

a. OTHER INSURED'S POLICY OR GROUP NUMBER

a. EMPLOYMENT? (CURRENT OR PREVIOUS)   YES   NO

a. INSURED'S DATE OF BIRTH MM | DD | YY   SEX   M   F

b. OTHER INSURED'S DATE OF BIRTH MM | DD | YY   SEX   M   F

b. AUTO ACCIDENT?   PLACE (State)   YES   NO

b. EMPLOYER'S NAME OR SCHOOL NAME

c. EMPLOYER'S NAME OR SCHOOL NAME

c. OTHER ACCIDENT?   YES   NO

c. INSURANCE PLAN NAME OR PROGRAM NAME

d. INSURANCE PLAN NAME OR PROGRAM NAME

10d. RESERVED FOR LOCAL USE

d. IS THERE ANOTHER HEALTH BENEFIT PLAN?   YES   NO   *If yes*, return to and complete item 9 a-d.

READ BACK OF FORM BEFORE COMPLETING & SIGNING THIS FORM.
12. PATIENT'S OR AUTHORIZED PERSON'S SIGNATURE I authorize the release of any medical or other information necessary to process this claim. I also request payment of government benefits either to myself or to the party who accepts assignment below.

SIGNED _____   DATE _____

13. INSURED'S OR AUTHORIZED PERSON'S SIGNATURE I authorize payment of medical benefits to the undersigned physician or supplier for services described below.

SIGNED _____

PATIENT AND INSURED INFORMATION

14. DATE OF CURRENT: MM | DD | YY   ILLNESS (First symptom) OR INJURY (Accident) OR PREGNANCY(LMP)

15. IF PATIENT HAS HAD SAME OR SIMILAR ILLNESS. GIVE FIRST DATE MM | DD | YY

16. DATES PATIENT UNABLE TO WORK IN CURRENT OCCUPATION FROM MM | DD | YY   TO MM | DD | YY

17. NAME OF REFERRING PHYSICIAN OR OTHER SOURCE

17a. I.D. NUMBER OF REFERRING PHYSICIAN

18. HOSPITALIZATION DATES RELATED TO CURRENT SERVICES FROM MM | DD | YY   TO MM | DD | YY

19. RESERVED FOR LOCAL USE

20. OUTSIDE LAB?   YES   NO $ CHARGES

21. DIAGNOSIS OR NATURE OF ILLNESS OR INJURY. (RELATE ITEMS 1,2,3 OR 4 TO ITEM 24E BY LINE)

1. |___.__   3. |___.__
2. |___.__   4. |___.__

22. MEDICAID RESUBMISSION CODE   ORIGINAL REF. NO.

23. PRIOR AUTHORIZATION NUMBER

24. A DATE(S) OF SERVICE From / To MM DD YY MM DD YY	B Place of Service	C Type of Service	D PROCEDURES, SERVICES, OR SUPPLIES (Explain Unusual Circumstances) CPT/HCPCS	MODIFIER	E DIAGNOSIS CODE	F $ CHARGES	G DAYS OR UNITS	H EPSDT Family Plan	I EMG	J COB	K RESERVED FOR LOCAL USE
1											
2											
3											
4											
5											
6											

25. FEDERAL TAX I.D. NUMBER   SSN   EIN

26. PATIENT'S ACCOUNT NO.

27. ACCEPT ASSIGNMENT? (For govt. claims, see back)   YES   NO

28. TOTAL CHARGE $

29. AMOUNT PAID $

30. BALANCE DUE $

31. SIGNATURE OF PHYSICIAN OR SUPPLIER INCLUDING DEGREES OR CREDENTIALS (I certify that the statements on the reverse apply to this bill and are made a part thereof.)

SIGNED _____   DATE _____

32. NAME AND ADDRESS OF FACILITY WHERE SERVICES WERE RENDERED (If other than home or office)

33. PHYSICIAN'S, SUPPLIER'S BILLING NAME, ADDRESS, ZIP CODE & PHONE #

PIN#   GRP#

PHYSICIAN OR SUPPLIER INFORMATION

(APPROVED BY AMA COUNCIL ON MEDICAL SERVICE 8/88)   ***PLEASE PRINT OR TYPE***   APPROVED OMB-0938-0008 FORM CMS-1500 (12-90),   FORM RRB-1500,
APPROVED OMB-1215-0055 FORM OWCP-1500,   APPROVED OMB-0720-0001 (CHAMPUS)

Figure 13-3 CMS-1500 claim form. This is known as the *universal claim form.*

TABLE **13-1**	Frequent Causes for Claim Denial and Corrective Actions
Causes for Claim Denial	**Corrective Actions**
The patient cannot be identified as a covered person.	Confirm that coverage information on file is current, including insurance company and group number, and that the Social Security number is accurate.
Coding is deemed inappropriate necessary.	Review provided services and recode as for services provided.
The patient is no longer covered by the plan.	Bill the patient for the charges. The patient may provide confirmation of new coverage.
The data are incomplete.	Complete the required data and resubmit the claim. Flag it as a resubmission.
Services are not covered by the plan.	Bill the patient for the charges unless there is a basis for an appeal.

AFF LEGAL TIP

SIGNATURE ON FILE

Keeping patient information confidential is a primary concern in all medical practices. To adhere to HIPAA's regulations, you should not release any information about the patient to any party, including the claims administrator, without the written authorization of the patient or the patient's guardian. Obtain a written authorization to release information to the patient's insurance company from each patient on his or her first visit to the practice. Keep this signature in the patient's file. Any claims submitted by the physician's office should have "signature on file" on the claim form. A new authorization should be signed at the beginning of each year. This written authorization for the release of information only pertains to the insurance company specified. Only such information as is pertinent to the claim and necessary for the processing of that claim should be released. Releasing any patient information without written consent is a breach of confidentiality and a HIPAA violation.

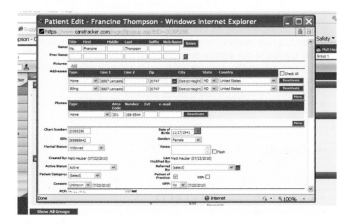

Figure 13-4 Screen shot of insurance information "form" in an electronic version. Courtesy of Ingenix® CareTracker™.

COG Reimbursement

Diagnosis-Related Groups

In Chapter 15, you will learn to assign diagnosis codes. The diagnosis code is provided to a third-party payer to tell them why a service or procedure was provided. **Diagnosis-related groups (DRGs)** categorize inpatients according to the similarity of their diagnoses, treatments, and length of hospital stays. Initially, these categories were developed by researchers at Yale University in the mid-1970s to aid the process of UR. Some 13,000 codes were run through a computer and grouped according to their clinical similarities (including similarities in resources used). Today, DRGs are used to determine reimbursement for Medicare patients' inpatient services. The fee attached to each DRG is based on the national average of all Medicare charges and is adjusted for regional differences in hospital wages and updates. Hospitals are paid a set amount for each DRG regardless of actual costs for treating the patient. For example, if a hospital uses fewer resources to care for a patient and discharges that patient in less time, it may keep the difference between its actual cost and the DRG payment. Conversely, if the patient stays longer than usual and requires more services, the hospital absorbs the loss. A patient who has an unusually long stay or a complicated case is considered an *outlier*, and the hospital may be paid more than the standard DRG rate if the added expenses can be justified. The hospital coder uses ICD-9-CM codes to pick the appropriate DRG. The more information the hospital has prior to admission, the more accurate the coding; for example, for a patient admitted with chest pain, the hospital coder needs to know that the patient also has hypertension and diabetes.

You may be asked to schedule a patient for admission to the hospital. Assigning the correct ICD-9-CM code from the outpatient practice will influence the DRG to which the patient will be assigned. The hospital coder selects the proper DRG based on these factors:

- Principal diagnosis
- Surgeries
- Complications and comorbid conditions

Explanation of Benefits

Employee Name:　Joe Doe
SSN: 555-55-5555　(1)
Group No. 55555
Patient Name: Joe Doe

Date of Service: 6-15-2013
Provider: Dr. Jones
Provider TIN: 35-5555555

Date of Service (2)	Comment Code (3)	Amount of Charge (4)	Amount Allowed (5)	At (6)	Amount Paid (7)
6-15-2009	57	87.00	82.00	80%	65.60
			Total (8)		65.60
			Less Deductible (9)		25.00
			Amount Paid (10)		40.60

Payable to:　　Dr. Jones
　　　　　　　　Address

Comment Code:
57 - The amount charged exceeds Usual and Customary

Figure 13-5 Explanation of benefits.

Reading the EOB (Explanation of Benefits)

After the claim has been processed, an EOB will be issued. Although each payer has his or her own EOB format, this sample EOB illustrates the key points included in an EOB. The terms used may differ, and the formats differ widely.

1. The top section typically includes the name of the employee and the Social Security number (SSN) or other identifying number, as well as the name of the patient, the group number, the date of service and provider name, and employer identification number (EIN) (Federal identification number assigned to the physician).

2. The date of service is included and is shown as the date the service is actually rendered, not the date that was posted or billed.

3. The Comment Code is a tool used on many EOBs to indicate a coded comment that is on the bottom as exceeding "Usual and Customary." In this situation, the claim will be processed on the Usual and Customary amount. The difference between the amount charged ($87.00) and the amount allowed ($82.00) is $5.00. Unless the physician is contractually bound by an agreement with a managed care plan that forbids the practice of balance billing, that difference of $5.00 may be billed to the patient.

4. Amount of Charge shows the amount that the physician's office billed for the service.

5. Amount Allowed shows the amount of charge upon which the claim processing will be based (in this example, it is the amount of Usual and Customary).

6. This indicates the percentage of co-insurance payable by the plan.

7. Amount Paid shows the amount payable by the plan after co-insurance has been applied, but is not necessarily the amount that is actually paid (see #10).

8. The Total shows the total submitted and payable after the claim has been processed.

9. After all processing on the claim has been completed, any deductible is applied. In this example, Joe still had $25.00 to be applied to his annual deductible. Therefore, $25.00 is deducted from the amount paid and the actual reimbursement to the physician is $40.60. The amount applied to the deductible should be billed to the patient.

10. The amount actually reimbursed.

Physicians can help with coding in the following ways:

- Record the appropriate documentation to identify each patient's problems, complaints, or other reasons for the encounter or visit.
- Work with the medical records or the office coding and billing staffs to determine the proper diagnosis to code, using terminology that includes specific diagnoses, symptoms, problems, or reasons for the encounter (ICD-9-CM codes describe all of these).

AFF ETHICAL TIP

When a Provider is Unethical

The following scenario may occur in a medical office:

While you are filing an insurance claim, the physician tells you to "adjust" the laceration length from 4 cm to 9 cm. (The physician can bill more for a 9-cm laceration.) When you question him about this, he says, "Don't worry. The patient isn't paying the difference, the insurance company is, and they have plenty of money."

How should you handle this situation?

Ethically and legally, you cannot change the length of a laceration on the medical record or the bill. This is fraud. You must explain to the physician that you are uncomfortable with this request and that you are ethically and legally bound to truthful billing. Any requests to alter or misrepresent the medical records or claims of a patient must be firmly denied.

A physician who operates in an unethical manner should be reported. If he or she is a partner in a practice, alert the other physicians about the suspect actions. You can also contact your state medical association, the American Medical Association, or the institutional review board at the hospital where your physician is affiliated.

Resource-Based Relative Value Scale

As part of the 1989 Omnibus Budget Reconciliation Act (OBRA), the U.S. Congress stipulated that reimbursement to physicians for Medicare services is based on a fee schedule. This fee schedule sets a maximal fee for each service with the **resource-based relative value scale (RBRVS)**. The goal of RBRVS is to reduce Medicare Part B costs and to establish national standards for payment based on CPT-4 codes. (Remember, Part B of Medicare covers physicians' services; Part A covers hospital expenses.)

Fee calculations are based on the following factors:

- Intensity of the service
- Time required
- Skills needed
- Overhead expenses
- Malpractice premiums

The particular fee is adjusted by a geographical practice cost index (GPCI), which reflects the difference in health care costs in different parts of the country. This determines the relative value unit (RVU). Finally, a national conversion factor is assigned yearly. The formula looks like this: CPT code 99205 has an RVU of 4.58, and the national conversion factor is 36.7856. The Medicare allowed charge would be $168.48. RVU × national conversion factor = Medicare allowed amount.

 CHECKPOINT QUESTION

7. Why are DRGs used?

COG Policies in the Practice

Managed care contracts and negotiated services affect many practice policies. You must be knowledgeable and precise in administering practice policies, especially with regard to assignment of benefits and balance billing.

Assignment of benefits is a service the practice may provide. If assignment of benefits is accepted, the patient's signature must be on file, authorizing the claims administrator to reimburse the physician. Managed care plans require physicians to accept assignment, although many physicians do not accept assignment for non–managed care patients. If assignment is not accepted, the patient is responsible for paying all charges and filing a claim with the claims administrator for reimbursement directly to the patient.

Balance billing is prohibited by most managed care contracts. The physician cannot charge the patient the difference between the physician's usual charge and the allowable charge specified by the contract. For other types of plans, however, balance billing is not restricted, and the practice may bill the patient for any difference between the physician's charged fee and the amount allowable by the plan according to **usual, customary, and reasonable (UCR)** tables.

A few national firms provide UCR data to claims administrators who use that information to determine the maximum amount payable for any given service (the **plan maximum**). UCR data are calculated from surveys of the amount physicians charge for each service or procedure. That amount is calculated on a geographic basis to reflect regional variations in health care costs. Non–managed care plan physician reimbursements are based on a maximum allowable charge as specified in the UCR data. The physician may choose to bill the patient for the difference between the amount charged and the UCR amount.

español SPANISH TERMINOLOGY

¿Tiene usted seguro médico?
Do you have medical insurance?

¿Cuál es el nombre del seguro?
What is the name of the insurance?

¿Cuál es el número de su póliza?
What is the number of your policy?

¿Cubre el hospital?
Will it pay for the hospital?

¿Tiene Medicare?
Do you have Medicare?

¿Tiene su tarjeta de Medicare?
Do you have your Medicare card?

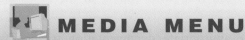

MEDIA MENU

- Student Resources on thePoint
  - CMA/RMA Certification Exam Review
- Internet Resources

Centers for Medicare and Medicaid Services
http://www.cms.gov

Medicare for Recipients
http://www.Medicare.gov

BlueCross BlueShield Association
http://www.bluecares.com

Local Medical Review Policies
http://www.lmrpdata.com

American Medical Association
http://www.ama-assn.org

All Government Agencies, Federal and State
http://www.usa.gov

PSY PROCEDURE 13-1: ## Completing a CMS-1500 Claim Form

Purpose: To ensure competency in completing a CMS-1500 claim form accurately and completely using managed care policies and procedures and third-party guidelines

Equipment: Case scenario, completed encounter form, blank CMS-1500 claim form, pen

Scenario: Naomi A. Dishman is an established leukemia patient who was seen in your office on June 20, 2008, 30 minutes after falling down the steps of her home. She is complaining of pain and swelling in her right ankle. Her charges and codes for the visit are: Established Patient Office Visit Level III (99213) and x-ray, right ankle, two views (73600). Her diagnosis is listed as ankle sprain.

Steps	Purpose
1. Using the information provided in Figure 14-5, complete the demographic information in lines 1 through 11d.	This section includes vital information to identify the policyholder and start the process of paying the claim.
2. Insert "SOF" (signature on file) on lines 12 and 13. Check to be sure there is a current signature on file in the chart and that it is specifically for the third-party payer being filed.	It is fraudulent to say there is a signature on file if there is not one in the chart. Patients should sign a separate authorization for each recipient of their information. If there is no SOF, you must call the patient to come in and sign one or mail them a form to be signed and sent back.
3. If the services being filed are for a hospital stay, insert information in lines 16, 18, and 32.	These fields are used for hospital services only.
4. If the services are related to an injury, insert the date of the accident in line 14.	If the date of accident field is not completed and an ICD-9 code for an injury is used, the payer's computer system will reject the claim.
5. Insert dates of service. Each line may be a different date of service.	You must be accurate with the dates of service.
6. Using the encounter form, place the CPT code listed for each service and procedure checked off in column D of lines 21–24 on the form.	The codes on the encounter form are current and accurate because the form has been reviewed before using any revised or new codes every January.
7. List the reason for the encounter on line 21.1 and any other diagnoses listed on the encounter form that relate to or affect the services or procedures.	All diagnoses or concurrent conditions that will affect the current treatment should be communicated to the third-party payer. For example, diabetes should be listed for a podiatric service.
8. Reference the codes placed in lines 21 (1–4) to each line listing a different CPT code by placing the corresponding one digit in line 24, column E.	Each line that lists a CPT code must also list a reason for that particular service or procedure. This reason will justify the medical necessity of the service or procedure.
9. **AFF** You notice that Ms. Dishman has no signature on file, but the box on line 12 of her claim form says she does. Explain how you would respond.	Correct the error immediately. Do not file the claim until the signed form is in her record. Mail the patient an authorization with a self-addressed, stamped envelope and a letter explaining that you need this for her record. You could also flag her account with a note to obtain a signed authorization at her next visit.

- Most patients in the physician's office have some type of health care plan.
- Types of plans include group, individual, and government-sponsored health benefits, such as Medicare or Medicaid.
- Many physicians have contracts with managed care plans, such as HMOs and PPOs.
- Each type of plan has certain requirements regarding eligibility and claims submission, and you must be knowledgeable about those requirements.

- In particular, one of your primary duties is to file claims in a timely and accurate manner to ensure appropriate reimbursement for the physician.
- When filing claims, you must be careful to maintain patient confidentiality and to avoid fraud.

Warm Ups for Critical Thinking

1. Jane and Joe are married, and both are employed and cover themselves and their two children on their health plans. Jane's birthday is July 23, and Joe's birthday is August 9. Joe is 2 years older than Jane. When claims are submitted for their two children, which spouse's plan is primary? Show which plan is primary and secondary for each family member.

	Primary	Secondary
Jane		
Joe		
Child 1		
Child 2		

2. The requirements for Medicaid vary from state to state. How do you determine the Medicaid requirements for your particular state? Locate the name, address, and telephone number of your state's resource.

3. As discussed in Chapter 8, HIPAA requires certain procedures and practices when transmitting insurance claims electronically. Search the HIPAA law for these guidelines and create a procedure for ensuring compliance regarding electronic claims filing. You can find this information by going to http://www.hhs.gov/news/press/2002pres/hipaa.html.

   See also Appendix A for excerpts from HIPAA's Administrative Simplification section.

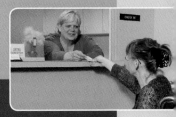

14

Diagnostic Coding

Outline

Learning Outcomes

Cognitive Domain

*Note: AAMA/CAAHEP 2008 Standards are
italicized.*

1. Spell and define the key terms
2. Describe the relationship between coding
   and reimbursement
3. Name and describe the coding system used
   to describe diseases, injuries, and other reasons for encounters with a medical provider
4. Explain the format of the ICD-9-CM
5. Give four examples of ways E codes are
   used
6. *Describe how to use the most current
   diagnostic coding classification system*
7. Describe the ICD-10-CM/PCS version and its
   differences from ICD-9

Psychomotor Domain

*Note: AAMA/CAAHEP 2008 Standards are
italicized.*

1. *Perform diagnostic coding* (Procedure 14-1)
2. *Apply third-party guidelines*

Affective Domain

*Note: AAMA/CAAHEP 2008 Standards are
italicized.*

1. *Work with physician to achieve the
   maximum reimbursement*

ABHES Competencies

1. Apply third-party guidelines
2. Perform diagnostic and procedural coding
3. Comply with federal, state, and local health
   laws and regulations

advance beneficiary
notice (ABN)
audit
conventions
cross-reference
E-codes

eponym
etiology
inpatient
International
Classification of
Diseases, Ninth

Revision, Clinical
Modification
(ICD-9-CM)
late effects
main terms
medical necessity

outpatient
primary diagnosis
service
specificity
V-codes

Coding, at its simplest, is the assignment of a number to a verbal statement or description. Medical coding is anything but simple. The **International Classification of Diseases, Ninth Revision, Clinical Modification (ICD-9-CM)** is a system for transforming verbal descriptions of disease, injuries, conditions, and procedures into numeric codes. The Centers for Medicare and Medicaid Services (CMS) has mandated that all physicians must begin using ICD-10-CM/PCS by October 1, 2013. It is essential that the physician and medical assistant work together to achieve accurate documentation, code assignment, and reporting of diagnoses and procedures. Use of standardized codes makes it easier for third-party payers to understand the reason for the patient's encounter with the health care provider and increases the likelihood of timely processing of claims and prompt payment when appropriate.

Coding is a way to standardize medical information for purposes such as collecting health care statistics, performing a medical care review, and indexing medical records. It is also used for health insurance claims processing (see Chapter 13). Because coding is the basis for reimbursement, it is imperative that you code patient visits accurately and precisely. Incorrect, insufficient, or incomplete coding on claims forms can lead to nonpayment for the physician as well as incorrect information in the insurance companies' databases, which may affect the patients' insurability. For example, if a patient complaining of chest pain is coded as having "acute myocardial infarction" instead of "chest pain," that patient may be incorrectly labeled as having heart disease. The Current Procedural Terminology (CPT) codes, which are used to report services and procedures performed by health care providers, determine the amount paid (see Chapter 15), but the code assigned to the diagnosis or reason for the service or procedure proves the medical necessity for the services or procedures so that claims are paid. The third-party payer needs to know why the service was performed to assess **medical necessity**. Medical necessity means the procedure or service would have been performed by any reasonable physician under the same or similar circumstances. The ICD-9 and ICD-10 diagnostic codes convey this information. Is a chest radiograph medically necessary for a patient who has gout? No, but it may be necessary for a patient with acute bronchitis. The diagnosis justifies the procedure.

Since Medicare considers certain procedures medically necessary only at certain intervals, having the patient sign an **advance beneficiary notice (ABN)** will ensure payment of treatments and procedures that will likely be denied by Medicare. An example is a Pap smear for a low-risk woman, which will be paid for once every 2 years. If the physician considers it *not* to be medically necessary, but the patient wants a Pap test, the patient will be responsible for payment and must sign an ABN.

CHECKPOINT QUESTION

1. What is meant by medical necessity?

COG Diagnostic Coding

The ICD-9-CM is a statistical classification system based on the ICD-9, developed by the World Health Organization (WHO). The CM, which stands for *clinical modification*, addresses the intent of these codes to describe the clinical picture of the patient. These codes are much more precise than those needed for statistical grouping and trend analysis found in the ICD-9 and used in hospital coding.

The new ICD-10-CM/PCS classification system provides significant improvements over ICD-9 with more detailed and current information. The new system will provide for expansion as new technologies are implemented. The new coding system consists of two parts: ICD-10-CM and ICD-10-PCS, which is used for hospital or inpatient coding.

The ICD-9-CM, which is now mandated by the Health Insurance Portability and Accountability Act of 1996 (HIPAA), is the most comprehensive statistical classification of its kind. Containing more than

10,000 diagnostic codes and 1,000 procedure codes, it consists of three volumes:

- Volume 1: Tabular List of Diseases
- Volume 2: Alphabetic Index of Diseases
- Volume 3: Tabular List and Alphabetic Index of Procedures

The ICD-9-CM code books are available from several publishers, and although the presentation of the material may be different, the content must be the same. Depending on the publisher, these three volumes may be included within one book. In the physician's office, only Volumes 1 and 2 are used. Volume 3 is used by hospitals.

The diagnostic classification systems in Volumes 1 and 2 are maintained by a federal government agency, the National Center for Health Statistics (NCHS); the procedure classification (Volume 3) is maintained by the CMS, the federal agency that regulates health care financing. All three volumes are updated regularly, with codes being added, revised, and sometimes deleted. Changes in the ICD-9-CM are published by NCHS and CMS with the approval of WHO. Both the American Health Information Management Association (AHIMA) and the American Hospital Association (AHA) advise and assist in keeping the classification system current.

 CHECKPOINT QUESTION

2. What organization must approve any changes in the disease classification system?

 AFF LEGAL TIP

DOES EVERYONE NEED TO KNOW?

Remember that the ICD-9 codes placed on the CMS-1500 are confidential and should be protected as much as any other medical information. Forms left lying in common areas in the office may be seen by other patients. Keep printers and copies of these forms in a private place, and share the diagnosis codes only with those who need the information to carry out their duties. Patients have the right to keep their diagnoses private.

Inpatient Versus Outpatient Coding

There is a big difference between coding medical claims in a hospital or other inpatient facility and coding for the physician in an outpatient medical practice. The systems and references used to assign codes to third-party claims is only one difference in the coding requirements and practices of the physician and the inpatient medical facility. Volumes 1

and 2 of the ICD-9-CM are used to report the diagnostic code that justifies physician services whether those services are provided in the office or in the hospital. Hospital coders use Volume 3 to report inpatient procedures, services, and supplies, as well as the reasons for the services.

The UB-04 (uniform bill) is used by institutions to report inpatient admissions and outpatient and emergency department services and procedures. These charges are for nursing services, building maintenance, and all costs associated with running the institution. These charges do not include physician services. The CMS-1500 (universal claim form) is used to report physician services, whether the physician sees the patient in the office, emergency department, hospital, or nursing home, because even though the physician may have been in the hospital, it is his **service** for which we are billing in the medical office.

The term **outpatient** is used to describe patients treated in the following places:

- Health care provider's office
- Hospital clinic
- Emergency department
- Hospital same-day surgery unit or ambulatory surgical center that releases the patient within 23 hours
- Observation status in a hospital (the patient is admitted for a short time for observation only, and the physician bills for his or her service during the stay)

The term **inpatient** refers to a patient who is admitted to the hospital for treatment with the expectation that the patient will remain in the hospital for 24 hours or more.

Hospital coders code only services provided by the hospital and hospital employees. Coders who are employed by the physician practice are concerned with the services provided by the physician no matter where the services are provided. For example, the hospital room, meals, and laboratory testing that a patient receives are billed and coded by the hospital billing department. The daily visits the physician makes to the patient are billed and coded by the physician's office.

Since the focus of this textbook is medical assisting, we concentrate on outpatient coding.

 CHECKPOINT QUESTION

3. Name and give uses for the three volumes of the ICD-9-CM.

COG ICD-9-CM: The Code Book

Coding books are available from several publishers, such as Ingenix and Medicode. The AMA (American Medical Association) Press also publishes coding books and training materials. The classification system is also available as part of a medical software package; one of these packages is CodeManager from the AMA. Although each publisher offers special features and helpful aids, the format remains the same. Some coders become comfortable with certain special features (i.e., AMA publications are spiral bound) and, since the content is the same, can choose among the various publications based on organization, illustrations, tabs, bullets, and color coding.

To become an expert medical coder, you need general knowledge of human anatomy and medical terminology. In addition to using a code book, you will need reference materials such as a medical dictionary and/or medical dictionary software.

To ensure accurate coding, update your ICD-9-CM coding books and software as needed. (Updates and addenda can be purchased from the publisher of your coding book.) You must update codes on superbills (preprinted bills listing a variety of procedures) or any other forms you use. Experts have estimated that millions of dollars in reimbursement have been lost because an incorrect code was taken from a standardized form that had not been updated. New codes are published each October, and third-party payers require their use after January 1.

 CHECKPOINT QUESTION

4. How often is the ICD-9-CM updated? When is the use of the new codes required?

Volume 1: Tabular List of Diseases

Volume 1 contains the classification of diseases (conditions) and injuries by code numbers. Figure 14-1 shows the table of contents from this volume. These 17 chapters cover groupings of diseases and injuries by **etiology** or cause (e.g., infectious diseases) and by anatomic system (e.g., digestive, respiratory). Figure 14-2 is a sample page from the tabular list showing each level of classification. Note that each chapter has a heading or title [e.g., 16, Symptoms, Signs, and Ill-Defined Conditions (780–799)]. Following the title in parentheses is the range of three-digit categories included in that chapter. In each chapter, you will find subtitles in large type followed by a range of three-digit categories in parentheses [e.g., 16, Symptoms (780–789)]. These sections describe general disease. Three-digit codes followed by a title, the category codes, describe specific diseases (e.g., 780, general symptoms). The fourth digit further breaks down the category (e.g., 780.0, alteration of consciousness), and the fifth digit is the highest level of definition (e.g., 780.01, coma).

You must always code a diagnosis to its highest definition. Volume 1 tells you how many digits are required to code a diagnosis correctly and to a level that most third-party payers will accept. Volume 1 also includes five appendices, which are outlined in Table 14-1.

Supplementary Classifications

Supplementary classifications in Volume 1 include V- and E-codes.

V-Codes

V-codes, which range from V01 to V82, provide a means of indexing the reason for hospital or physician office care for other than current or genuine illness, such as a history of illness, immunizations, or live-born infants according to type of birth. An example of a V-code is V10.04, which is used for a person with a personal history of a malignant neoplasm of the stomach. Because of this history, it would be important for this patient to have regular checkups. You would not want to code the visit 230.2, neoplasm of the stomach, because that would imply the patient has the malignant neoplasm at this visit. V-codes may be used alone if no disease diagnosis is appropriate or as the second or third code to help better explain the reason for the visit.

E-Codes

E-codes, which range from E800 to E999, are used to classify external causes of injuries and poisoning. Specificity is limited to the fourth-digit level. E-codes are used in conjunction with codes in Chapters 1 to 17. They help to provide information of interest to industrial medicine, insurance underwriters, national safety programs, public health agencies, and others concerned with causes of injuries (e.g., auto accidents, accidents caused by heavy industrial machinery). These codes do not affect reimbursement.

Volume 2, Section 3, has a separate index to access E-codes, the Alphabetic Index to External Causes of Injury and Poisoning.

 CHECKPOINT QUESTION

5. List four reasons for using E-codes.

Volume 2: Alphabetic Index to Diseases

Volume 2, the Alphabetic Index to Diseases, contains many diagnostic terms that do not appear in Volume 1. For example, itch, barbers, beard, and scalp are all listed under *Itch* in Volume 2. In Volume 1, they are all listed under code 110.0. The index is arranged by condition. Always check all indentations in the index under the condition to ensure that you have the one most appropriate to the diagnosis you intend to code.

The alphabetic index is organized into three sections:

• Section 1, Alphabetic Index to Diseases and Injuries, is organized by **main terms** printed in boldface type. Section 1 is used for reporting the reason for patient

TABLE OF CONTENTS

Figure 14-1 Table of contents from ICD-9-CM, Volume 1.

encounters for most insurance claims. Following the main term is a code number, which refers you to the tabular listing (Volume 1). You must not accept this number as the correct code without a **cross-reference** or check of the tabular list. Never code directly from the alphabetic index. This could result in an incomplete or incorrect coding assignment. For example, if you have a patient with fluid overload and you look under fluid, it may seem logical to code the first code under fluid, which is abdomen, 789.5, but your patient is generally retaining fluid. If you use the alphabetic

index only, you do not know that the correct code is 276.6, fluid overload, which excludes ascites, 789.5, and localized edema, 782.3. Box 14-1 outlines several exceptions to the main term rule.

- Section 2, Table of Drugs and Chemicals, includes an extensive listing of drugs, chemical substances, and toxic agents. It also shows E-codes and American Hospital Formulary Service (AHFS) list numbers, which are in the table under the main term *Drug*.
- Section 3, Alphabetic Index to External Cases of Injuries and Poisonings, leads you to codes that describe

✓5ᵗʰ **780.5** **Sleep disturbances**

> **EXCLUDES** *that of nonorganic origin (307.40-307.49)*

780.50 **Sleep disturbance, unspecified**

780.51 **Insomnia with sleep apnea**

DEF: Transient cessation of breathing disturbing sleep.

780.52 Other insomnia

Insomnia NOS

DEF: Inability to maintain adequate sleep cycle.

780.53 **Hypersomnia with sleep apnea**

DEF: Autonomic response inhibited during sleep; causes insufficient oxygen intake, acidosis and pulmonary hypertension.

780.54 Other hypersomnia

Hypersomnia NOS

DEF: Prolonged sleep cycle.

780.55 **Disruptions of 24-hour sleep-wake cycle**

Inversion of sleep rhythm

Irregular sleep-wake rhythm NOS

Non-24-hour sleep-wake rhythm

780.56 **Dysfunctions associated with sleep stages or arousal from sleep**

780.57 Other and unspecified sleep apnea

780.59 Other

✓4ᵗʰ **780** **General symptoms**

✓5ᵗʰ **780.0** **Alteration of consciousness**

> **EXCLUDES** *coma:*
> *diabetic (250.2-250.3)*
> *hepatic (572.2)*
> *originating in the perinatal period (779.2)*

780.01 **Coma**

DEF: State of unconsciousness from which the patient cannot be awakened.

780.02 **Transient alteration of awareness**

DEF: Temporary, recurring spells of reduced consciousness.

780.03 **Persistent vegetative state**

DEF: Persistent wakefulness without consciousness due to nonfunctioning cerebral cortex.

780.09 Other

Drowsiness   Stupor

Semicoma   Unconsciousness

Somnolence

780.1 **Hallucinations**

Hallucinations: Hallucinations:

NOS   olfactory

auditory   tactile

gustatory

> **EXCLUDES** *those associated with mental disorders, as functional psychoses (295.0-298.9)*
> *organic brain syndromes (290.0-294.9, 310.0-310.9)*
> *visual hallucinations (368.16)*

DEF: Perception of external stimulus in absence of stimulus; inability to distinguish between real and imagined.

✓5ᵗʰ **779.8** **Other specified conditions originating in the perinatal period**

779.81 **Neonatal bradycardia**

> **EXCLUDES** *abnormality in fetal heart rate or rhythm complicating labor and delivery (763.81-763.83)*
> *bradycardia due to birth asphyxia (768.5-768.9)*

779.82 **Neonatal tachycardia**

> **EXCLUDES** *abnormality in fetal heart rate or rhythm complicating labor and delivery (763.81-763.83)*

779.89 Other specified conditions originating in the perinatal period

Figure 14-2 Sample page from ICD-9-CM, Volume 1, showing categories, subheadings, and so on.

TABLE 14-1 ICD-9-CM Appendices	
The following five appendices are found in Volume 1.	
Title	**Description**
Appendix A: Morphology of Neoplasms	This appendix is used in conjunction with Chapter 2 in ICD-9-CM when coding neoplasms. It lists the five-digit alphanumeric codes used to identify the morphology of a neoplasm. For example, in the morphology code M8070/3, the 8070 indicates that the morphology is squamous cell carcinoma. The "/3" indicates that it is the primary site.
Appendix B: Glossary of Mental Disorders	Alphabetic list of mental disorders, including detailed descriptions of each disease.
Appendix C: Classification of Drugs by American Hospital Formulary Service (AHFS) List Number and the ICD-9-CM Equivalents	This appendix lists the AHFS list number (e.g., 24:04 for cardiac drugs) and the ICD-9-CM code number for each one (e.g., 24.04 cardiac drugs would be equivalent to category 972.9, the ICD-9-CM category of "other and unspecified agents primarily affecting the cardiovascular system").
Appendix D: Classification of Industrial Accidents by Agency	This includes codes that can be used as a supplement to describe types of equipment or materials that may be responsible for an industrial accident or illness.
Appendix E: List of Three-Digit Categories	This is a list of all three-digit categories in ICD-9-CM.

Note: Appendices A through D are not recognized by most government programs, such as Medicare and Medicaid. As previously mentioned, ICD-9-CM has other uses, however, and you may find that you need the appendices to track such things as disorders treated.

BOX 14-1

EXCEPTIONS TO THE MAIN TERM RULE

Sometimes, you have to think outside the box. Most of the time, locating the condition instead of the location works well, but sometimes a diagnosis will stump you.

1. Obstetric conditions may be found under the main terms *Delivery, Pregnancy,* and *Puerperal.*
2. Complications of medical or surgical procedures or primary diagnoses can be found under complications. For example, complications of pneumonia would be found under *Complications*—not *Pneumonia.*
3. Conditions arising from an earlier problem or procedure are called "late effects" and can be found under the words *Late effects, Due to ..., As a result of ..., Residual,* etc.
4. Lacerations can be found under *Wounds.*
5. V-Codes are codes used for patients who are not sick. They may be found by looking for terms such as *Admission, Examination, History of ..., Observation, Problem with ..., Status, Vaccination, Encounter for ..., Follow-up,* etc.

circumstances of injuries, accidents, and violence. These codes are not used for medical diagnoses. Main entries in this section usually are a type of accident or violence (e.g., assault, fall, collision). These codes can supplement the diagnostic code, but they should never be used alone or as principal diagnosis codes. E-codes are frequently used with these codes. For example, a person who fractured a tibia in a fall off a sidewalk curb would be given a code from Chapter 17, Volume 1, in the ICD-9-CM for the injury (e.g., fracture of tibia, closed, is 823.80), and an additional code, E880.0, indicates that the accident was a fall off a sidewalk curb.

 CHECKPOINT QUESTION

6. What are V-codes used for?

Volume 3: Inpatient Coding

Volume 3, the Tabular List and Alphabetic Index of Procedures, is used in inpatient facilities and is based on anatomy, not surgical specialty. There are no alphabetic characters in these procedure codes. The codes are two-digit categories with a maximum of two decimal digits where necessary. Most refer to surgical procedures, and the rest cover miscellaneous diagnostic and therapeutic

A

INJURY AND POISONING   **807–808.49**

☑4th **807 Fracture of rib(s), sternum, larynx, and trachea**

The following fifth-digit subclassification is for use with codes 807.0-807.1:

0 rib(s), unspecified
1 one rib
2 two ribs
3 three ribs
4 four ribs
5 five ribs
6 six ribs
7 seven ribs
8 eight or more ribs
9 multiple ribs, unspecified

☑5th **807.0** **Rib(s), closed**   `MSP`
☑5th **807.1** **Rib(s), open**   `MSP`
807.2 **Sternum, closed**   `MSP`
DEF: Break in flat bone (breast bone) in anterior thorax.

807.3 **Sternum, open**   `MSP`
DEF: Break, with open wound, in flat bone in mid anterior thorax.

807.4 **Flail chest**   `MSP`
807.5 **Larynx and trachea, closed**   `MSP`
  Hyoid bone   Trachea
  Thyroid cartilage

807.6 **Larynx and trachea, open**   `MSP`

B

Fracture — *continued*
  multiple — *continued*
    skull, specified or unspecified bones, or
      face bone(s) with any other bone(s) —
        continued

> *Note — Use the following fifth-digit subclassification with categories 800, 801, 803, and 804:*
>
> *0   unspecified state of consciousness*
> *1   with no loss of consciousness*
> *2   with brief [less than one hour] loss of consciousness*
> *3   with moderate [1-24 hours] loss of consciousness*
> *4   with prolonged [more than 24 hours] loss of consciousness and return to pre-existing conscious level*
> *5   with prolonged [more than 24 hours] loss of consciousness, without return to pre-existing conscious level*
> *Use fifth-digit 5 to designate when a patient is unconscious and dies before regaining consciousness, regardless of the duration of the loss of consciousness*
> *6   with loss of consciousness of unspecified duration*
> *9   with concussion, unspecified*

  with
    contusion, cerebral 804.1 ▬5▬
    epidural hemorrhage 804.2 ▬5▬
    extradural hemorrhage 804.2 ▬5▬
    hemorrhage (intracranial) NEC
      804.8 ▬5▬
    intracranial injury NEC 804.4 ▬5▬
    laceration, cerebral 804.1 ▬5▬
    subarachnoid hemorrhage 804.2 ▬5▬
    subdural hemorrhage 804.2 ▬5▬

Figure 14-4 Samples of fifth-digit classifications from ICD-9-CM. (**A**) Volume 1. (**B**) Volume 2.

Primary Codes

In outpatient coding, the **primary diagnosis** is simply the patient's chief complaint or the reason the patient sought medical attention today. It may be a routine follow-up visit, or there may be a new problem. The primary code is listed first on the CMS-1500.

When More Than One Code is Used

Each CMS-1500 form allows the reporting of four different ICD-9 codes. In many cases, more than one code is used for a single patient visit. When patients have more than one diagnosis, it is necessary to convey an accurate picture of the patient's total condition. For example, an elderly patient may have the following diagnoses listed each time she visits the doctor: degenerative arthritis, type 2 diabetes mellitus, macular degeneration, hypertension, and pernicious anemia. If any of these conditions is related to or affects her treatment, they should be listed as supplementary information. If she visits the doctor because she has influenza and her other diagnoses are not addressed at the visit, it is not necessary to list all the diagnoses given. The primary diagnosis is her reason for coming to the office (symptoms of influenza). But the fact that she is diabetic will affect her treatment and makes her visit medically necessary. Multiple codes should be sequenced with the proper service or procedure code on the proper line of the CMS-1500. Figure 14-5 shows the proper sequencing for another patient's CMS-1500. On Line 1 of Section 24 on the CMS-1500, you place the code and charge for the visit. In Block 24E, the diagnosis code for the ankle injury appears first because that is what brought the patient to the office today. On Line 2 of 24A, the laboratory work is listed but is also referenced to the diagnosis on Line 21, Item 2, which is the proper code for the patient's diabetes; this is referenced to Item 2 on Line 24. If the patient did not have diabetes, the laboratory work would not be considered reasonable for a patient with an ankle injury. If this procedure were not followed, the laboratory work would be seen as medically unnecessary, and the physician would not be reimbursed.

Late Effects

Late effects are symptoms or conditions arising from an acute illness. The effects are present after treatment for the acute illness or injury has ended. Proper coding sequence requires that you list the code number identifying the residual or current condition first, with the code number identifying the cause or original illness or injury listed second. Key words used in the patient's medical records defining late effects include "late," "due to an old injury," "due to a previous illness/injury," "due to an illness or injury occurring a year or more ago," "sequela of ...," "as a result of ...," "resulting from ...," and so on. Patients who are status post cerebrovascular accident (CVA) may have residual effects from their original stroke, for example, and may have a diagnosis of left hemiparesis as a result of CVA 3 years ago. Figure 14-6 is a sample listing of a late effect from the ICD-9-CM.

Coding Suspected Conditions

In the inpatient setting, coders list conditions after the patient's testing is complete. In other words, they are coding with complete information. In outpatient settings, however, the coder reports the reason for the patient visit as it occurs. When filing claims, the coder is limited by the information and documentation on hand at the time of the patient visit. If at the end of the visit the diagnosis is not confirmed, the physician may indicate "rule out," "suspected," or "probable." For example, a patient who comes in complaining of headache may be sent for magnetic resonance imaging (MRI) of the head because the physician suspects a serious disorder. On the patient's encounter form, the physician may list the diagnosis as "rule out brain tumor." It is not accurate to code the visit as brain tumor before it is confirmed by MRI. On this first visit to the physician's office, the reason for being seen is headache. The patient's symptom (headache) is the only confirmed reason for the encounter at this point. On the second visit to the doctor, the MRI has confirmed a glioma in the frontal lobe. For the second and all subsequent visits, glioma is coded as the reason for the encounter. Refer back to Figure 14-2 which shows a page from the ICD-9-CM that includes many of the symptom codes.

PSY LEGAL TIP

DON'T GIVE PATIENTS A DISEASE THEY DON'T HAVE!

It is important that you use the code that explains the patient's situation accurately. Coding AIDS before that diagnosis is made could be construed as defamation of character and even libel. Some patients just want to be tested for HIV, but there are no signs or symptoms.

The ICD-9-CM offers a variety of codes for HIV testing. For a patient who has the test simply because he or she wants to know, you will use V72.6, which is simply "laboratory examination." The code used for a patient who has known exposure is V01.79, which is "contact with or exposure to communicable diseases, other viral diseases." For patients who want to be tested because they are worried about exposure, V69.2 is used. This code is "high-risk sexual behavior." In this case, two codes would be used: V69.2 and V01.79. This approach will ensure that a patient is not assigned a diagnosis code for a problem he or she does not have.

PLEASE
DO NOT
STAPLE
IN THIS
AREA

CARRIER

HEALTH INSURANCE CLAIM FORM

PICA | | PICA

1. MEDICARE MEDICAID CHAMPUS CHAMPVA GROUP HEALTH PLAN FECA BLK LUNG OTHER	1a. INSURED'S I.D. NUMBER (FOR PROGRAM IN ITEM 1)
X (Medicare #) (Medicaid #) (Sponsor's SSN) (VA File #) (SSN or ID) (SSN) (ID)	000-00-0000A

2. PATIENT'S NAME (Last Name, First Name, Middle Initial)	3. PATIENT'S BIRTH DATE MM DD YY SEX	4. INSURED'S NAME (Last Name, First Name, Middle Initial)
Naomi A Dishman	04 14 24 M☐ F☒	Same

5. PATIENT'S ADDRESS (No., Street)	6. PATIENT RELATIONSHIP TO INSURED	7. INSURED'S ADDRESS (No., Street)
405 Carolina Ave	Self☐ Spouse☐ Child☐ Other☐	
CITY STATE Danville VA	8. PATIENT STATUS Single☐ Married☒ Other☐	CITY STATE
ZIP CODE TELEPHONE (Include Area Code) 24540 (434) 555-5555	Employed☐ Full-Time Student☐ Part-Time Student☐	ZIP CODE TELEPHONE (INCLUDE AREA CODE) ( )

9. OTHER INSURED'S NAME (Last Name, First Name, Middle Initial) NONE	10. IS PATIENT'S CONDITION RELATED TO:	11. INSURED'S POLICY GROUP OR FECA NUMBER
a. OTHER INSURED'S POLICY OR GROUP NUMBER	a. EMPLOYMENT? (CURRENT OR PREVIOUS) YES☐ NO☒	a. INSURED'S DATE OF BIRTH MM DD YY SEX M☐ F☐
b. OTHER INSURED'S DATE OF BIRTH SEX MM DD YY M☐ F☐	b. AUTO ACCIDENT? PLACE (State) YES☐ NO☒	b. EMPLOYER'S NAME OR SCHOOL NAME
c. EMPLOYER'S NAME OR SCHOOL NAME	c. OTHER ACCIDENT? YES☒ NO☐	c. INSURANCE PLAN NAME OR PROGRAM NAME
d. INSURANCE PLAN NAME OR PROGRAM NAME	10d. RESERVED FOR LOCAL USE	d. IS THERE ANOTHER HEALTH BENEFIT PLAN? YES☐ NO☐ If yes, return to and complete item 9 a-d.

READ BACK OF FORM BEFORE COMPLETING & SIGNING THIS FORM.

12. PATIENT'S OR AUTHORIZED PERSON'S SIGNATURE I authorize the release of any medical or other information necessary to process this claim. I also request payment of government benefits either to myself or to the party who accepts assignment below.

SIGNED Signature on File   DATE 010513

13. INSURED'S OR AUTHORIZED PERSON'S SIGNATURE I authorize payment of medical benefits to the undersigned physician or supplier for services described below.

SIGNED

14. DATE OF CURRENT: ILLNESS (First symptom) OR INJURY (Accident) OR PREGNANCY(LMP) MM DD YY 05 28 13	15. IF PATIENT HAS HAD SAME OR SIMILAR ILLNESS. GIVE FIRST DATE MM DD YY	16. DATES PATIENT UNABLE TO WORK IN CURRENT OCCUPATION MM DD YY MM DD YY FROM TO
17. NAME OF REFERRING PHYSICIAN OR OTHER SOURCE	17a. I.D. NUMBER OF REFERRING PHYSICIAN	18. HOSPITALIZATION DATES RELATED TO CURRENT SERVICES MM DD YY MM DD YY FROM TO
19. RESERVED FOR LOCAL USE		20. OUTSIDE LAB? $ CHARGES YES☐ NO☐

21. DIAGNOSIS OR NATURE OF ILLNESS OR INJURY. (RELATE ITEMS 1,2,3 OR 4 TO ITEM 24E BY LINE)

1. 845.03   3. ___ . ___
2. 250.00   4. ___ . ___

22. MEDICAID RESUBMISSION CODE   ORIGINAL REF. NO.

23. PRIOR AUTHORIZATION NUMBER

24. A. DATE(S) OF SERVICE From To MM DD YY MM DD YY	B. Place of Service	C. Type of Service	D. PROCEDURES, SERVICES, OR SUPPLIES (Explain Unusual Circumstances) CPT/HCPCS MODIFIER	E. DIAGNOSIS CODE	F. $ CHARGES	G. DAYS OR UNITS	H. EPSDT Family Plan	I. EMG	J. COB	K. RESERVED FOR LOCAL USE
1 05 28 13 05 28 13	11		99213	1	100 00	1				
2 05 28 13 05 28 13	11		82947	2	25 00	1				
3										
4										
5										
6										

25. FEDERAL TAX I.D. NUMBER SSN EIN 54-0000000 ☐☐	26. PATIENT'S ACCOUNT NO. 1234	27. ACCEPT ASSIGNMENT? (For govt. claims, see back) X YES☐ NO	28. TOTAL CHARGE $ 125 00	29. AMOUNT PAID $	30. BALANCE DUE $ 125 00
31. SIGNATURE OF PHYSICIAN OR SUPPLIER INCLUDING DEGREES OR CREDENTIALS (I certify that the statements on the reverse apply to this bill and are made a part thereof.) SIGNED DATE	32. NAME AND ADDRESS OF FACILITY WHERE SERVICES WERE RENDERED (If other than home or office)		33. PHYSICIAN'S, SUPPLIER'S BILLING NAME, ADDRESS, ZIP CODE & PHONE # JOSEPH G NORTH, MD 1111 GRAYSON STREET DANVILLE VA PIN# GRP#		

PHYSICIAN OR SUPPLIER INFORMATION

PATIENT AND INSURED INFORMATION

(APPROVED BY AMA COUNCIL ON MEDICAL SERVICE 8/88)   **PLEASE PRINT OR TYPE**   APPROVED OMB-0938-0008 FORM CMS-1500 (12-90), FORM RRB-1500, APPROVED OMB-1215-0055 FORM OWCP-1500, APPROVED OMB-0720-0001 (CHAMPUS)

Figure 14-5 Sample CMS-1500 claim form indicating proper sequencing.

A　**LATE EFFECTS OF INJURIES, POISONINGS, TOXIC EFFECTS, AND OTHER EXTERNAL CAUSES (905-909)**

Note: These categories are to be used to indicate conditions classifiable to 800-999 as the cause of late effects, which are themselves classified elsewhere. The "late effects" include those specified as such, or as sequelae, which may occur at any time after the acute injury.

✓4ᵗʰ **905 Late effects of musculoskeletal and connective tissue injuries**

905.0　**Late effect of fracture of skull and face bones**
Late effect of injury classifiable to 800-804

905.1　**Late effect of fracture of spine and trunk without mention of spinal cord lesion**
Late effect of injury classifiable to 805, 807-809

905.2　**Late effect of fracture of upper extremities**
Late effect of injury classifiable to 810-819

905.3　**Late effect of fracture of neck of femur**
Late effect of injury classifiable to 820

905.4　**Late effect of fracture of lower extremities**
Late effect of injury classifiable to 821-827

905.5　**Late effect of fracture of multiple and unspecified bones**
Late effect of injury classifiable to 828-829

905.6　**Late effect of dislocation**
Late effect of injury classifiable to 830-839

905.7　**Late effect of sprain and strain without mention of tendon injury**
Late effect of injury classifiable to 840-848, except tendon injury

905.8　**Late effect of tendon injury**
Late effect of tendon injury due to:
open wound [injury classifiable to 880-884 with .2, 890-894 with .2]
sprain and strain [injury classifiable to 840-848]

905.9　**Late effect of traumatic amputation**
Late effect of injury classifiable to 885-887, 895-897
EXCLUDES　*late amputation stump complication (997.60-997.69)*

B

Late

Late — *continued*
　effect(s) (of) — continued
　　tuberculosis — *continued*
　　　genitourinary (conditions classifiable to 016) 137.2
　　　pulmonary (conditions classifiable to 010-012) 137.0
　　　specified organs NEC (conditions classifiable to 014, 017-018) 137.4
　　viral encephalitis (conditions classifiable to 049.8, 049.9, 062-064) 139.0
　　wound, open
　　　extremity (injury classifiable to 880-884 and 890-894, except .2) 906.1
　　　　tendon (injury classifiable to 880-884 with .2 and 890-894 with.2) 905.8
　　　head, neck, and trunk (injury classifiable to 870-879) 906.0

Figure 14-6 Sample section of late effects in ICD-9-CM. (**A**) Volume 1. (**B**) Volume 2.

 CHECKPOINT QUESTION

7. When coding a visit on a date before a definitive diagnosis is made, what is coded?

Documentation Requirements

As discussed throughout this chapter, you should choose the code assigned to any given claim for a service or procedure based on the documentation available in the patient's record at the time of the service. An **audit** is conducted by the government, a managed care company, and a health care organization to determine compliance and to detect fraud. Remember, if it's not in the chart, it did not happen. Auditors verify the codes used based on information recorded in the chart on the date of service.

AFF ETHICAL TIP

Don't Break the Rules

Imagine an unethical patient asking a physician to break the rules. Unfortunately, it happens. Some insurance companies still offer limited coverage when the patient is not sick. Routine exams and tests may be covered at a reduced rate or not at all. For this reason, some patients may think that if the doctor codes the claim with a diagnosis, then that makes the service medically necessary, and their insurance will pay. Coding based on anything other than what the documentation proves is wrong. It is not only unethical, it is illegal. If a patient asks you to be dishonest, explain that this would be unethical. Tell the patient that random audits are often carried out by the CMS to ensure that the medical chart indicates that the services and procedures on claims were actually performed and the reasons were legitimate.

COG The Future of Diagnostic Coding: International Classification of Diseases, Clinical Modification, Tenth Revision

A new edition of the ICD, the International Classification of Diseases, Tenth Revision (ICD-10), is scheduled to be implemented on October 1, 2013. The WHO was responsible for revising the ICD to improve the quality of data input into clinical databases. The ICD-10-CM includes more codes and will be used by every type of health care provider for all encounters, including hospice and home health care. ICD-10 codes are alphanumeric, but the format of the index is similar to the ICD-9-CM. Two new chapters relating to disorders of the eye and the ear have been added to the ICD-10. Computer software will be revised, and the ICD-9-CM code books will be obsolete. Let's look at some of the differences between ICD-9-CM and ICD-10-CM.

Format of Codes

Diagnosis coding under the new system uses 3–7 alpha and numeric characters and full code titles, but the format is very much the same as ICD-9-CM. For example, In ICD-9 the code for a laparoscopic appendectomy would be 470.1. In ICD-10-CM, the code will be 0DTJ4ZZ. Each character contained within the seven-character system can contain up to 34 possible values that include the numbers 0–9 or the letters A–H, J–N, and P–Z. The letters O and I are not used to avoid being confused with the numbers 0 and 1. This longer combination of numbers and letters allows for expanding of the system as new technologies are discovered and used.

Conventions

Many of the same conventions will be used. One major difference deals with the use of "Excludes" notes. With ICD-10-CM there will be two types of excludes notes: *Excludes1* and *Excludes2*. "Excludes1" means not coded here and does not allow for exceptions. It means that the two codes in question cannot be used together. "Excludes2" indicates that if medical documentation supports both conditions, both may be coded. For example,

Excludes1:   intestinal malabsorption (K90)
sequelae of protein-calorie malnutrition (E64.0)
Excludes2:   nutritional anemias (D50–D53)
starvation (T73.0)

In the above example, you are told that for the malnutrition codes in the range of E40–E46, you *cannot* use codes in the K90-category or in the E64.0 category. However, for the malnutrition codes in the range of E40–E46 you *can* include nutritional anemias in the range of D50–D53 and starvation, T73.0, provided that both conditions exist and are well documented by physician in the medical record.

Extra Digits

In ICD-9-CM, coders are instructed to use a fifth digit. With the addition of more characters, some disorders will require a seventh character in ICD-10-CM. In some cases, there will be no fifth or sixth digit used, and there must be a placeholder, "X." For example,

032.1 Maternal care for breech presentation

The seventh character is either 1 for a single gestation or 1–9 for multiple gestations. Each fetus must be identified in the record so that consistent designation can be made to the correct fetus.

0: not applicable or unspecified
1: fetus 1
2: fetus 2
3: fetus 3
4: fetus 4
5: fetus 5
9: other fetus

Therefore, if the maternal care is for a single gestation, the correct code is 032.1XX0. If the "X" placeholder is not there and 032.10 is assigned, the code is incorrect.

Special Codes

E-Codes and V-Codes are no longer located in a supplemental listing. In ICD-10-CM, these types of codes have been placed into the main classification system but no longer begin with Es and Vs. Category Y93 includes activity codes, which are used only on the initial visit for treatment of an injury. These new codes are used together with an external cause code and place of occurrence code. Seventh characters specify if the activity was work related, non–work related, student activity, or military activity.

In ICD-10-CM, the codes for diabetes mellitus will change considerably. They provide more detail than the current 250 category in ICD-9-CM. Box 14-3 outlines the new, more specific diabetes codes.

Medical coders must learn to use the new ICD-10-CM code books and will find training opportunities through the various coding professional organizations and the CMS. It will be a challenge to learn, but the new system promises to enhance efficiency and accuracy and will ultimately improve the important process of coding claims.

BOX 14-3

DIABETES MELLITUS CODES IN ICD-10

Categories E08–E13 are as follows:

E08	Diabetes mellitus due to underlying conditions
E09	Drug- or chemical-induced diabetes mellitus
E10	Type 1 diabetes mellitus
E11	Type 2 diabetes mellitus
E13	Other specified diabetes mellitus

As you can see, these three-character codes do not provide full information. To provide further detail, a fourth digit describes underlying conditions, and the fifth and sixth digits provide even more specificity. Just as in ICD-9-CM, you must take the code to the last character provided within the category.

For example, for a diagnosis of diabetes mellitus type 2 with moderate nonproliferative retinopathy without macular edema, the code will be chosen from the following:

E11.3	Type 2 diabetes mellitus with ophthalmic complications
E11.33	Type 2 diabetes mellitus with moderate nonproliferative diabetic retinopathy
E11.331	Type 2 diabetes mellitus with moderate nonproliferative diabetic retinopaty with macular edema
E11.339	Type 2 diabetes mellitus with moderate nonproliferative diabetic retinopathy without macular edema

Source: Excerpted from Falen, TJ. *Learning to Code with ICD-9-CM 2011.* Lippincott Williams and Wilkins, Baltimore: 2010.

 CHECKPOINT QUESTION

8. How will the implementation of ICD-10-CM improve the coding of reasons for services?

---

 español

SPANISH TERMINOLOGY

¿Qué son todo estos números? ¿Esta es la factura?
    What are all these numbers? Is that my bill?

No, estos números son códigos para su seguro.
    No, these numbers are used for your insurance.

Se les llaman números de codificación.
    These are called coding numbers.

MEDIA MENU

- **Student Resources on thePoint**
  - **CMA/RMA Certification Exam Review**
- **Internet Resources**
  World Health Organization
  http://www.who.int/en
  U.S. Department of Health and Human Services
  http://www.hhs.gov
  Centers for Medicare and Medicaid Services
  http://www.cms.gov
  American Health Information Management Association
  http://www.ahima.org

PSY PROCEDURE 14-1: **Locating a Diagnostic Code**

Purpose: To quickly and accurately locate a code based on reasonableness for the medical service or procedure performed
Equipment: Diagnosis, ICD-9-CM Volumes I and II Code Book, medical dictionary

Steps	Purpose
1. Using the diagnosis "chronic rheumatoid arthritis," choose the main term within the diagnostic statement. If necessary, look up the word(s) in your dictionary (main term is *Arthritis*).	In a diagnosis that has more than one word, choosing the condition, not the location, helps find the code quickly. If you don't know what the word(s) means, you cannot make the most accurate choice.
2. Locate the main term in Volume 2.	The alphabetic list is in Volume 2.

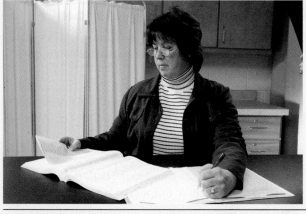

Step 2. Locate the main term.

Steps	Purpose
3. Refer to all notes and conventions under the main term.	These notes and conventions are there for a reason. In order to find the correct code, you should pay close attention to them.
4. Find the appropriate indented subordinate term (appropriate indented subordinate term is *rheumatoid*).	The indented terms go with the terms above them.
5. Follow any relevant instructions, such as "See also."	If the book wants you to see another code, you should go there to determine if the code you have chosen is the correct code.
6. Confirm the selected code by cross-referencing to Volume 1. Make sure you have added any necessary fourth or fifth digits.	Volume 1 will tell you if there is a fourth or fifth digit to further specify a diagnosis. Remember, if there is a fifth digit, it must be used.
7. Assign the code.	Without an appropriate code to explain the medical necessity of a service, insurance will not pay!
8. **AFF** Your office manager instructs you to assign a diagnosis code to a claim for a patient that you know does not have the diagnosis. What would you do?	

- Medical outpatient diagnostic coding involves the use of numbers to describe diseases, injuries, and other reasons for seeking medical care. ICD-9-CM provides an index to report and track diseases. Diagnostic coding is linked to reimbursement because it assures that the physician's service or procedure was medically necessary.

- As a medical assistant, you must understand the format and guidelines for assigning a code or reason for each encounter, treatment, and/or service.
- ICD-10-CM will be implemented in October 2013 and will replace the current version with different code formatting.

Warm Ups   for Critical Thinking

1. Tom Barksdale has been seen by the physician for controlled non–insulin-dependent type 2 diabetes mellitus for about 10 years. While being seen for a routine check of his blood sugar, he complains of numbness and tingling in his left lower leg and foot. An x-ray of both legs is performed because poor circulation in the extremities can be a complication of diabetes. The x-ray confirms the diagnosis of peripheral neuropathy. Which ICD-9 code should be listed with the office visit? Which code indicates the reason for the x-ray? Which code should be placed on the CMA-1500 first as the primary diagnosis or reason for the visit?

2. Determine the main term for the following multiple word diagnoses: gestational diabetes; amyotrophic lateral sclerosis; benign, localized hyperplasia of prostate; and nursemaid's elbow.

3. A patient calls complaining of pain and swelling in the right hand since awakening this morning. The patient comes in, sees the doctor, and returns to the front desk with an encounter form that states his diagnosis is "gout." In order to make this diagnosis, the physician would need to know the patient's uric acid level. You know that the patient just had blood drawn for the test. It is a test that must be sent to an outside lab. Do you still code today's visit as "gout?" What would you do?

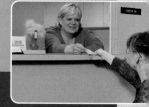

CHAPTER

15

Outpatient Procedural Coding

Outline

Healthcare Common Procedure Coding System

Physician's Current Procedural Terminology

Performing Procedural Coding
The Layout of CPT-4
The Alphabetic Index
Reading Descriptors
Place of Service

Section Guidelines
Primary and Add-on Codes
Unlisted Procedures and Special Reports

Evaluation and Management Codes
Key Components

Other Categories of Evaluation and Management Codes

Anesthesia Section
Surgery Section
Radiology Section
Pathology and Laboratory Section
Medicine Section

CPT-4 Modifiers

Fraud and Coding

ICD-10-PCS

Learning Outcomes

Cognitive Domain

Note: AAMA/CAAHEP 2008 Standards are italicized.

1. Spell and define the key terms
2. Explain the Healthcare Common Procedure Coding System (HCPCS), levels I and II
3. Explain the format of level I, Current Procedural Terminology (CPT-4) and its use
4. Describe the relationship between coding and reimbursement
5. *Describe how to use the most current procedure coding system*
6. *Define upcoding and why it should be avoided*
7. *Describe how to use the most current HCPCS coding*
8. *Describe the concept of RBRVS*
9. *Discuss all levels of governmental legislation and regulation as they apply to medical assisting practice, including FDA and DEA regulations*
10. *Define both medical terms and abbreviations related to all body systems*

Psychomotor Domain

Note: AAMA/CAAHEP 2008 Standards are italicized.

1. *Perform procedural coding (Procedure 15-1)*
2. *Apply third-party guidelines*

Affective Domain

Note: AAMA/CAAHEP 2008 Standards are italicized.

1. *Work with physician to achieve the maximum reimbursement*
2. *Demonstrate assertive communication with managed care and/or insurance providers*
3. *Apply ethical behaviors, including honesty/integrity in performance of medical assisting practice*

ABHES Competencies

1. Apply third-party guidelines
2. Perform diagnostic and procedural coding
3. Comply with federal, state, and local health laws and regulations

Key Terms

add-on code
Current Procedural
    Terminology (CPT)

descriptor
Healthcare Common
    Procedure Coding
    System (HCPCS)

key component
modifiers
primary code

procedure
upcoding

As discussed in Chapter 14, coding is a way to standardize medical information for purposes such as collecting health care statistics, performing a medical care review, and indexing medical records. It is also used for health insurance claims processing (see Chapter 13 for more information). Because coding is linked to reimbursement, you must code accurately and precisely. Incorrect, insufficient, or incomplete coding on claims forms can lead to improper reimbursement for the physician as well as recording and possibly passing along inaccurate patient information. Because learning to code is an ongoing process, continuing education is vital. This can be accomplished by attending workshops in your geographic area or by joining a local association of coders, which may also sponsor coding clinics. Two organizations are the American Academy of Professional Coders (AAPC) and the American Health Information Management Association (AHIMA). Other sources are local medical societies and your school.

COG Healthcare Common Procedure Coding System

The **Healthcare Common Procedure Coding System (HCPCS)** is divided into two principal subsystems, referred to as level I and level II. Level I of the HCPCS comprises Current Procedural Terminology (CPT), a numeric coding system maintained by the American Medical Association (AMA). Level II of the HCPCS is a standardized coding system that is used primarily to identify products, supplies, and services not included in the CPT codes, such as ambulance services and durable medical equipment, prosthetics, orthotics, and supplies when used outside a physician's office. Box 15-1 describes level II codes. Level III codes, also referred to as local codes, were established when an insurer preferred that suppliers use a local code to identify a service, for which there was no level I or level II code. In the interest of standardizing code sets, The Health Insurance Portability and Accountability Act of 1996 (HIPAA) required the elimination of level III local codes, which took effect on December 31, 2003.

 CHECKPOINT QUESTION

1. What are level II codes? List their sections.

COG Physician's Current Procedural Terminology

HCPCS level I codes, or the Physician's **Current Procedural Terminology (CPT)**, is a comprehensive listing of medical terms and codes for the uniform coding of procedures and services provided by physicians. The fourth edition, CPT-4, contains more than 7,000 new codes. CPT-4 is updated annually, with the newest version available each October. Providers are required to use the updated codes by January of each year. The CPT-4 allows insurance companies to:

- Communicate easily with one another
- Compare reimbursable amounts for procedures
- Speed claims processing

BOX 15-1

HCPCS LEVEL II CODES

Because Medicare and other insurers cover a variety of services, supplies, and equipment that are not identified by CPT codes, the level II HCPCS codes were established for submitting claims for these items. The development and use of level II of the HCPCS began in the 1980s. Level II codes are also referred to as alpha-numeric codes because they consist of a single alphabetical letter followed by four numeric digits, whereas CPT codes are identified using five numeric digits. The HCPCS level II code listing comes out once a year in the National Coding Manual, which can be ordered from the American Hospital Association, American Medical Association, or other publishers of the CPT coding book. It includes the following sections:

- Chemotherapeutic drugs
- Dental services
- Durable medical equipment
- Injections
- Ophthalmology services
- Orthotics
- Some pathology and laboratory and rehabilitation supplies
- Vision care

COG Performing Procedural Coding

Every code means something unique and is used only to describe a specific **procedure**, service, or medical supply provided by physicians to their patients. This is true for inpatients and outpatients. Codes and descriptions are updated, revised, or changed yearly. If your physician's office uses an encounter form or preprinted routing slip that lists the procedures performed, you must update this form yearly and work with your software vendor to update your computer software. The CPT-4 code selected will be placed on the CMS-1500 universal claim form in Section 24, Box D, along with any modifiers used. Procedure 15-1 outlines the steps in performing procedural coding. Figure 15-1 is a sample universal claim form showing the proper placement of codes for consultation and chest radiography. The general layout and features of the CPT-4 book published by the American Medical Association are user-friendly. There are definitions, diagrams, simple explanations, examples, and instructions.

PLEASE DO NOT STAPLE IN THIS AREA

PICA **HEALTH INSURANCE CLAIM FORM** PICA

CARRIER

1. MEDICARE [X] (Medicare #) MEDICAID [ ] (Medicaid #) CHAMPUS [ ] (Sponsor's SSN) CHAMPVA [ ] (VA File #) GROUP HEALTH PLAN [ ] (SSN or ID) FECA BLK LUNG [ ] (SSN) OTHER [ ] (ID)
1a. INSURED'S I.D. NUMBER (FOR PROGRAM IN ITEM 1): 654321987A

2. PATIENT'S NAME (Last Name, First Name, Middle Initial): Labosky, Theodore P
3. PATIENT'S BIRTH DATE MM DD YY: 05 10 1936 SEX M [X] F [ ]
4. INSURED'S NAME (Last Name, First Name, Middle Initial): Same

5. PATIENT'S ADDRESS (No., Street): 1313 Mockingbird Lane
6. PATIENT RELATIONSHIP TO INSURED: Self [X] Spouse [ ] Child [ ] Other [ ]
7. INSURED'S ADDRESS (No., Street)

CITY: Philadelphia STATE: PA
8. PATIENT STATUS: Single [ ] Married [ ] Other [X]; Employed [ ] Full-Time Student [ ] Part-Time Student [ ]
CITY STATE

ZIP CODE: 19103 TELEPHONE (Include Area Code): (215)123-3456
ZIP CODE TELEPHONE (INCLUDE AREA CODE) ( )

9. OTHER INSURED'S NAME (Last Name, First Name, Middle Initial): Labosky, Theodore P
10. IS PATIENT'S CONDITION RELATED TO:
11. INSURED'S POLICY GROUP OR FECA NUMBER

a. OTHER INSURED'S POLICY OR GROUP NUMBER: Medigap 67891237777
a. EMPLOYMENT? (CURRENT OR PREVIOUS) [ ] YES [X] NO
a. INSURED'S DATE OF BIRTH MM DD YY SEX M [ ] F [ ]

b. OTHER INSURED'S DATE OF BIRTH MM DD YY SEX M [ ] F [ ]
b. AUTO ACCIDENT? [ ] YES [X] NO PLACE (State)
b. EMPLOYER'S NAME OR SCHOOL NAME

c. EMPLOYER'S NAME OR SCHOOL NAME: Retired
c. OTHER ACCIDENT? [ ] YES [X] NO
c. INSURANCE PLAN NAME OR PROGRAM NAME: Medicare

d. INSURANCE PLAN NAME OR PROGRAM NAME
10d. RESERVED FOR LOCAL USE
d. IS THERE ANOTHER HEALTH BENEFIT PLAN? [ ] YES [ ] NO *If yes,* return to and complete item 9 a-d.

READ BACK OF FORM BEFORE COMPLETING & SIGNING THIS FORM.
12. PATIENT'S OR AUTHORIZED PERSON'S SIGNATURE I authorize the release of any medical or other information necessary to process this claim. I also request payment of government benefits either to myself or to the party who accepts assignment below.
SIGNED Signature on File DATE 8/12/13
13. INSURED'S OR AUTHORIZED PERSON'S SIGNATURE I authorize payment of medical benefits to the undersigned physician or supplier for services described below.
SIGNED SOF

PATIENT AND INSURED INFORMATION

14. DATE OF CURRENT: ILLNESS (First symptom) OR INJURY (Accident) OR PREGNANCY(LMP) MM DD YY: 08 12 2013
15. IF PATIENT HAS HAD SAME OR SIMILAR ILLNESS. GIVE FIRST DATE MM DD YY
16. DATES PATIENT UNABLE TO WORK IN CURRENT OCCUPATION FROM MM DD YY TO MM DD YY

17. NAME OF REFERRING PHYSICIAN OR OTHER SOURCE: John Mahan MD
17a. I.D. NUMBER OF REFERRING PHYSICIAN: 54-0000000
18. HOSPITALIZATION DATES RELATED TO CURRENT SERVICES FROM MM DD YY TO MM DD YY

19. RESERVED FOR LOCAL USE
20. OUTSIDE LAB? [ ] YES [ ] NO $ CHARGES

21. DIAGNOSIS OR NATURE OF ILLNESS OR INJURY. (RELATE ITEMS 1,2,3 OR 4 TO ITEM 24E BY LINE)
1. 466.0
2. ___.__
3. ___.__
4. ___.__
22. MEDICAID RESUBMISSION CODE ORIGINAL REF. NO.
23. PRIOR AUTHORIZATION NUMBER

24.	A DATE(S) OF SERVICE From MM DD YY	To MM DD YY	B Place of Service	C Type of Service	D PROCEDURES, SERVICES, OR SUPPLIES (Explain Unusual Circumstances) CPT/HCPCS MODIFIER	E DIAGNOSIS CODE	F $ CHARGES	G DAYS OR UNITS	H EPSDT Family Plan	I EMG	J COB	K RESERVED FOR LOCAL USE
1	08 12 13	08 12 13			99243	1	150 00	1				
2	08 12 13	08 12 13			71020	1	110 00	1				
3												
4												
5												
6												

25. FEDERAL TAX I.D. NUMBER SSN EIN: 54-0111111 [ ] [X]
26. PATIENT'S ACCOUNT NO.: 1234
27. ACCEPT ASSIGNMENT? (For govt. claims, see back) [X] YES [ ] NO
28. TOTAL CHARGE: $ 260 00
29. AMOUNT PAID: $ 00 00
30. BALANCE DUE: $ 260 00

31. SIGNATURE OF PHYSICIAN OR SUPPLIER INCLUDING DEGREES OR CREDENTIALS (I certify that the statements on the reverse apply to this bill and are made a part thereof.)
SIGNED DATE
32. NAME AND ADDRESS OF FACILITY WHERE SERVICES WERE RENDERED (If other than home or office)
33. PHYSICIAN'S, SUPPLIER'S BILLING NAME, ADDRESS, ZIP CODE & PHONE #: 215 123-0000
Donald Myers MD PC
233 South Sixth Street
Philadelphia PA 19106
PIN# GRP#

PHYSICIAN OR SUPPLIER INFORMATION

(APPROVED BY AMA COUNCIL ON MEDICAL SERVICE 8/88) *PLEASE PRINT OR TYPE* APPROVED OMB-0938-0008 FORM CMS-1500 (12-90), FORM RRB-1500, APPROVED OMB-1215-0055 FORM OWCP-1500, APPROVED OMB-0720-0001 (CHAMPUS)

Figure 15-1 Sample CMS claim form for consultation and chest radiography.

The Layout of CPT-4

CPT-4 is divided into six major sections: Evaluation and Management, Anesthesia, Surgery, Radiology, Pathology and Laboratory, and Medicine. These sections are followed by explanations and listings of the Category I and Category II codes, which are explained in Box 15-2.

Next are the appendices. The appendices most widely used in the outpatient arena are Appendices A through C. Appendix A is a listing of the modifiers available to help further explain a code. Appendix B is a summary of the additions, deletions, and revisions made since the last edition of the CPT-4. Appendix C includes clinical examples designed to assist providers in the selection of Evaluation and Management levels. Appendices D through I are seldom used in the medical office. You may refer to the CPT-4 code book to see their content.

The Alphabetic Index

The CPT alphabetic index is located in the back of the book and is organized by main terms like the ICD-9-CM book (Fig. 15-2). Unlike the ICD-9 index, you can locate codes by finding the procedure, the location, or the condition. For example, the code for removal of a colon polyp could be found under *Removal, Colon,* or *Polyp.* When you find the service or procedure, you will see either one code or a range of codes. Cross-reference by finding this section in the tabular section to be sure you have the correct code.

Reading Descriptors

When reading a code's **descriptor**, or description, you will read up to the semicolon and then look down for any indentations using the same words before the semicolon. Figure 15-2 is a sample page from a CPT-4 book. Refer to Figure 15-2, and locate the code for incision and drainage of an infected bursa. The proper code is 27604. It is indented under the code 27603. Read up to the semicolon in the code above. The descriptor for 27603 reads, "Incision and drainage, leg or ankle; deep abscess or hematoma." If the incision and drainage was done in an infected bursa of the leg or ankle, then the code is 27604. This descriptor is "Incision and drainage, leg or ankle; infected bursa." You would use 27603 for an incision and drainage of a leg or ankle for a deep abscess or a hematoma. Use of the indentation and the semicolon organizes the codes in a way that also saves space and keeps the CPT books from becoming too large. Although the manual coding process is still widely used, CPT software is available and is growing in popularity.

 CHECKPOINT QUESTION

2. What is the significance of the semicolon in a CPT descriptor?

Place of Service

The CPT-4 book begins with "Place of Service Codes for Professional Claims." Most payers require that place of service codes be placed on each line of Section 24, Column B of the CMS-1500 claim form. Because the CMS maintains these place of service codes, you should make sure that a certain payer recognizes the codes listed in CPT-4. For example, if a procedure is performed in the physician's office, the place of service code recognized by Medicare and Medicaid is 11. The most commonly used place of service codes are found in Table 15-1.

BOX 15-2

CPT-4 CATEGORIES

CPT-4 includes three categories of codes. Category I codes include all current U.S. Food and Drug Administration–approved physicians' procedures and services. The AMA developed it in collaboration with various other health organizations.

Category I CPT codes describe a procedure or service identified with a five-digit CPT code and descriptor nomenclature. The inclusion of a descriptor and its associated specific five-digit identifying code number in this category of CPT codes is generally based upon the procedure being consistent with contemporary medical practice and being performed by many physicians in clinical practice in multiple locations.

Category II CPT codes are intended to facilitate data collection by coding certain services and/or test results that are agreed upon as contributing to positive health outcomes and quality patient care. This category of CPT codes is a set of optional tracking codes for performance measurement. These codes may be services that are typically included in an E/M service or other component part of a service and are not appropriate for Category I CPT codes. The use of tracking codes for performance measures will decrease the need for record abstraction and chart review, thus minimizing administrative burdens on physicians and survey costs for health plans.

Once approved by the Editorial Panel, the newly added Category III CPT codes will be made available on a semiannual (twice a year) basis via electronic distribution on the AMA/CPT Web site. The full set of Category III codes will be included in the next published edition for that CPT cycle.

Source: http://www.ama-assn.org/ama/pub/category/12886.html.

Leg (Tibia and Fibula) and Ankle Joint

Incision

27600   Decompression fasciotomy, leg; anterior and/or lateral compartments only

27601   posterior compartment(s) only

27601   anterior and/or lateral, and posterior compartment(s)

     (For incision and drainage procedures, superficial, see 10040-10160)

     (For decompression fasciotomy with debridement, see 27892-27894)

27603   Incision and drainage, leg or ankle; deep abscess or hematoma

27604   infected bursa

27605   Tenotomy, percutaneous, Achilles tendon (separate procedure); local anesthesia

27606   general anesthesia

27607   Incision (eg, osteomyelitis or bone abscess), leg or ankle

27610   Arthrotomy, ankle, including exploration, drainage, or removal of foreign body
     CPT Assistant Nov 98:9

27612   Arthrotomy, posterior capsular release, ankle, with or without Achilles tendon lengthening
     CPT Assistant Nov 98:8

     (See also 27685)

Excision

27613   Biopsy, soft tissue of leg or ankle area; superficial

27614   deep (subfascial or intramuscular)
     CPT Assistant Nov 98:8

     (For needle biopsy of soft tissue, use 20206)

27615   Radical resection of tumor (eg, malignant neoplasm), soft tissue of leg or ankle area

27618   Excision, tumor, leg or ankle area; subcutaneous tissue

27619   deep (subfascial or intramuscular)

27620   Arthrotomy, ankle, with joint exploration, with or without biopsy, with or without removal of loose or foreign body

27625   Arthrotomy, with synovectomy, ankle;
     CPT Assistant Nov 98:8

27626   including tenosynovectomy

27630   Excision of lesion of tendon sheath or capsule (eg, cyst or ganglion), leg and/or ankle

27635   Excision or curettage of bone cyst or benign tumor; tibia or fibula;

27637   with autograft (includes obtaining graft)

27638   with allograft

27640   Partial excision (craterization, saucerization, or diaphysectomy) bone (eg, osteomyelitis or exostosis); tibia

27641   fibula

27645   Radical resection of tumor, bone; tibia

27646   fibula

27647   talus or calcaneus

Introduction or Removal

27648   Injection procedure for ankle arthrography

     (For radiological supervision and interpretation, use 73615. Do not report 76003 in addition to 73615)

     (For ankle arthroscopy, see 29894-29898)

Repair, Revision, and/or Reconstruction

27650   Repair, primary, open or percutaneous, ruptured Achilles tendon;

27652   with graft (includes obtaining graft)

27654   Repair, secondary, Achilles tendon, with or without graft

27656   Repair, fascial defect of leg

27658   Repair, flexor tendon, leg; primary, without graft, each tendon
     CPT Assistant Nov 98:8

27659   secondary, with or without graft, each tendon

27664   Repair, extensor tendon, leg; primary, without graft, each tendon
     CPT Assistant Nov 98:8

27665   secondary, with or without graft, each tendon
     CPT Assistant Nov 98:8

27675   Repair, dislocating peroneal tendons; without fibular osteotomy

27676   with fibular osteotomy

27680   Tenolysis, flexor or extensor tendon, leg and/or ankle; single, each tendon
     CPT Assistant Nov 98:8

27681   multiple tendons (through separate incision(s))
     CPT Assistant Nov 98:8

27685   Lengthening or shortening of tendon, leg or ankle; single tendon (separate procedure)
     CPT Assistant Nov 98:8

27686   multiple tendons (through same incision), each
     CPT Assistant Nov 98:8

= Revised code   = New code   = Contains new or revised text   = References: see p xv for details

Figure 15-2 Sample page of 2010 CPT book.

Section Guidelines and Symbols

Each section begins with its own specific guidelines and a listing of specific procedures and services applicable in that field. The guidelines contain definitions, explanatory notes, a listing of the previously unlisted procedures found in that particular section, directions on how to file a special report, modifiers for use in that particular section, and definitions to assist the coder.

There are many publishers of CPT-4 books, but they all use symbols to help the coder. When a code has one of these symbols beside it, the coder can look at the bottom of the page to see what the symbol

TABLE 15-1 Place of Service Codes Used in Physician Coding

Place of Service	Code
Physician's office	11
Patient's home	12
Assisted living facility	13
Urgent care facility	20
Inpatient hospital	21
Outpatient hospital	22
Emergency room–hospital	23
Ambulatory surgical center	24
Skilled nursing facility	31
Hospice	34

These two-digit codes are placed on each line of Section 24, Column B.
Source: Current Procedural Terminology, CPT 2006 Professional Edition; American Medical Association.

means. Some of the most common symbols found in CPT are:

- ● New code
- ▲ Revised code
- ◄► New or revised text
- ⊞ Add-on code

Primary and Add-on Codes

Most of the CPT codes are used alone; but in some cases, **add-on codes** are used for procedures or services that are always perfomed in addition to the primary procedure. A plus sign (+) appears next to an add-on code. These codes are never used alone. The **primary code** is the one that represents the most resource-intense procedure or service performed at an encounter. The primary code is listed first on the CMS-1500 form. The add-on code is listed on the line under the primary code. For example, a dermatology coder uses the code 11100 for a biopsy on a lesion. If the doctor biopsies more than one lesion, 11100 is listed on the first line, and the add-on code +11101 is used to report each additional lesion.

Unlisted Procedures and Special Reports

CPT provides unlisted codes at the beginning of each section for use when an unusual, variable, or new procedure is done. When an unlisted code is used, however, you must submit a copy of the procedure report with the claim. Each section's guidelines list the information to be included in a special report. This information includes:

1. Definition or description of the nature, extent, and need for the procedure
2. Time, effort, and equipment necessary to provide the service

3. Complexity of symptoms
4. Final diagnosis
5. Pertinent physical findings
6. Diagnostic and therapeutic procedures
7. Concurrent problems
8. Follow-up care

COG Evaluation and Management Codes

Evaluation and Management (E/M) codes are five-digit numbers that begin with the number 9. These are the most frequently used codes. E/M codes describe various patient histories, examinations, and decisions physicians must make in evaluating and treating patients in various settings (e.g., office, outpatient, hospital). In essence, the E/M codes address what the physician does when interacting with the patient. For this reason, the physician's documentation must meet standards so the physician and coder (medical assistant) can decide which level or type of code to use for a specific patient–physician encounter.

Key Components

To code the services described in the E/M section, you must be sure that the patient's medical record indicates that certain **key components** are present. Two of three key components are required for established patients, and three of three are required for new patients. These components are the elements that make up the visit. All E/M codes contain the following components:

- History
- Physical examination
- Medical decision making
- Counseling
- Coordination of care
- Nature of presenting problem
- Time

History, physical examination, and medical decision making are three key components for a visit.

Mr. Fowler was seen today for follow-up of his bacterial pneumonia. He has finished his course of antibiotics and reports feeling much better. His sputum culture on the day of his discharge shows no growth. On exam, his chest is clear, there is no wheezing, and he is breathing well. I explained to the patient that his pneumonia was probably contracted when he was exposed to a co-worker with the same illness. He was reminded of the importance of frequent handwashing. He will return in 3 months.

Key: Red = history; green = physical exam; yellow = medical decision making

Charting example showing history, physical exam, and medical decision making.

History

The amount of history documented in a patient's record determines which of the four classifications or levels is assigned. The classifications of the type of history taken from the patient are:

- Problem focused
- Expanded problem focused
- Detailed
- Comprehensive

Table 15-2 lists the classifications and gives a general description and examples of each. The provider must select one of these based on the documentation in the patient's record. Note that the times listed in the table are not regulated; they are used only for describing a typical level.

Examination

The examination levels are the same as for the history taken. A review of systems is a systematic way to assess the body when doing a physical exam. The level of an examination depends on how many body systems were examined. CPT recognizes the following body systems: eyes; ears, nose, mouth, and throat; cardiovascular; respiratory; gastrointestinal; genitourinary; musculoskeletal; skin; neurologic; psychiatric; and hematologic/immunologic (laboratory tests). Analyze the following chart note to assign the proper level of exam.

> *Patient presents with complaints of runny nose and sore throat x 3 days. Patient states the urinary tract infection we treated two weeks ago is better. On examination her eyes are red, nose is boggy, throat is red and swollen. Patient reports no more urinary problems since finishing the Bactrim DS. Urinalysis is clear.*

Charting example showing examination level.

TABLE 15-2	History and Physical Examinations		
The physician or provider must select which history and physical examination code to use. You, however, should have a basic understanding of each category. It is important to note that there are separate codes for each category and separate codes for both new and established patients.			
Type of History and Physical Examination	**Patient Problems and Physician Time Required**		**Examples**
Problem focused	Patient problems are self-limited and minor. Physician time: usually 10 minutes		9-month-old patient with diaper rash 40-year-old patient with sunburn 18-year-old patient with poison ivy 60-year-old patient with a routine blood pressure check
Expanded problem focused	Patient problems are mild to moderate. Physician time: 15–20 minutes		55-year-old patient with recurrent urinary tract infection 16-year-old patient with chronic asthma presenting with a cold 76-year-old patient with osteoarthritis 56-year-old patient with a stomach ulcer
Detailed	Patient problems are moderate to severe. Physician time: usually 30 minutes		18-year-old patient with first Pap smear and contraceptive education 67-year-old patient with the new onset of dysuria 18-month-old patient with delayed motor skill development 34-year-old patient with diabetes requiring insulin dose changes
Comprehensive	Patient problems are moderate to severe. Physician time: usually 45 minutes		36-year-old patient with infertility 8-year-old patient with new onset of diabetes 65-year-old patient with history of left-sided weakness and confusion

At this visit, the patient had an expanded problem-focused examination. The doctor examined her eyes, nose, and throat (her problem area) and also did a urinalysis to confirm that an earlier treatment took care of her previous urinary tract infection. Note that, even if the doctor examined the patient's skin, arm strength, etc., if it is not in the chart note, it cannot be considered in the selection of the level of her examination.

Medical Decision Making

The third key component, medical decision making, is defined in CPT-4 as:

- Straightforward
- Low complexity
- Moderate complexity or
- High complexity

Medical decision making refers to the kinds of things the physician must do to establish a diagnosis for the patient. A provider must consider and determine the number of diagnoses and/or management options available, the amount and complexity of any data to be reviewed, and the risk of complications or other problems the patient has. To use a particular decision-making level, the physician must document the information to justify his level selection. For example, a doctor may write a chart note like this:

> *Mr. Jones presents today for follow-up of his severe back pain. He is no better. I offered him several options, including physical therapy, anti-inflammatories, and surgery. I reviewed 35 pages of records from his surgery in Baltimore, MD, five years ago. He has cardiac problems that may make another surgery too risky.*

Charting example showing medical decision making.

This visit would qualify for a level of moderate complexity. The documentation states the number of management options and the amount of data reviewed and lists the patient's other problems.

Time

Time is not considered a key component unless more than half of the visit is spent counseling the patient. Time spent with a patient (e.g., counseling or coordinating care) is sometimes the key component in determining E/M codes. When time spent with the patient is more than 50% of the typical time for the visit, time becomes the deciding factor in choosing an E/M code. For example, if a physician spends an additional 15 minutes counseling a patient in what would normally be only a 10-minute expanded

problem-focused history and physical examination, the counseling was more than 50% of the typical 25-minute face-to-face time. The appropriate E/M code is one with a 25-minute time frame (10 minutes and an extra 15 minutes for counseling).

WHAT IF?

What if a patient's visit turns out to be mostly counseling?

A 42-year-old established patient with a family history of alcoholism sees her family doctor for an annual exam. She tells the doctor that she is doing fine, but her exam reveals some tenderness over her liver, and there is a faint odor of vodka on her breath. After a few minutes, the patient admits to the doctor that she is having marital problems and has been drinking excessively lately. The rest of the visit is spent explaining the dangers of drinking and the effects of alcohol on the liver. The doctor spends time giving her information about Alcoholics Anonymous and other resources. The chart notation reads: "Visit began at 9:15 a.m. Patient states she is doing well. On palpation of the liver, there is guarding and tenderness. There is a faint odor of ETOH. I spent 30 minutes of a 45-minute appointment counseling the patient and arranging a referral to Southside Drug and Alcohol Rehabilitation Center. Her husband was given several brochures, information about Al-Anon (an arm of Alcoholics Anonymous for family members of alcoholics), and hints about finding online resources. She left in the care of her husband who was instructed to take the patient to the rehab center now. Time 10:00 a.m."

Time is the only factor when selecting the level for this office visit. Remember, the documentation must clearly state that more than half of the visit was spent counseling a patient face to face. According to CPT, the time counted can be with the patient and/or family members or caretaker. Using the times listed in the descriptors in CPT, locate the proper category (office visit for established patient), and find the level that describes the amount of time the physician spent with the patient. The chart states the entire visit was 45 minutes; therefore, the correct code would be 99215.

 CHECKPOINT QUESTION

3. List three things a physician must consider when assigning a level of medical decision making.

Other Categories of Evaluation and Management Codes

As a medical assistant, you will be responsible for billing for your provider-employer. Although many of these services are performed in the medical office, physicians also visit and care for patients in other places. You will assist the physician in assigning codes for these visits and procedures. Other categories in the E/M section include observation codes and hospital inpatient services including initial care and subsequent care. There is a section for consultations ordered by other physicians.

Emergency department service codes are used only when the service is rendered in a 24-hour hospital-based facility that specializes in providing treatment of unscheduled events. Nursing homes, rest homes, and home visits are listed. Critical care, preventive medicine, and newborn care are other sections used by physicians for their direct care of patients. For a complete list of the subsections and categories, refer to the CPT code book.

 CHECKPOINT QUESTION

4. To code for a service in the E/M section, what three key elements are considered?

Anesthesia Section

Anesthesia codes are five-digit codes that begin with 0. Anesthesia codes are divided by anatomic site and by specific type of procedure. For example, head, neck, and thorax are anatomic sites, and the codes in each section represent the specific procedure, such as plastic repair of cleft lip. Medical assistants in an anesthesiology practice code anesthesia procedures provided in the hospital setting, even though the office is an outpatient facility.

Two types of **modifiers** (letters or numbers added to a code to add detail to the code) are used in the anesthesia section. One type is the standard modifier that is found in all sections of CPT. The other type is the physical status modifier, a two-digit code beginning with the letter P and ending in a number from 1 to 6. These physical status modifiers indicate the patient's condition at the time of anesthesia and the corresponding complexity of services (e.g., P1 indicates a normal, healthy patient, and P5 indicates a patient who is not expected to survive without the procedure).

Surgery Section

The surgery section is organized by body systems. Surgery codes begin with numbers 1 through 6. The CPT-4 codes in this section include surgery packages. When an operation is performed, CPT requires that the doctor's fee includes

the following: the surgical procedure; normal, uncomplicated follow-up care; and local infiltration, metacarpal, metatarsal, or digital block or topical anesthesia. General anesthesia must be given by an anesthesiologist.

You cannot bill separately for preoperative and postoperative visits unless you use a modifier to explain the circumstances. For example, a patient has a cholecystectomy (gallbladder removal). The fee charged for the surgery covers three office visits after the surgery. Between the first and second visit, the patient develops symptoms associated with appendicitis. The doctor can charge for this office visit because it is not related to the cholecystectomy. The surgery package does not apply.

The Centers for Medicare and Medicaid Services (CMS) has defined the surgical package for Medicare recipients somewhat differently. According to CPT-4, no complications or problems related to the surgery are included in the surgical package. If additional procedures are performed to correct or alleviate these problems, they should be coded separately. According to CMS, however, complications that do not require a revisit to the operating room are included in the price of surgery.

Third-party payers have different rules about what constitutes a surgery package, so the coder must check with the relevant third-party payers. Some insurance carriers have a set number of follow-up days that is consistent for all surgical services. Check with the carrier to learn what these are so you can bill for the additional office, outpatient, or hospital visits. The fees for fracture care and deliveries also include the care given before and after the service.

 CHECKPOINT QUESTION

5. What items are included in a surgical package?

Content of the Surgery Section

The subheadings in the surgery section are as follows: integumentary system, musculoskeletal system, respiratory system, cardiovascular system, hemic and lymphatic system, urinary system, digestive system, male genital system, intersex surgery, female genital system, maternity care and delivery, endocrine system, nervous system, eye and ocular adnexa, and auditory system. Each subheading contains subsections that organize the procedures by location and type. For example, in the musculoskeletal system section, the subcategories begin with the head and move down the body. The first heading is "Head." Under this heading are the following procedures that are done to the head: incision; excision; introduction or removal; repair, revision, and/or reconstruction; skull, facial, and nasal fractures and/or dislocations, etc. The next heading is "Neck (Soft Tissues) and Thorax," which begins with incision, excision, and so on.

TABLE 15-3	Medical Terminology Refresher	
Words that end in the following suffixes are related to surgical procedures.		
CPT Subcategory	**Suffix**	**Meaning**
Incision	-tomy	Incision into
Excision	-ectomy	Surgical removal
Repair, revision, or reconstruction	-pexy	Surgical fixation
	-plasty	Surgical repair
	-rrhaphy	Suture

It is helpful to be familiar with the suffixes and definitions related to surgical procedures. Table 15-3 provides a refresher on these words and word parts.

Radiology Section

The radiology section of CPT-4 is divided into the following four subsections:

- Diagnostic radiology/diagnostic imaging
- Diagnostic ultrasound
- Radiation oncology
- Nuclear medicine

All radiology codes are five-digit numbers that begin with 7. They are generally arranged by anatomic site, from the top of the body to the bottom. Many radiology codes indicate the number of views for a particular study. Obviously, the facility must be reimbursed for film, developer, and the radiology technologist's time and service.

Some radiologic tests require the administration of a contrast medium that enhances the image. The descriptors for such tests specify "with contrast" or "without contrast." "With contrast" refers to contrast medium that is given intravascularly. If the contrast medium is given orally or rectally, you use the code "without contrast."

If a physician performs the procedure and supervises and interprets a procedure (e.g., injects contrast medium and then supervises and interprets), two codes should be used. A written report in the patient's medical record is necessary for billing these codes. The code for the procedure can be found in the surgery, medicine, or radiology section, and the code for supervision and interpretation is found in the radiology section. If two physicians are participating (e.g., a surgeon and radiologist), the radiology portion is billed by the radiologist.

Pathology and Laboratory Section

All codes in pathology and laboratory work are five-digit numbers that begin with 8. These codes are divided into sections for panels of tests, drug testing,

consultations with pathologists, urinalysis, chemistry testing, antibody testing, cytopathology, and so on. The last part of the pathology and laboratory section includes services and procedures provided by a pathologist, including gross (can be seen by the naked eye) and microscopic examination of tissue removed in surgery. Each tissue specimen is submitted under a different identifying code for diagnosis by the pathologist. The codes represent the level of the physician's work. Postmortem examination or autopsy is performed by a pathologist, and CPT-4 provides codes to report such examinations.

A subsection, automated multichannel tests, deserves a special note. When coding, check that the tests performed are included in the lists under this subsection. For example, the physician may perform the following three tests for a patient: Bilirubin, direct; Cholesterol; and Blood urea nitrogen (BUN). To code this, you assign the code 80003, three clinical chemistry tests, because all of these tests are listed under the automated multichannel test subsection. If the tests performed were Bilirubin, direct; cholesterol; and Blood acetaldehyde, however, you would code 80002, two clinical chemistry tests, and 82000, Blood acetaldehyde. That is because "Blood acetaldehyde" was not on the list of clinical chemistry tests in the automated multichannel test subsections.

Also of note are the terms *qualitative* and *quantitative* used in the drug screening section. Patients who are on certain medications, such as digoxin for the heart or Dilantin for seizures, have regular drug levels tested to be sure the amount of drug in the blood is at the proper therapeutic level. These tests are quantitative because the doctor is looking for the amount of drug in the blood. When testing for illegal drugs, however, the amount does not matter. The mere presence of the drug makes the test positive and provides the information wanted. This is qualitative information.

Medicine Section

Like the E/M codes, medicine codes are five-digit numbers that begin with 9. Like the other five sections of the CPT-4, this section includes guidelines for appropriate coding.

The first subsection in the medicine section is for immunization injections and includes codes from 90701 to 90749. Typically, immunization injections are given when the patient comes to the physician's office for either a routine physical examination or for a minor problem, such as a sore throat. When the injection is given at the time of such a visit, use two codes—one for the service (usually an E/M code) and one for the immunization injection. For example, an established patient may come into the physician's office for a brief examination for a minor problem (e.g., controlled hypertension blood pressure check). The patient may be examined briefly by a nurse or medical assistant while the physician is in the office and may also be given an immunization for poliomyelitis. The codes for this are:

1. 99211, office and other outpatient visit for the evaluation and management of an established patient, which may not require the presence of a physician. Usually, the presenting problems are minimal. Typically, 5 minutes are spent performing or supervising services. (This code is generally used for examination by employees of the practice while a physician is in the office but not performing the examination.)
2. 90713, poliomyelitis vaccine.

Next, CPT lists codes for therapeutic or diagnostic injections (codes 90782–90799). Consider the code 90782, therapeutic injection of medication (specify); subcutaneous or intramuscular. This code is the same for most injectable therapeutic substances. In order to be reimbursed for the medication itself, an additional, more specific code is necessary. Injection codes begin with a J and can be found in the HCPCS level II codes. Other injections in this section include infusions and chemotherapy (see Box 15-1). Using the most specific codes for injectable substances and supplies while keeping invoices to document actual cost helps verify charges submitted for these services.

The medicine section also includes codes used by psychiatrists and codes for biofeedback; dialysis; esophageal procedures; eye surgery and other ophthalmologic services; speech and hearing services including cochlear implants; cardiac diagnostic testing, such as electrocardiography and echocardiography; CPR; vascular studies like cardiac catheterization; allergy testing; electroencephalography; sleep studies; and other miscellaneous services and procedures.

 CHECKPOINT QUESTION

6. Why is it necessary to use two codes for an injection?

COG CPT-4 Modifiers

CPT-4 provides a way to give additional information about a procedure through the use of additional two-digit numbers called modifiers.

There are two ways to write modifiers. You can write the five-digit code with a hyphen followed by the two-digit modifier (e.g., 28702-22). Any modifier can be added to 999 and placed on a separate line on the CMS-1500. If multiple modifiers are used, write the five-digit code with the first modifier as -99 (multiple modifiers), followed by the additional modifiers (e.g., 28702-99922). Of course, the modifier can never appear on the claim form by itself because it refers to the procedure and must be directly below it on the claim form.

Box 15-3 provides a few examples of modifiers. The modifiers used for certain sections are listed in the section guidelines. A separate listing of available modifiers

---

BOX 15-3

EXAMPLES OF CPT-4 MODIFIERS

Here are just a few examples of CPT-4 modifiers. A complete list can be found in Appendix A of CPT-4.

- *20 microsurgery or 99920:* This modifier signifies that the surgeon used an operating microscope to perform a procedure.
- *23 unusual anesthesia or 99923:* This modifier signifies that anesthesia was used in a procedure that normally would not require it.
- *26 professional component or 99926:* This modifier signifies that there are two components to the procedure, a professional one and a technical one; for example, a physician who does not perform a particular test, but interprets the test and dictates a report.

can be found in Appendix A of CPT-4. Check Appendix A first; then go to the guidelines of the appropriate section to verify that the modifier may be used with the specific CPT code. Failure to use an appropriate modifier causes database and reimbursement errors.

 CHECKPOINT QUESTION

7. What are modifiers?

ETHICAL TIP

Be Diligent About Accuracy

Even if you pay attention to detail and strive for accuracy, there are still times when you will make mistakes. In some cases, you will learn to code by trial and error. It is important, however, not to make the same error twice. Examine every explanation of benefits for problems. Develop a system to remember and track rejected claims. Do what it takes to correct any coding problems in order to get reimbursement. When a claim is pending, patients usually receive a letter from their insurance company telling them that they have asked for additional information from their doctor. Often, patients receive this letter before you receive the request for information. Be as prompt as possible in answering these requests. Patients will depend on you to assist them with their claims. It is your ethical responsibility to take care in getting the proper reimbursement.

Fraud and Coding

Billing for services not performed, using another patient's coverage to receive reimbursement, and falsifying records are examples of blatant fraud. Millions of dollars have been budgeted to investigate fraud and abuse. The attorney general of the United States has jurisdiction over such cases, and in most states, the Office of the Inspector General investigates reports of possible fraud. In cases of suspected fraud, peer review organizations have been authorized by CMS to obtain medical records of Medicare beneficiaries for review.

Less severe and nondeliberate fraudulent practices also cause misuse of health care dollars, and CMS remains vigilant by conducting audits. Fiscal intermediaries (organizations under contract with the U.S. government to handle Medicare claims) randomly review and compare the documentation in the record with the information and codes received and report their findings on the particular providers.

Even though the physician may already have been paid for a claim, the medical office may still be audited. As a federal program, Medicare has the same authority as the Internal Revenue Service to audit claims and may do so retroactively. This means that an audit can occur even a couple of years after payment has been received for claims. If the medical practice is found to be in error, the physician may be required to repay an amount owed plus interest. Even worse, such errors can jeopardize the physician's ability to participate in Medicare-funded programs.

When submitting Medicare or other insurance claims, do not bill for services the physician has not performed, and do not bill more than the proper fee for a service (**upcoding**). Many citations have been handed down for upcoding.

LEGAL TIP
BE CAREFUL

To avoid costly errors, be certain that you can justify your coding:

- Keep adequate, accurate, and complete documentation in medical and billing records.
- Use the proper tools to code. Code books are updated yearly. Always use the most recent book.
- Follow the coding rules.
- Stay abreast of new rules, and keep up to date on any changes to existing ones. Medicare has regional updates, usually at no charge, and provides one of the best sources of information.
- Work closely with the provider, and never code anything about which you are not sure.

ICD-10-PCS

The Procedure Classification System developed by the CMS is a replacement for Volume 3 of the ICD-9 and is used in the United States exclusively for inpatient hospital settings. The new procedure coding system uses seven alpha or numeric characters, whereas the ICD-9-CM coding system uses only three to five numeric digits. The use of this new system will roll out in conjunction with the ICD-10-CM requirements.

SPANISH TERMINOLOGY

¿Qué son todo estos números? ¿Esta es la factura?
  What are all these numbers? Is that my bill?

No, estos números son códigos para su seguro.
  No, these numbers are used for your insurance.

Se les llaman números de codificación.
  These are called coding numbers.

MEDIA MENU

- **Student Resources on thePoint**
  - **CMA/RMA Certification Exam Review**
- **Internet Resources**

  Medical Billing Association
  http://www.e-medbill.com

  American Health Information Management Association
  http://www.ahima.org

  American Medical Association
  http://www.ama-assn.org

PSY PROCEDURE 15-1: Locating a CPT Code

Purpose: To assign the most accurate code for services and procedures rendered by a physician or other provider in order to communicate with a third-party payer

Equipment: CPT-4 code book, patient chart

Steps	Purpose
1. Identify the exact procedure performed (*Muscle biopsy, deep*).	This will ensure accuracy.
2. Obtain the documentation of the procedure in the patient's chart.	The documentation must match the code assigned.
3. Choose the proper code book.	CPT level I and II codes are listed separately.
4. Using the alphabetic index, locate the procedure.	The alphabetic index is a quick reference.
5. Locate the code or range of codes given in the tabular section.	The index lists ranges of codes in many cases. You must select the correct code by cross-referencing to the codes themselves.
6. Read the descriptors to find the one that most closely describes the procedure.	Reading the descriptors carefully ensures accuracy.
7. Check the section guidelines for any special circumstances.	These guidelines are helpful in staying within the coding rules for each section.
8. Review the documentation to be sure it justifies the code.	In the event of a chart audit, the documentation must match the code.
9. Determine if any modifiers are needed.	If there are any unusual circumstances, the modifier will explain.
10. Select the code and place it in the appropriate field of the CMS-1500 form (accurate code is 20205).	Accurate completion of the CMS-1500 form produces clean claims.
11. **AFF** Your physician is helping you find a code in the CPT-4 code book. He chooses a code based on what the surgery entailed, but the operative report does not support what he says he did. How would you advise the physician to correct the problem and proceed?	

Chapter Summary

- Medical coding involves the use of numbers to describe diseases, injuries, and procedures.
- The purposes of coding include indexing medical records, performing medical care reviews, deriving health statistics, and reimbursing physicians and hospitals for services.
- As a medical assistant, you are responsible for knowing the format and usage of CPT-4, the system used to report services and procedures by the physician.
- Accurate and thorough coding is essential to ensure appropriate reimbursement.

- You must assist the physician in making sure the proper documentation is available to substantiate the codes used on a claim.
- As in all other aspects of patient contact and care, coding of patients' records is covered by the Health Insurance Portability and Accountability Act of 1996 (HIPAA). Only those with a need to know should have access to patient records.

Warm Ups for Critical Thinking

1. How would you handle a physician who you think overbills for procedures? To whom would you report this? How might you collect documentation of fraud?

2. Using a CPT-4 code book, find as many different main terms as you can for "Removal of ear wax" (69210). Remember, the medical term for ear wax is *cerumen*. Hint: When thinking of the ear, think, "auditory canal."

3. By attempting to locate the code for the procedure in the scenario that follows, make a list of any further information needed to select the correct code. A 12-year-old girl presents for headaches. She reports that when she has a headache, she cannot see well. The physician orders an electroencephalogram.

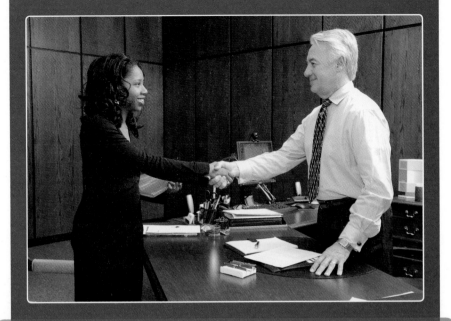

PART

III

Career
Strategies

Competing in the Job Market

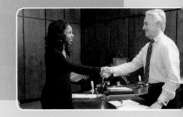

Congratulations! You have reached a pivotal point in your medical assisting career. This unit prepares you to make the transition from student to employee. The first chapter introduces you to the externship program. Your externship is the springboard to starting your career. The remainder of chapter 16 focuses on how to acquire the job that you have worked so hard to prepare for. The last chapter is a mock certification examination. You will now prepare for the next phase in your goal of becoming a medical assistant. You will be prepared to enter this fascinating and exciting career with confidence and professionalism while enjoying the rewards and accepting the challenges that face you. Good luck in your new adventure! Make it more than a job. Make it a profession and a career.

CHAPTER 16

Making the Transition: Student to Employee

Outline

Externships
Types of Facilities
Externship Benefits
Externship Responsibilities
Guidelines for a Successful
Externship
Externship Documentation
Externship Evaluations
Graduate Surveys
Employer Surveys

Establish the Job for You
Setting Employment Goals
Self-Analysis
Finding the Right Job
Applying for the Job
Answering Newspaper
Advertisements
Preparing Your Résumé
Preparing Your Cover Letter
Completing an Employment
Application

The Interview
Preparing for the Interview
Completing a Portfolio
Crucial Interview Questions
Follow-Up
Leaving a Job
Be a Lifelong Learner
Recertification
Professionalism

Learning Outcomes

Cognitive Domain

AAMA/CAAHEP 2008 Standards are italicized.

1. Spell and define the key terms
2. Explain the purpose of the externship experience

3. Understand the importance of the evaluation process
4. List your professional responsibilities during your externship
5. List personal and professional attributes necessary to ensure a successful externship

6. Determine your best career direction based on your skills and strengths
7. Identify the steps necessary to apply for the right position and be able to accomplish those steps
8. Draft an appropriate cover letter
9. List the steps and guidelines in completing an employment application
10. List guidelines for an effective interview that will lead to employment
11. Identify the steps that you need to take to ensure proper career advancement
12. Explain the process for recertification of a medical assisting credential
13. Describe the importance of membership in a professional organization
14. *Recognize elements of fundamental writing skills*
15. *List and discuss legal and illegal interview questions*
16. *Discuss all levels of governmental legislation and regulation as they apply to medical assisting practice*

Psychomotor Domain

AAMA/CAAHEP 2008 Standards are italicized.

1. Write a résumé to properly communicate skills and strengths (Procedure 16-1)
2. *Compose professional/business letters*

Affective Domain

AAMA/CAAHEP 2008 Standards are italicized.

1. *Apply local, state, and federal health care legislation*

ABHES Competencies

1. Comply with federal, state, and local health laws and regulations
2. Perform fundamental writing skills including correct grammar, spelling, and formatting techniques when writing prescriptions, documenting medical records, etc.

Key Terms

externship
networking
portfolio

preceptor
résumé

Graduation from a medical assisting program is an important milestone in your life. It is normal to have conflicting emotions ranging from excitement to anxiety. The purpose of this chapter is to help you make this transition from student to employee. The first part of the chapter discusses externships. An externship is your first opportunity to use your knowledge in a clinical setting. The chapter also discusses the benefits of externship programs, how to get the most out of your externship, and the documentation that accompanies an externship. The later part of the chapter prepares you to begin searching for employment. Résumé preparation is discussed along with successful interviewing techniques. An introduction to key employment laws is also discussed.

COG Externships

Accredited medical assisting programs are required to provide an **externship** as part of the course requirement. An externship is a training program that gives you the experience of working in a professional medical office under the supervision of a preceptor or supervisor who will help you to apply the theories and procedures you learned during classroom training. This is the opportunity for you to perform and perfect the skills that you have learned during the academic portion of your program.

In an externship, you will discover areas of interest in certain types of practices or health care specialties

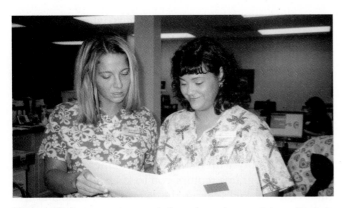

Figure 16-1 By working side by side with practicing allied health professionals, you will prepare for the real world in your extern site.

(Fig. 16-1). Rotating through clinical sites will expose you to different offices you may pursue as possible opportunities for future employment. The length and schedule of your externship will depend on your school's curriculum and the medical site where you will be working, but most externships range from 160 to 240 hours in a semester. You are not paid for this externship experience, but you will receive curriculum credit based on the hours earned.

Types of Facilities

The health care industry is diversified, with a wide variety of specialty offices and clinics. As a medical assisting student, you will experience an extensive scope of procedures during an externship in a general or family practice clinic or office. Family practices are generally referred to as primary care providers. Patients range in age from newborns to the elderly and typically have a broad range of complaints and illnesses. General practice facilities provide the best exposure to all types of procedures performed by medical assistants.

Your externship may be more limited in specialty practices. For example, staff members in obstetric offices usually do not perform electrocardiograms, and staff members in orthopedic offices wouldn't perform gynecologic examinations. Working in these types of practices, however, will give you experience in special examinations and procedures in areas that you might not observe in a general practice setting. Each specialty has advantages and disadvantages as a site, but all offer invaluable experience that cannot be adequately simulated in the classroom.

Extern Sites

Most schools have extern sites they have used for years. Based on the experience of former students, personnel in these sites know what the student must do to complete the clinical experience. An ideal site should provide a variety of experiences, both in administrative (front office) and clinical (back office) procedures.

A **preceptor** works with externship students the same as the instructor in the classroom. Preceptors typically are graduate medical assistants who have been through a similar externship program.

The school is careful to choose externship sites with preceptors who are willing to work with you and help you feel comfortable in the medical setting. They understand that all of your experience up to this point has been with fellow students in a protected classroom. They understand how nervous you are and will help you to ease the transition from classroom to the medical office. Your clinical sites are usually chosen within easy travel distance.

 AFF WHAT IF?

You notice that on several occasions your preceptor does not follow standard precautions. Why is this dangerous? Whom should you tell? Would you tell your instructor at school? Why or why not? How would you discuss this with your preceptor?

Not following standard precautions when handling body fluids may expose you to blood-borne pathogens like HIV and hepatitis. When you see dangerous practices, it is usually best to confront the employee first. As an extern, you may or may not feel comfortable doing that. You will have a faculty member who has been designated as the externship coordinator. This person needs to be notified. He or she will help you decide the best way to handle the situation. If necessary, the office manager or clinical supervisor might address the issue with everyone in an office meeting rather than singling out particular employees.

 CHECKPOINT QUESTION

1. What is the role of the preceptor?

Externship Benefits

Benefits to the Student

Externship is a vital part of medical assisting training. You will develop self-confidence and professionalism during the externship portion of your training. No amount of classroom training can compare with the experience of applying skills and knowledge in a medical facility. An externship also allows you to broaden your knowledge base by learning new and different equipment and techniques. You will adapt your base of knowledge to your environment.

Benefits to the Medical Assisting Program

As you gain experience from the externship, the school also benefits from the affiliation, or connection, with the medical community. Many sites have a long history of training students. Schools rely on good training sites to enhance the medical assisting curriculum. Medical assisting programs also rely on the medical profession to aid in updating and revising the curriculum and course content to ensure that the methods and procedures presented to the students from year to year are current.

The school, the program director, and externship preceptors review students' extern experiences to change the program to reflect the needs of the community and the profession as health care constantly changes, such as with new technology. If students are routinely required to perform a procedure or examination that is not a part of the curriculum, for example, this will usually be considered for an addition to future lectures and laboratory sessions. If the accepted practice of a procedure has changed, changes will be made in the way it is taught to ensure that students are kept abreast of health care advances.

Benefits to the Externship Site

The student and the school are not the only ones to benefit from the externship period. The site also gains information about how well different areas of the facility are functioning. Site personnel may discover through the presence and questions of students that they should review certain policies or add others to help the office run more smoothly. Medical facilities must be updated on a continuing basis. Items may be deleted or added to policy, and procedure manuals or parts may have to be revised to provide clearer instructions.

As a student, you will be looking at the office as a newcomer, with a fresh perspective, and you may have many questions for the staff. As you become more familiar with the office routine, you will be more comfortable asking questions without the fear of appearing inexperienced. These questions may help point out to the office personnel things that should be changed or clarified.

Externship Responsibilities

Responsibilities of the Student

You will develop many attributes, or characteristics, of a professional health care worker during the externship program. You should foster characteristics during this time to ensure that you continue to grow professionally and are an asset to the profession.

You must be dependable. Dependability is a good sign of maturity. Students who are not at the site on time, who take excessive numbers of breaks, or who do not follow through on assignments cannot properly provide for the needs of the patients who rely on the medical staff of the facility.

You must act in a professional manner. All concepts of professionalism include a positive, pleasant, confident attitude with a sincere desire to help the physician, the patient, and the staff.

You must be well groomed and meet the program's dress code. If the medical facility requires clothing that differs from your school's requirements, you are usually asked to comply with the site's requirements.

Many programs require you to keep a journal listing the events of each day at the extern site. Students will be expected to assist in the completion of the evaluation form and must therefore keep records of dates and procedures observed and performed. You will also keep a record of the time you spent at the site.

 CHECKPOINT QUESTION

2. List three responsibilities that you have during your externship.

ETHICAL TIP

HIPAA and Students

The Health Insurance Portability and Accountability Act of 1996 (HIPAA) Privacy Rule does not prohibit students accessing patient medical information as part of their education. The wording of the privacy rules defines "health care operations" in a way that includes training of health care providers and professionals. Students are part of the covered entity's workforce for HIPAA compliance purposes. The rule does require that students receive training about the organization's policies and procedures related to protected health information. This training must be completed within a reasonable period of time after the student begins the externship. Documentation of this training must be kept for 6 years.

Responsibilities of the Medical Assisting Program

The primary responsibility of the program is to arrange for the best possible clinical experience for students. The program usually has a coordinator who matches students to appropriate sites. Once a site has been chosen, you will meet with the externship coordinator to discuss the particulars of the medical facility. An interview is sometimes held to acquaint you with your preceptor before the externship begins.

After your site rotation has begun, the program's externship coordinator will visit or call frequently to follow your progress. If either you or the site has concerns, the coordinator will mediate to eliminate problems or concerns as they arise.

The externship coordinator will make an evaluation, or appraisal, of your progress at the site. These evaluations, which are discussed later, will be used to determine whether you are prepared for the profession or your skills are deficient and need more reinforcement. The school is also responsible for maintaining liability insurance for students during clinical hours. You may pay a small premium when you pay your tuition. Students are required in most instances to provide proof of general immunizations and vaccination for hepatitis B. Some schools may provide the vaccine for students. Most programs require a current physical examination, a serology profile, and a tuberculin skin test before students are admitted to the program or before they make contact with patients.

Responsibilities of the Externship Site

The medical facility is, of course, responsible for providing opportunities for training. The staff will help orient you to the office and its policies. In some sites, students are allowed only to observe certain procedures but are given permission to perform some basic or routine procedures. Even if you are not allowed to perform specific procedures, the opportunity to observe and ask questions will be useful. In this way, you will become as familiar as possible with all clinical areas and functions. In many cases, the site preceptor will plan and oversee your externship experience, verify time sheets and other documentation generated at the extern site, and report to the externship coordinator from your school.

Guidelines for a Successful Externship

Success in your externship is important for you to obtain employment. Your success in your externship is evaluated according to certain standards, or criteria. The person or persons evaluating you during your externship are professional medical personnel who know the standards for the health care field as they relate to medical assisting. These areas include the following:

- Procedural performance
- Preparedness
- Attendance
- Appearance
- Attitude

Procedural Performance

You will be judged on your ability to measure up to the standard of care for an entry-level medical assistant. This means you are expected to perform at the level of a new employee in the field. Your preceptor is there to assist you, not to teach you the basics that you should have learned in the classroom. Come to your externship prepared. Ask questions, when in doubt, before starting any procedure. Ask questions outside the patient's room. Never perform a procedure alone, unless otherwise directed by your instructor.

Preparedness

Preparation is the best insurance for success, regardless of the goal. Personal preparation for the externship helps prevent losing time because of other extracurricular obligations. Make sure in advance that you have prepared:

- Reliable transportation
- Reliable day care services
- Backup systems for a sick child, snow cancellations of school, or early dismissals from school
- Financial coverage and support for any hours that you are unable to work at your usual job because of your extern site hours

Attendance

If you have planned well for transportation, family considerations, and finances, you are more likely to attend all sessions at the clinical sites. You must also be healthy. A good diet, regular exercise, and proper rest help you maintain good health. Careful attention to hygiene and medical asepsis help ensure that you do not bring illnesses home from the clinical sites.

If at any time you will be late or will not be able to attend the site for any reason, you must notify both the externship coordinator and the site preceptor. Never be a no-call or no-show. Almost all sites have an answering service for leaving messages, as do most schools. There is no excuse for not notifying all parties involved if you will be unavoidably late or will not be able to attend the scheduled session.

Office hours vary from site to site; it is always a good practice, however, to arrive a few minutes before the scheduled opening. This allows time to check for telephone messages, arrange the day's appointments, turn on office equipment, and generally get into the routine of the office. Plan your transportation, leaving plenty of time for any problems that may occur. Arriving in a flurry, frustrated by traffic or home problems, with no time to ease into your day causes a high level of tension and anxiety. This makes it more difficult to have the caring and compassionate attitude necessary to deal with the complex problems in the medical office.

Appearance

You have only one opportunity to make a first impression, which is usually based on appearance. Appearance is much more than looks. A beautiful face on a poorly groomed person is not seen as professional and does not inspire trust and confidence in patients or co-workers. The key to a professional appearance is careful preparation and planning.

If you wear a uniform for your externship, it must be freshly laundered and pressed; clean but wrinkled is not acceptable. Plan your wardrobe for ease of care and a professional appearance. Fad or trendy clothing, suggestive clothing, and flashy clothing are not appropriate for clinical sites. All clothing should be in good repair, with no missing buttons, hanging hems, tears, rips, or stains. Duty shoes should be clean, polished frequently, and kept in good condition. Laced shoes look better with fresh, clean shoelaces. Check nylon hosiery for runs and snags and replace them as needed. You may wear laboratory coats in some programs; uniforms may be worn in others. The clinical preceptor or the externship coordinator will inform you of the dress code in advance.

Professional appearance includes hair and makeup. Your hair should be conservatively styled, and long hair must be kept away from the face. Wash it frequently so that it is fresh and clean. Makeup should be minimal and tastefully applied. Never use perfume or cologne, which may be irritating to co-workers and patients. Keep fingernails short to avoid transferring pathogens or ripping gloves when you perform procedures.

Wear only minimal, tasteful jewelry. Rings can puncture gloves, possibly causing exposure to a pathogen. Therefore, it is a good idea to avoid wearing them in the clinical site.

 CHECKPOINT QUESTION

3. Describe the proper attire for your externship.

Attitude

Attitude is also part of appearance. Most patients and co-workers will see your emotions through facial expressions and body language. A person who looks eager is usually perceived as a good, diligent worker. Attitude is determined by how well you handle change and direction and how adaptable and flexible you are during difficult assignments.

The medical profession is constantly changing, making it imperative for all professionals to stay flexible. In the classroom, you learn generic methods for treatments and procedures. Because of the constantly changing technology, you may have to adjust to other methods in the field. If you learned a procedure one way in the classroom training but find that it is performed differently in the clinical site, the new method must be accepted and performed as well as possible. Frequently, there is more than one right way to do a procedure, and the classroom method you learned may be just one of

---

BOX 16-1

STRATEGIES FOR A SUCCESSFUL EXTERNSHIP

Your externship will be successful if you:

- Show enthusiasm and interest in learning.
- Are a team player.
- Offer to assist with as many tasks as possible.
- Ask questions or for clarification before doing any procedures or tasks about which you are unsure.
- Immediately admit to any errors or mistakes that you make.
- Accept corrections and suggestions by staff members.
- Anticipate tasks that need to be done, and do them before you are asked.
- Do not make remarks such as: "I can't believe that you don't have that on the computer." "This office is outdated." "Don't you know about these new regulations?"

---

the accepted methods. The next physician or clinical site may use yet another equally correct procedural method.

Your attitude determines your altitude. Students who work with a positive attitude during their externship are likely to reach higher levels of the profession than those who see the externship as an imposition or a burden. Box 16-1 offers some additional suggestions.

 LEGAL TIP

YOU'RE IN THE REAL WORLD NOW!

In Chapter 2, you learned that a medical assistant practices under the license of a physician. As an extern, you are not an employee of the physician; therefore, the legal doctrine of respondeat superior does not apply. Since you are participating in a college activity, any liability issues are covered by the college's liability or malpractice insurance. Most colleges have a blanket policy to cover students who are taking courses conducted in a medical facility that has entered into a clinical affiliation with the college. Students pay a fee at the beginning of the semester of the clinical experience. Malpractice insurance covers any issues with patient care in the medical site. It is important that you identify yourself as a student. You must be wearing a name tag with your student status clearly visible. Patients have the right to know who is participating in their care. The Joint Commission requires that licensed medical facilities that participate in student learning must screen students as if they were employees. Most extern sites will require criminal background and drug testing before allowing a student to begin an externship. In other words, students are put through the same hiring process as the permanent employees. Licensure and certification are discussed in Chapter 2.

Externship Documentation

Most programs use a time sheet or record of some sort to document your hours in the externship (Fig. 16-2). The beginning and ending hours of each day are recorded. How breaks are handled depends on the externship coordinator, program requirements, and specific site. Some sites allow half an hour for lunch, and others allow an hour; some close for an hour or more midday, while others are open and staffed from morning until evening. Some programs make students responsible for time sheet signatures; others delegate the responsibility to the site preceptor. However the form is handled, it is used to validate your time in the externship and is a requirement for completion of most programs.

Journals are required by many programs. These provide proof that tasks are performed and learning takes place. The student will list each day's activities, and this is reviewed by the externship coordinator. Checklists serve as further documentation of tasks observed and performed. In many cases, the site supervisor actually assigns a grade to the student using criteria provided by

---

**CLINICAL EXPERIENCE
STUDENT'S TIME REPORT**

To obtain proper credit, an account of time and days in attendance must be recorded by each intern student. This report must be verified by the job supervisor and attached to the final 55-day roster. This information is kept strictly confidential.

Student's Name: _____   Course No.: _____

Program: _____   Course Title: _____

Minimum Contact Hrs. Required: _____   Quarter/Year: _____

WEEK OF (DATES)	TIME OF DAY							TOTAL HOURS	SITE SUPERVISOR
	M	T	W	TH	F	S			

TOTAL HOURS FOR QUARTER: _____

I certify that the above time report is a true statement of the hours worked.

I approve this statement of hours in attendance for the quarter covered.

_____   _____   _____   _____
Student's Signature   Date   Externship Coordinator's Signature   Date

Figure 16-2 Sample extern time sheet.

the college. Site evaluations performed by the student are another form of externship documentation and are discussed in the next section.

Every accredited school will use surveys to gather information from students. Sample evaluations are available through The American Association of Medical Assistants' (AAMA's) Web site. Evaluations are used to improve performance and services offered to students. Most medical assisting programs have advisory boards whose members use the results of such surveys to make necessary changes to existing programs. Your input is vital to this ongoing quest for excellence. Take these evaluations seriously and be honest. Do not take the opportunity to complain about individual problems that may have been encountered. It is more appropriate to address these concerns under comments. For example, if a particular instructor's grading criteria are more strict than others' criteria, your evaluation of that instructor should not be based on the fact that you got a lower grade in his or her class. You should be fair and objective and evaluate the instructor on his or her actual performance in the classroom. Evaluations are not designed to prove popularity but to report strengths and deficiencies in areas that can be improved.

Externship Evaluations

The preceptor or office manager at your site will evaluate you on a completed form that contains detailed areas to be graded; these are equivalent to grades on a test or examination. The externship coordinator is responsible for compiling evaluations and keeping you abreast of your progress. Frequent conferences with your coordinator usually help accomplish this. After your externship is completed, your input in the quality of your experience helps program administrators choose the best extern sites in the future.

Most schools use a site evaluation form to gather impressions of the program's extern sites and the students' overall externship experience (Fig. 16-3). This form helps determine the effectiveness of the site for training and whether any issues should be addressed before assigning other students. Be objective and honest in your evaluation of the site. When completing a site evaluation, consider these questions:

- Was the overall experience positive or negative?
- Were opportunities for learning abundant and freely offered or hard to obtain?
- Were staff personnel open and caring or unwelcoming?
- Was the preceptor available and easily approachable or preoccupied and distant?

If the site is not providing a positive learning experience, the program should discontinue using it.

Graduate Surveys

When you graduate, the college will want to know your opinion of its instruction and services. You will be asked to evaluate your experience at the college in general, your course work, and your extern experience. Take the time to think back over your overall experience at the school. Information provided is tabulated and distributed to those evaluated. This is an integral part of the quality improvement and planning processes of educational institutions. Figure 16-4 illustrates a sample graduate survey.

Employer Surveys

After you have been on a job for awhile, the college will survey your employer to assess his/her satisfaction with your performance, skills, and professionalism. Figure 16-5 is a sample of an employer evaluation. You must always do your best. Your performance is not only a reflection of you but also of your medical assisting program and the college you attended.

 CHECKPOINT QUESTION

4. What is the purpose of having students evaluate their externship experience?

COG **Establish the Job for You**

Once your externship is complete, you are one step closer to getting the job that you desire. Take an inventory of your qualifications, strengths, and weakness. Preparation will help you search for and find the perfect job.

Setting Employment Goals

Before beginning to search for a job, decide what you want and need from a job and make that your goal. People who do not set employment goals too often accept only what is presented to them. They often end up unhappy in their work because they did not choose their job in the first place. The average person approaches the job search with the attitude, "I wonder what is available," rather than, "Here is what I would like to do, and here is the facility where I would like to work." *That* is setting a goal. It is also a positive, proactive approach to the job market rather than a reactive position to what is available. In general, the medical field is looking for proactive people. You will work harder and more enthusiastically if you choose your workplace.

The best way to set a goal and eventually get what you want is to study your strengths and weaknesses and, from that self-knowledge, design the best job for you. Goal setting means describing the ideal job for you and deciding that this is the job that you will someday have.

Externship Site Evaluation

Pittsylvania Community College

Medical Assisting Program

Name of externship site being evaluated: ____________________________

INSTRUCTIONS: Consider each item separately and rate each item independently of all others. Circle the rating that indicates the extent to which you agree with each statement. Please do not skip any rating.
5 = Strongly Agree 4 = Generally Agree 3 = Neutral (acceptable) 2 = Generally Disagree
1 = Strongly Disagree N/A = This activity is Not Available at this site

At this externship site, I was:

1. Provided orientation to the office/facility	5	4	3	2	1	N/A
2. Assigned to a supervisor/preceptor who actively participated in my learning experience	5	4	3	2	1	N/A
3. Allowed to perform the entry-level skills I had learned in school	5	4	3	2	1	N/A
4. Given the opportunity to perform administrative skills	5	4	3	2	1	N/A
5. Given the opportunity to perform clinical skills	5	4	3	2	1	N/A
6. Adequately supervised and knew who to ask for help if I needed it	5	4	3	2	1	N/A
7. Treated respectfully by healthcare providers and other staff	5	4	3	2	1	N/A
8. Provided with adequate personal protective equipment (e.g. gloves) to protect my health and safety	5	4	3	2	1	N/A
9. Able to communicate effectively with						
a. supervisory personnel	5	4	3	2	1	N/A
b. staff and co-workers	5	4	3	2	1	N/A
c. physicians/health care professionals	5	4	3	2	1	N/A
d. patients/clients/family members	5	4	3	2	1	N/A
10. Not used to replace paid employees	5	4	3	2	1	N/A
11. Provided regular constructive verbal feedback from by supervisor	5	4	3	2	1	N/A
12. Provided a final written performance evaluation	5	4	3	2	1	N/A

13. Were you asked to perform any skills for which you were not prepared by your medical assisting program?
_______Yes _______No

If yes, please identify: ____________________________

14. Would you recommend this site for future externship students? ___Yes ___No Why? __________

____

15. What part of the externship experience did you like best and/or least? ______________

____

Student's name and signature ____________________________ Date __________

Figure 16-3 Sample site evaluation form.

On a sheet of paper, describe the best job for you if you had your choice. For example, you might describe these elements:

- Specialty area (e.g., obstetrics, pediatrics, surgery)
- Duties (clinical or administrative)
- Type of employer and supervisor
- Other employees and co-workers
- Type of facility
- Desired atmosphere (casual or formal)
- Ideal hours
- Availability of flextime (a system of scheduling that allows for a personal choice in hours or days worked)

Next, write down where you expect to be in 2 years and in 5 years, in terms of both position and income. Now you are more focused on where you want to work, what you want to do, and the direction you want to be going. The next question is how to get there.

To win the position you want, you have to learn to sell yourself. Generally, employers will not come looking for you; you will have to go to them. They will compare you with all of the other equally well-qualified candidates who are interested in the same position. If 25 people interview for a job, even if you are second best, you still lose. The one who is best suited for a job does not necessarily get it; instead, frequently the one who

---

GRADUATE SURVEY

Pittsylvania Community College
MEDICAL ASSISTING PROGRAM

The primary goal of a Medical Assisting Education program is to prepare its graduates to function as competent Medical Assistants. This survey is designed to help your program faculty determine the strengths of your program as well as those areas that need improvement. All data will be kept confidential and will be used for program evaluation purposes only.

BACKGROUND INFORMATION:

Job Title: _____ If not working, what are you doing? _____

Current Salary (optional): _____

Place of employment: _____

Length of employment at time of survey: _____ years and/or _____ months.

Name of graduate (Optional): _____

Certification/Registration Status (check all that apply): ☐ CMA ___ RMA

INSTRUCTIONS: Consider each item separately and rate each item independently of all others. Circle the rating that indicates the extent to which you agree with each statement. Please do not skip any rating.
5 = Strongly Agree   4 = Generally Agree   3 = Neutral (acceptable)   2 = Generally Disagree   1 = Strongly Disagree

I. KNOWLEDGE (Cognitive Learning Domain)
THE PROGRAM:

A. Helped me acquire the medical assisting knowledge appropriate to my level of training.	5	4	3	2	1
B. Helped me acquire the general medical knowledge base appropriate to my level of training	5	4	3	2	1
C. Prepared me to collect patient data effectively.	5	4	3	2	1
D. Prepared me to perform appropriate diagnostic and medical procedures.	5	4	3	2	1
E. Trained me to use sound judgment while functioning in the healthcare setting.	5	4	3	2	1

Comments:_____

II. SKILLS (Psychomotor Learning Domain)
THE PROGRAM:

A. Prepared me to perform all clinical skills appropriate to entry level medical assisting	5	4	3	2	1
B. Prepared me to perform all administrative skills appropriate to entry level medical assisting.	5	4	3	2	1

Comments: _____

February 2006, 2013   1

III. BEHAVIORS (Affective Learning Domain)
THE PROGRAM:

A. Prepared me to communicate effectively in the healthcare setting.	5	4	3	2	1
B. Prepared me to conduct myself in an ethical and professional manner.	5	4	3	2	1
C. Taught me to manage my time efficiently while functioning in the healthcare setting.	5	4	3	2	1
D. Strongly encouraged me to apply for and pass my:					
CMA	5	4	3	2	1
RMA	5	4	3	2	1

Comments: _____

IV. GENERAL INFORMATION *(Check yes or no)*

A. I have attained CMA certification.	☐ YES	☐ NO
B. I have attained RMA registry.	☐ YES	☐ NO
C. I am a member of the American Association of Medical Assistants	☐ YES	☐ NO
D. I am a member of the American Medical Technology Association	☐ YES	☐ NO
E. I actively participate in continuing education activities.	☐ YES	☐ NO

If you answered NO to any of the above questions, please explain why: _____
_____

V. ADDITIONAL COMMENTS

OVERALL RATING:
Please rate and comment on the OVERALL quality of your preparation as a medical assistant:
5 = Excellent   4 = Very Good   3 = Good   2 = Fair   1 = Poor

Comments: _____

Please identify two or three strengths of the program.
_____

Please make two or three suggestions to further strengthen the program.
_____

What qualities/skills were expected of you upon employment that were not included in the program?
_____

Please provide comments and suggestions that would help to better prepare future graduates.
_____

Thank You!   Date: _____

February 2006, 2013   2

Figure 16-4 Sample graduate survey.

---

performs best in the interview does. Marketing yourself takes real effort.

Self-Analysis

A good presentation of your qualifications begins with self-analysis. You must know what strengths you have to offer a potential employer as well as your weaknesses. Make an honest list of your strengths and weaknesses. Each of your strengths presents an opportunity to sell yourself and your value as an employee. When you are interviewing for a position, concentrate on projecting your strengths to the interviewer.

Just as your strengths give you a special advantage, each weakness is a reason someone may not want to offer you the position. Recognize and work to resolve your weaknesses. Recognizing your weaknesses as a threat to securing the position you want will help you develop strategies to eliminate these problems or turn them into strengths. As long as you are aware of your weaknesses, you are better prepared to handle them.

Once you know the type of job you want and have identified your positive and negative qualities, it is time to begin to look for the right job.

 CHECKPOINT QUESTION

5. What is the purpose of self-analysis?

COG Finding the Right Job

The internet offers employment services that allow you to search for a certain type job in a specific geographic location. Even though searching the internet is easier and less time consuming than the traditional ways of looking for a job, an internet search may not be the best way to find a job. For jobs in your hometown, it is helpful to begin with the newspaper. Keep in mind that many of the most desirable job openings are never advertised; they are posted internally and filled from within. Membership in your professional organization is an excellent way to network.

Many studies show that most positions are never advertised in the media. Open positions that are posted internally are often filled with current employees or by referrals from current employees. Any organization that looks within and obtains a recommendation from a current employee to fill an available position accomplishes two things: (1) it saves the cost of advertising, and (2) the recommendation itself is usually a good one because it comes from someone who presumably knows the demands and special needs of that particular organization.

It is important for someone seeking employment in the medical field to build as many contacts within the field as possible. These contacts help you with **networking**. Networking is using friends, family members, and professional colleagues to advance or obtain

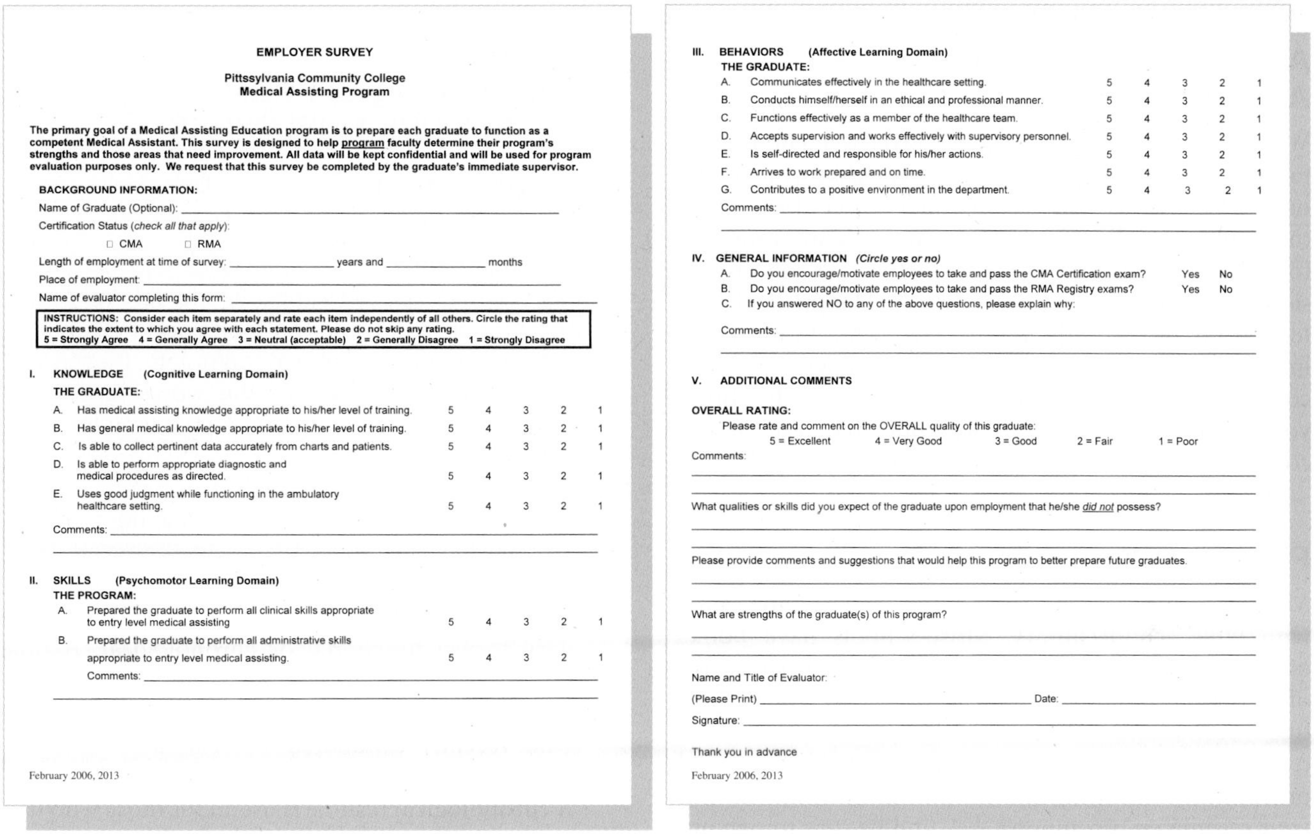

Figure 16-5 Sample employer evaluation.

information in the workplace. It is impossible to have too many contacts. Everyone with whom you associate should know that you are looking for employment. Friends and acquaintances cannot tell you about a job or recommend you for a job if they do not know that you are searching.

Traditional sources of information for job openings:

- *Local, state, or federal government employment offices.* These agencies are designed to find work for the unemployed. They frequently have listings of positions that are not found anywhere else. Rather than calling the office with inquiries, make an appointment to visit. Register with the service. Get to know the contact person with whom you will be contacting frequently.

- *School placement office.* If your school has a placement office, contact the coordinator or personnel officer and outline what you are looking for and where you want to work. Their job is to assist you in securing the position you want. If you establish a working relationship with a contact person, you will probably have better results.

- *Medical facilities.* Do not wait for an advertisement. Go to the office or facility where you would like to work and leave a résumé—a document summarizing your professional qualifications—and a cover letter explaining how much you want to work there. Find

out the name of the office manager or personnel officer and call first for an appointment. This shows better planning and foresight and is more professional than dropping by unannounced.

- *Private agencies.* Many medical facilities solicit privately to avoid being swamped by applications from unqualified applicants. A fee is charged for the service but is usually paid by the employer. Call the agency to make an appointment with a representative who will interview you and tell you what steps to follow.

- *Temporary services.* These agencies fill short-term vacancies for medical offices. If you are new in an area, this is a good way to learn which facilities would be good choices for you. You may be assigned for several days or several weeks. If you work well as a temporary replacement and like the site, leave your résumé and let the appropriate individuals know that you would like to work in this place if an opening occurs. Check with the temporary agency regarding any fees that you may be charged or that the medical office may have to pay if it hires you, often called a finder's fee.

CHECKPOINT QUESTION

6. List four resources that you may use to identify potential job opportunities.

COG **Applying for the Job**

Answering Newspaper Advertisements

When responding to a newspaper advertisement, be sure to do exactly what the advertisement asks you to do; one of the qualities that many interviewers look for is the ability to follow directions. At the same time, try to make your response more distinctive (yet still professional) than others they may receive. The medical profession rarely responds well to those who do not fit its image and almost never accepts someone who does not conform at the entry level. Most employers will require you to submit a résumé. A well-prepared résumé and cover letter are essential to job hunting.

Preparing Your Résumé

Many resources can help you write your **résumé**. Start with your school library. Most schools have books on how to create résumés. Numerous Web sites also offer this information. Caution: Many Web sites have free information, but some charge fees. Focus on free resources before paying for these services. Many word processing programs have templates for résumés. Put your résumé on a computer disk and be sure to personalize it for the position you are seeking. For example, if you give a career objective, try putting in the title a description of the particular job you are seeking. Keep changing this for every different position so that your résumé is personalized for each interview.

The résumé is a flash picture of yourself; if it is neat and professional, the reviewer will presume that it is a reflection of you. Procedure 16-1 outlines the steps in writing a résumé. Here are some guidelines that will help you create a résumé that will capture the reviewer's interest.

1. Evaluate your skills, goals, and what you have to offer. With this list in hand, you can better concentrate on highlighting your strengths.
2. Confine your résumé to one page, selecting carefully what you want to include. The résumé must state just what the reviewer needs to know and no more.
3. Include the following key information:
   - Name, address, and telephone number: Include these at the top of your résumé (usually centered). (Because you are including your telephone number, you should expect calls from prospective employers. Box 16-2 offers some tips for handling such calls.)
   - Education: Start with the most recent and work backward.
   - Affiliations or volunteer work (if appropriate): If this information shows that you have good organizational skills or have held an office for the group, you should include it.

BOX 16-2

HANDLING CALLS FROM PROSPECTIVE EMPLOYERS

Here are some tips for handling calls from prospective employers:

- Tell family members or other household members that you are expecting important telephone calls.
- Keep a pen and paper by the telephone.
- Instruct people to take a complete message. Ask them to write down the person's name, phone number, message, and what time the call was received.
- Leave a professional message on your answering machine. Avoid leaving cute or silly messages.

   - Experience: This may be listed in either of two standard forms: functional or chronological. A functional résumé focuses on skills and qualifications rather than employment and works well for those who recently graduated or who are re-entering the job market after a period of years (Fig. 16-6). A chronological résumé is useful for those who have an employment history, particularly if the history is relevant to the position being sought. Start with the most recent employment and work backward. Include your title, position, and a few of your key responsibilities (Fig. 16-7). Explain any gaps such as pregnancy, schooling, relocations, and so on.
   - References: You may or may not include your references on a separate sheet. When you have chosen the people you want to use as references, be sure to ask their permission. Start by asking your instructors if you can use them as references. Other medical professionals (physicians or nurses) will also make strong references. Previous employers also make very good references. You should have a minimum of three references. Do not bring a list of more than five people. Prospective employers are not interested in your neighbors, pastor, or relatives as references.
4. Do not include hobbies and personal interests unrelated to work. It is not relevant that you play the guitar, but it would be impressive to know that you volunteer at a free clinic.
5. Use action words (Box 16-3).
6. Center the résumé on white or off-white heavy bond or high rag content paper, 8.5 × 11 inches. (Colors are not acceptable, and cheap paper will not convey the professional impression you hope to make.) Keep a 1-inch margin around the text. Single space within the sections of information, but leave a blank line between the sections.

Tina Elmwood C.M.A.
22 Brandy Drive
Dayton, Ohio 00000
444-777-6666

Employment Objective: To use my medical assisting skills in a challenging position. My goal is to work with children. (*Change this sentence to reflect the type of office that you are applying to.*)

Experience:

Externship (160 hours) at Family Practice Associates, Bayview Drive, Dayton, Ohio (*If you have a positive evaluation from your preceptor, bring it with you to the interview. Do not attach it to the résumé.*)

Education:

Medical Assisting Program, Diploma. Graduated June 2008. West County Community College, Dayton Ohio (*Bring a copy of your diploma and transcripts to the interview. Do not attach them unless employer has specifically requested them.*)
Dayton High School, Diploma. Graduated June 2006. Dayton, Ohio

Skills:

Clinical and Laboratory skills listed on Role Delineation for Medical Assisting

Administrative skills listed on Role Delineation for Medical Assisting

Comfortable using all types of standard office equipment

Familiar with XYZ software programs (*List software programs that you are comfortable with. If you know what type of software the office uses, list that as well.*)

Certifications:

Certified Medical Assistant, American Association of Medical Assistants (*Bring copy to interview or attach to résumé.*)
Cardiopulmonary Resuscitation, American Heart Association (*Bring copy to interview or attach to résumé.*)

Figure 16-6 Sample functional résumé.

7. Use regular type. Avoid fonts that are cute or fancy. Use black ink. Do not print your résumé in color.
8. Have someone proofread your work. It is difficult to find your own errors or see areas that are not clearly worded.
9. Mail the résumé in an 8.5 × 11–inch manila envelope. This will present the interviewer with a résumé and cover letter that are smooth, with no fold lines. Many prefer to work with résumés that have not been folded for an envelope.
10. Many employers are now allowing applicants to send their résumés as an e-mail attachment. Use a well-known software to create your résumé, and keep it simple because some formatting may not transmit properly.
11. Be honest. Do not embellish your résumé or add fictional information. This could get you fired.

 CHECKPOINT QUESTION

7. What is the difference between a functional résumé and a chronological résumé?

Preparing Your Cover Letter

When contacting a prospective employer about a job, you need to send a résumé along with a cover letter. Keep your cover letter brief and meaningful. You want it to be read, and you want the reader to be impressed by what it says. Be sure that you mention the job itself in your letter. You may even consider a statement such as, "This is the type of position I would prefer." If you are applying to a pediatrician's office, you may write, "My goal is to work with children." If you know something favorable about the facility, include that in your letter. If you know anyone who works for the company, mention it. *Do not*

Beatrice Meza CMA
123 Main Street
West Harford, CT 00000
888-999-6666

Employment Objective: To use my medical assisting skills in a challenging position. My goal is to work in an obstetrical office. (*Change this sentence to reflect the type of office that you are applying to.*)

Education:

2013–2014 Medical Assisting Program; Mountain Laurel Community College, West Hartford, Connecticut (*Bring a copy of your diploma and transcripts to the interview. Do not attach them unless employer has specifically requested them.*)

Externship:

July 2014–(160 hours) Women's Health Care Center, Hartford, Connecticut (*If you have a positive evaluation from your preceptor, bring it with you to the interview. Do not attach it to the résumé.*)

Work Experience:

July 2013–present Receptionist, Dermatology Consultants, West Hartford, Connecticut. Worked part time while I was in school. Answered and triaged telephone calls. Assisted with various other medical administrative responsibilities. (*If you have a reference letter from this employer, bring it with you to the interview. Be prepared to answer questions about why you are leaving this position.*)
May 2010–July 2013 Cashier/Clerk for SuperMarket Grocers, West Hartford, Connecticut. Worked part time. Responsible for training new employees. Promoted to senior cashier.

Skills:

Clinical and Laboratory skills listed on the Role Delineation for Medical Assisting
Administrative skills listed on the Role Delineation for Medical Assisting
Comfortable using all types of standard office equipment
Familiar with XYZ software programs (*List software programs that you are comfortable with. If you know what type of software the office uses, list that as well.*)

Activities/Honors

Student Government representative
Most Improved Medical Assisting Student in 2013

Figure 16-7 Sample chronological résumé.

BOX 16-3

ACTION WORDS

Achieved	Established	Planned
Assisted	Filed	Prepared
Attained	Generated	Processed
Conducted	Handled	Scheduled
Completed	Implemented	Screened
Composed	Maintained	Selected
Created	Operated	Solved
Developed	Organized	Systemized
Directed	Participated	Wrote
Ensured	Performed	

---

mention the person by name unless you have secured his or her permission.

Make sure you address your letter to the right person. Call the personnel department or office manager and ask the name of the person handling the applications. Determine the correct spelling of the name and the preferred honorific, such as Mr., Ms., or Mrs.

The standard form for a cover letter has three brief paragraphs:

- First paragraph: State the position for which you are applying.
- Second paragraph: Stress your skills. Do not be redundant, since you will also send a résumé, but mention or highlight specifically the skills needed for this job.

- Third paragraph: Request an interview. Offer to call in a week to set up an interview (then do so). Keep a copy of your letter to refer to when calling.

Use the same good-quality paper for the cover letter that you use for your résumé. Include your name, address, and telephone number at the top of the page, centered or in block form. Single space the letter, and double space between paragraphs. Either block or modified block form is acceptable.

As mentioned earlier, many employers are now accepting résumés via e-mail. Although this may eliminate the need for a cover letter, the information included should still be communicated as an e-mail message. Accuracy is just as important in an electronic communication as in any other form. It is more professional to attach your résumé as a document instead of placing it in the body of an e-mail.

Completing an Employment Application

Some sites will have you fill out an employment application while you wait for your interview; others may mail one to you to be filled out and taken to the interview. Although résumés have their place and are indispensable, many facilities rely more on an application form. Many organizations accept online applications. The guidelines for completing an online application are similar to those of manual completion of an application:

1. Read through completely before beginning.
2. Follow the instructions exactly. Prospective employers notice neatness, erasures, evasions, and indecision.
3. Answer every question. If the question does not apply to you, draw a line or write N/A so that the interviewer will know that you did not overlook the question.
4. In the line for wage or salary desired, write "negotiable" or find out before the interview what is usual for the area for this type of position.
5. In spaces requesting your reason for leaving a previous position, try to sound positive. Answers such as "to explore a new career direction" are general enough to fill many needs. If the reason for leaving was relocation, schooling, or pregnancy, say so.
6. Type, or print legibly, being as neat as possible.
7. Use a black or blue pen. Never use a pencil or colored pen (red, green, purple) to complete the application. It does not portray a professional image.
8. You may attach your résumé to the application if you did not mail one already.

COG The Interview

Interviewing well is a skill that takes effort to develop. The résumé introduces you to potential employers, but the interview is how you "sell" yourself to them. As with any skill, if you want to stay proficient and keep your skills in good working order, you have to practice. Ask friends or family members to work with you to develop a relaxed approach to answering the questions most often asked during an interview. Have them try to trip you up or confuse you by throwing in tricky questions. Although the effect will not be the same with a friend or family member as with an interviewer, this practice can make a difference between getting the job and losing the chance. You can also rehearse in front of a mirror.

Usually, the person who interviews best is hired for the position. An excellent interview is absolutely crucial for obtaining any job. It is highly unlikely that you will get the job you want without doing well in the interview. Remember what the employer is looking for. Every employer is looking for something special from each employee. Medicine has special needs. The employer must believe that you possess a number of skills necessary to do the job:

- *Technical skills.* You must have the necessary proficiency to get the job done.
- *Confidentiality.* In medicine, you are exposed to sensitive information about patients. Is the interviewer convinced that you can be relied on to keep those confidences?
- *Human relations skills.* Will you get along with the others in the workplace?
- *Communication skills.* Do you have the verbal and writing skills that the job demands? Remember the importance of correct English. You will not be hired if your English and grammar are not exemplary.

If you fail to impress the interviewer with your grasp of these skills, you will never be considered for the position. The interviewer knows that whatever you display in the interview will also be displayed to the patients.

Preparing for the Interview

Before the day of the interview, find out all you can about the facility. What is its reputation? Does it have a big turnover of employees? Review your textbooks that cover the specialty so that you can ask informed questions about procedures performed at the site. Think of questions to ask and write them down. Anticipate questions that might be asked of you. Find out the name of the interviewer; if it is a difficult name, practice saying it. Go to the site ahead of time to be sure of its location and time the trip so that you will not be late for your appointment. Do this ideally at the same time of day as your appointment to judge traffic delays, parking problems, and so on.

Dress appropriately for the interview. The general rule is to dress one step above what is required for the job. Do not overdress, as if for a party; make sure your outfit is professional. Your personal hygiene must be

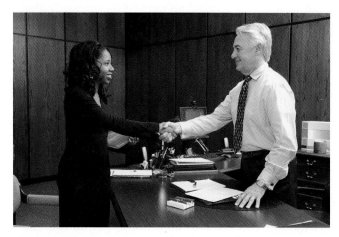

Figure 16-8 Dress and act professionally for the interview.

above reproach. If you normally smoke, avoid smoking before the interview. Those who do not smoke are acutely aware of the odor of smoke on one's clothes and breath. Avoid large jewelry and apply makeup carefully. Avoid perfumes; some people are very sensitive to scents.

Arrive on time or a few minutes early. Bring a few pens, a notepad, and your driver's license or official identification. Go alone; do not take a friend or family member for moral support. When you are introduced to the interviewer, offer your hand for a handshake and sit only when and where you are directed. Do not fidget, swing your foot, play with your hair, or tap your fingers on the chair arm. Make eye contact when the interviewer speaks with you and when you respond to the questions (Fig. 16-8). Sit up straight but relaxed, with your portfolio on your lap.

Completing a Portfolio

A **portfolio** is a folder or binder containing all of the information you will need to impress the interviewer. If you do not have a special folder or briefcase, a neat, new manila folder will be adequate. This folder or portfolio contains items that will verify the skills you have acquired. Procedure check-off sheets from your classes provide proof that you met the criteria needed to complete the tasks you will be expected to do on the job. Items known as "work product" in school are an excellent source as well. Assignments from the study guide and other graded work from instructors will show the quality of work. For example, a properly completed CMS-1500 from coding class will show an employer seeking a coder that you possess the knowledge to handle insurance claims.

Certificates of completion also make an impressive entry in a portfolio. They may be provided in your textbooks or from your instructors for specific training. For example, an instructor may give a certificate of completion for specific training for HIPAA, universal precautions, or blood-borne pathogens. Outside resources used

---

BOX 16-4

CONTENTS OF A PORTFOLIO

- Verification or at least the dates of immunizations (hepatitis B, TB test)
- Two copies of your résumé
- Two letters of reference
- Typed list of three references including names, phone numbers, and addresses
- Documentation of any special projects
- Copies of awards received

in your medical assisting program may also provide certificates, like the use of a fire extinguisher from the fire department or aging sensitivity training from an agency on aging. Other documentation that will help you present yourself to a prospective employer includes a copy of your current cardiopulmonary resuscitation certification, and letters of recommendation. The items usually included in your portfolio are listed in Box 16-4.

 WHAT IF?

You become tongue-tied during an interview. What should you do?

It's not unusual to feel nervous during the interview. To stay calm, take a deep breath and count to three before answering a question. Doing this also gives you time to think before you speak. Remember: Believe in yourself and your skills. Say to yourself, "I am going to get this job." Rehearse your answers to the common interview questions. Doing this exercise in front of a mirror is beneficial. Visit the Web sites listed in this chapter. Some of these sites offer virtual interviewing skills and have excellent tips for interviewing. Finally, arrive prepared and relaxed. Avoid excessive caffeine ingestion before the interview. Caffeine will increase your anxiety level.

Crucial Interview Questions

Every interviewer must have the answers to three basic questions. When you respond to the interviewer's questions, keep these in mind:

1. Do you have the necessary skills to do the job? (Don't forget to include any foreign language skills; Box 16-5.)
2. Do you have the necessary drive, energy, and commitment to get the job done?
3. Will you work well with the rest of the team?

BOX 16-5

KNOWLEDGE OF A FOREIGN LANGUAGE

If you are applying for a position that encourages bilingual applicants, be prepared for questions during the interview regarding your ability to speak another language. Know what languages are commonly spoken in your community. Whether it is Spanish, Polish, Italian, or any other language, take the time to become familiar with simple greetings: "Hello." "What is your name?" "Can I help you?" Tell the interviewer that you know a few words but are not fluent. It is not fair to the employer or to the patients to pretend otherwise if you are unable to communicate effectively. Most community colleges offer language courses. A local hospital may offer these courses with a focus on medical terms. Finally, the best way to learn a new language is to use it. If your classmates speak another language, ask them to tutor you. Being bilingual in the medical profession is always an asset.

A positive answer to all of these questions is not a guarantee that you will be offered the job, but a negative answer to any one of these will most assuredly mean that you will *not* get the job. Make sure that your comments make a positive impression regarding these three questions. In the medical field, the interviewer will need to establish your professionalism and ability to keep confidentiality. The interviewer will also want to know how interested you are in increasing and continuing your education and skills. Be sure that your answers will satisfy the interviewer.

Many interviewers use a prepared list of questions to direct the flow of the interview. Table 16-1 contains some commonly asked interview questions and guidance for responses. Be prepared with answers that will reflect well on your professionalism and qualifications.

When the interviewer finishes asking questions, he or she will usually ask if you have any questions. Refer to your notepad, on which you have listed questions such as these:

- What are the responsibilities of the position offered?
- If it is not personal, why is the current employee leaving?
- What are the opportunities for future advancement?
- How long is the training or probation period?
- How does the facility feel about continuing education? Do they pay membership dues to your professional organization? Is time off offered to employees to upgrade their skills? Does the facility subsidize the expense?
- Is there a job performance or evaluation process?
- What is the benefit package? Is there access to a 401(k) plan or other retirement plan? Health insurance? Life insurance?

Make notes of the answers for future reference. Avoid asking about time off or vacations during the interview. These questions imply that you are more interested in being paid to avoid work than you are in contributing to the work at hand.

Make sure the interviewer knows how important continuing education is to you. Talk about the types of continuing education courses you would like to attend and the subjects you would like to study. Show that you realize that the only constant in medicine is change and that you expect to keep abreast of the information in your area. Thank the interviewer for the opportunity to apply for the position and ask the time frame for a decision. As you leave, offer your hand for a handshake and ask if you may call again before the decision date to clear up any questions that the interviewer may have during the decision-making process.

Follow-Up

The day of the interview or no later than the day after, write a short thank you note for the opportunity to be interviewed and restate how interested you are in the job (Fig. 16-9). Remind the interviewer that you are available for additional questions. Call several days after the interview. Reintroduce yourself politely and add any new information or ask any questions that might have occurred to you after the interview. Thank the interviewer again for this opportunity.

Think back to your performance in the interview. Determine what skills you still need to develop or enhance in order to improve your interview skills. Remember that experience is the best teacher and each interview helps you continue to improve.

 CHECKPOINT QUESTION

8. What are the three basic questions in every interviewer's mind?

COG **Leaving a Job**

Should you leave, or should you stay? Almost everyone comes to this question at some point in his or her career. *Should I look for a new place to work and leave this place where I am safe and comfortable? Would another job be better or more satisfying? Would the benefits be better?*

An important factor in many relocations is salary. In addition to the financial aspects, however, employees today are looking for other elements that contribute to job satisfaction, such as:

- A sense of achievement
- Recognition
- Opportunity for growth and advancement

TABLE **16-1** Interview Questions and Responses	
Common Interview Questions	**Possible Responses and Points to Mention**
1. Tell me about yourself.	"I enjoy working with other people." Stress the good points you wrote on your self-analysis. Keep the comments professional. Do not give long explanations about personal topics. ("I have three brothers." "I like basketball.")
2. What are your strengths?	"My strengths are honesty and dependability." List any clinical or administrative skills in which you excel.
3. What are your weaknesses?	Be honest; everyone has a weakness. "My weakness is phlebotomy skills," and add, "but I have improved my skills by reading magazine articles about blood drawing and by practicing in the school laboratory." Do not say, "I am perfect" or "I have no weaknesses." State one weakness and explain how you are trying to improve it.
4. Why do you want this position?	"I like this office setting." "I always wanted to work for [as an example] a cardiologist." Mention that you are aware of the office's good reputation in the community, and if the location of the office is convenient, say so.
5. What are your goals?	List two or three immediate goals: "My priority is to acquire a medical assisting position that will be challenging and rewarding." Have at least two goals in your mind for where you want to be in 5 years.
6. Why did you leave your last position?	Always place a positive spin on why you left: "Looking for a new challenge." Never criticize past employers, their offices, or your co-workers.
7. What salary rate are you looking for?	Know the average pay in your area. Check with your placement office if you are unsure of the typical salaries. Never demand a certain pay rate.
8. How do you handle pressure?	Possible answers can include, "I set priorities" and "I remain calm and well organized." Avoid comments such as "I hate stress" or "I panic when I feel pressured."
9. Do you work better alone or as also part of a team?	Stress that you can work as a team member but that you can function independently.
10. Who was your best supervisor and why?	Possible remarks may include phrases such as "always fair," "supportive," and "encouraging." Avoid comments such as "She gave us long lunch breaks" or "She didn't make us work hard."
11. How do you handle conflict?	Indicate that you begin trying to resolve any problems in a professional manner. Indicate that you are always open to constructive criticism.
12. How would your classmates describe you?	Include remarks such as "good student," "team worker," and "helpful."
13. I noticed your grades in computer class were poor. Why?	Be honest: "It was a tough course" or "Although my grade was poor, I have restudied the course material, and my computer skills have improved." If you have taken any additional studies or tutoring to help in this subject area, mention that. Never say the teacher was unfair, the class was boring, or you didn't care about the class.
14. Describe the term "confidentiality" and how you would use it in our office.	Review the term. Stress to the interviewer that you know how important patient confidentiality is from a legal and ethical view point.

September 15, 2014

Dear Dr. Whitten,

I would like to thank you for the opportunity to meet with you today to discuss employment. I enjoyed meeting everyone. Your employees made me feel welcome. After meeting with you and spending some time in your office, I feel that I would be a good addition to your team. Thank you for considering me in filling your CMA position. I look forward to hearing from you.

Sincerely,

Jan Joyce, CMA

Figure 16-9 Sample thank you letter.

- Harmonious peer group relationships
- A good working relationship with supervisors
- Status
- Job security
- Comfortable working conditions
- Fair company policies

If you are no longer happy in your job, the reason probably lies in one or more of these elements. Before you make the decision to change jobs, do some internal soul searching to determine exactly what type of position would make you happy.

If you decide to leave your job, follow these steps:

- Always give adequate notice (minimum 2 weeks, optimal a month).
- Write a resignation letter. Keep the letter positive: "I am leaving this position to explore new opportunities." This is often the last item in your personnel file.
- Be positive during your exit interview. Do not criticize employees or the position.
- Clean and empty your locker, desk, and any other assigned space.
- Return your pager and any other equipment that has been assigned to you.
- Finish all duties and tie up any loose ends.
- Alert your supervisor to any unfinished business.
- Ask for a letter of reference.

COG Be a Lifelong Learner

You are about to embark on the career you have spent time, money, and energy to prepare for. Even though your formal schooling is coming to an end, you must continue to learn. Be a lifelong learner. In the medical field, changes occur frequently. You must stay abreast of new technologies, procedures, and legal issues. In addition to facility training, inservices, and seminars, you will need to stay current with your CPR certification and recertify your credential.

Recertification

You now face the process of acquiring certification in your field. As discussed in Chapter 1, whether you become a certified medical assistant or a registered medical assistant, you must keep your credential current. Both credentialing bodies require recertification. For AAMA, recertification is mandatory. A certified medical assistant (CMA) wishing to recertify must either retake the examination or complete 60 hours of continuing education units. A CMA who does not recertify by the end of the month of his or her birthday 5 years after the last date of certification loses the right to use the credential. Registered medical assistants (RMAs) are required to renew their certification each year by renewing their membership in the American Medical Technologists. If their membership lapses for more than 1 calendar year, the RMA must begin the process of becoming certified again. Both groups offer continuing education seminars and products. Information about the specific requirements and issues involving recertification is available on the organizations' Web sites.

To prepare for the process of recertifying, maintain a file with information about all educational sessions you attend. You should keep a brochure of the event with the following information: the topic, hours of session, learning objectives, and an outline of the program. You should also have proof of your attendance. When the time to apply for recertification comes, you will be prepared to complete the application.

Professionalism

Experts say that professionalism is the one quality all employers seek. An allied health care career holds excitement, variety, and prestige. But with that comes a responsibility to the patients you serve. This requires professionalism and a commitment to excellence. As a member of the health care team, you are expected to conduct yourself professionally. One sign of professionalism and seriousness of purpose is membership in your professional organization. Whether you are a member of AAMA or American Medical Technologists, the benefits of membership will be invaluable to you and your future. Participation in a professional organization keeps you abreast of changes and issues facing your profession. If you are a student member, continue as an active member. If not, consider joining. Many employers will pay dues and other expenses for professional activities. Information about joining these organizations can be found at their Web sites.

 CHECKPOINT QUESTION

9. What is the policy of the AAMA regarding recertification of the CMA credential?

 MEDIA MENU

- **Student Resources on thePoint**
  - **CMA/RMA Certification Exam Review**
- **Internet Resources**

  Careerspan.com
  http://www.careerspan.com/hc3.asp

  Resume.com
  http://www.resume.com

  ResumeWriters.com
  http://www.resumewriters.com

  Seeking Success.com
  http://www.seekingsuccess.com

  Resume Assistance
  http://www.resume-resource.com

  U.S. Equal Employment Opportunity Commission
  http://www.eeoc.gov

  American Medical Technologists
  http://www.amt1.com

  American Association of Medical Assistants
  http://www.aama-ntl.org

PSY PROCEDURE 16-1: Write a Résumé

Purpose: To summarize your skills and experience and to make yourself marketable in the medical assisting profession
Equipment: Word processor, paper, personal information

Steps	Reasons
1. At the top of the page, center your name, address, and phone numbers.	The reader should be able to contact you easily.
2. List your education, starting with the most current and working back. List graduation dates and areas of study.	Give the reader only the most vital information.
3. For the chronological format, list your prior related work exerpience with dates, responsiblities, company, and supervisor's name. The most recent should be first. For the functional format, list skills and qualifications (refer to Figs. 16-6 and 16-7 for examples).	If you have a long work history, include only jobs that used skills needed for the job for which you are applying. Otherwise, your résumé will be too long.
4. List any volunteer work with dates and places.	This will serve as proof of organizational and team-building skills. It will also show the reader that you are interesting in helping others.
5. List skills you possess including those acquired in your program and on your externship.	This will show the perspective employer exactly what skills you possess.
6. List any certifications or awards received.	This proves your competence.
7. List any information relevant to a certain position. For example, list competence in spreadsheet applications for a job in a patient billing department.	Supplying information specific to a certain position shows your interest and attention to detail.
8. After obtaining permission and/or notifying the people, prepare a list of references with addresses and phone contact information.	It is unprofessional to list someone for a reference without their knowledge and permission.
9. Carefully proofread the résumé for accuracy and typographical errors.	Many employers will automatically reject a résumé with errors.
10. Have someone else proofread the résumé for errors other than content.	Another set of eyes will ensure a perfect document.
11. Print the résumé on high-quality paper.	The appearance and professionalism of your résumé is a direct reflection of you.
12. **AFF** You have only had one job before finishing your medical assisting program. Should you try to "pad" your résumé by listing some anyway? Why or why not?	Honesty is one of the most important attributes sought by employers.

7. You receive an operative report addressed to Dr. Richard Adams on your fax machine, but your physician is Dr. Robert Adams. As soon as you see the cover sheet, you realize you received it by mistake. What should you do?

   Since you do not have a need to know, do not read the report. Call the number on the cover sheet, and tell them that you received the report in error. This alerts them to send another one to the correct Dr. Adams. Then shred the copy you received by mistake.

8. What if the last scenario was reversed? You sent a fax to the wrong number. You realize it just as you push the "Send" button.

   Call the party who received the information and ask them to shred it. Document the error in the patient's chart. If you do not know who received the misdirected fax, you should notify the patient of the possible breach.

9. Your boss asks you to check on the condition of his next door neighbor who is in the hospital. He tells you to let them know that he is the one requesting the information. Is this possible?

   Yes. A patient being admitted to a hospital may choose to be excluded from the hospital directory, and no information can be given out by the hospital. If the neighbor did not opt out of the directory, you will be given the patient's room number and general condition. Unless involved in the patient's care, your physician has no special privileges to protected health information.

10. You work in a busy pediatric office. You are the PA as he examines a 2-year-old boy with a possible concussion. He tells you that he suspects abuse. Can you report this without authorization?

    Not only can you report it, but you MUST report it. The Child Abuse Prevention and Treatment Act of 1974 (CAPTA) made reporting possible child abuse mandatory.

Adapted from Krager D, Krager C. HIPAA for Medical Office Personnel. New York: Thomson Delmar Learning; 2005.

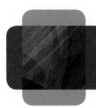

Appendix B

Key English-to-Spanish Health Care Phrases

Although English is the major language spoken in North America, a variety of languages are used in certain areas. Prominent among them is Spanish, representing Spain, the Caribbean Islands, Central and South America, and the Philippines. Rapport can be more easily established, and the patient and family will be at ease and feel more relaxed, if someone on the staff speaks their language. Some health care facilities, especially in areas with a large population of Spanish-speaking people, provide interpreters. In smaller hospitals or smaller communities this may not be possible.

It is to your advantage to learn the second most prominent language in your community. For this reason, the following table of English-to-Spanish phrases has been prepared. Instructions for using it are simple. Look for the phrase in English in the first column of the table. The second colulmn gives the phrase in Spanish. You can write this or point to it. The third column gives a phonetic pronunciation. The syllable in each word to be accented is printed in italic type. Even if you are not proficient in English-to-Spanish, your Spanish-speaking patients will appreciate your trying to converse in their language. Begin with "Buenos días. ¿Cómo se siente?" And remember "por favor."[a]

Introductory Phrases

please[a]	por favor	por fah-*vor*
thank you	gracias	*grah*-see-ahs
good morning	buenos días	*bway*-nos *dee*-ahs
good afternoon	buenas tárdes	*bway*-nas *tar*-days
good evening	buenas noches	*bway*-nas *noh*-chays
my name is	mi nombre es	me *nohm*-bray ays
yes/no	si/no	see/no
What is your name?	¿Cómo se llama?	¿Koh-moh say *jah*-mah?
How old are you?	¿Cuántos años tienes?	¿*Kwan*-tohs ahn-yos tee-*ayn*jays?
Do you understand me?	¿Me entiende?	¿Me ayn-tee-*ayn*-day?
Speak slower.	Habla más despacio.	*Ah*-blah mahs days-*pah*-see-oh
Say it once again.	Repítalo, por favor.	Ray-*pee*-tah-loh, por fah-*vor*
How do you feel?	¿Cómo se siente?	¿*Koh*-moh say see-*ayn*-tay?
good	bien	bee-ayn
bad	mal	*mah*l
physician	médico	*may*-dee-koh
hospital	hospital	*ooh*-spee-tall
midwife	comadre	koh-*mah*-dray
native healer	curandero	ku-ren-*day*-roh

From Rosdahl, C.B. [1995]. *Textbook of Basic Nursing*, 6th ed. Philadelphia: J.B. Lippincott.
[a]You should begin or end any request with the word PLEASE (POR FAVOR).

General

zero	cero	*se*-roh
one	uno	*oo*-noh
two	dos	dohs
three	tres	trays
four	cuatro	*kwah*-troh
five	cinco	*sin*-koh
six	seis	says
seven	siete	see-*ay*-tay
eight	ocho	oh-choh
nine	nueve	new-*ay*-vay
ten	diez	*dee*-ays
hundred	ciento, cien	see-*en*-toh, see-*en*
hundred and one	ciento uno	see-*en*-toh *oo*-noh
Sunday	domingo	doh-*ming*-goh
Monday	lunes	*loo*-nays
Tuesday	martes	*mar*-tays
Wednesday	miércoles	mee-*er*-cohl-ays
Thursday	jueves	*hway*-vays
Friday	viernes	vee-*ayr*-nays
Saturday	sábado	*sah*-bah-doh
right	derecho	day-*ray*-choh
left	izqierdo	ees-kee-*ayr*-doh
early in the morning	temprano por la mañana	tehm-*prah*-noh por lah mah-*nyah*-na
in the daytime	en el dìa	ayn el *dee*-ah
at noon	a mediodía	ah meh-dee-oh-*dee*-ah
at bedtime	al acostarse	al ah-kos-*tar*-say
at night	por la noche	por la *noh*-chay
today	ñoy	oy
tomorrow	mañana	mah-*nyah*-nah
yesterday	ayer	ai-*yer*
week	semana	say-*may*-nah
month	mes	mace

Parts of the Body

the head	la cabeza	la kah-*bay*-sah
the eye	el ojo	el *o*-hoh
the ears	los oídos	lohs o-*ee*-dohs
the nose	la nariz	la nah-*reez*
the mouth	la boca	lah *boh*-kah
the tongue	la lengua	la *len*-gwah
the neck	el cuello	el koo-*eh*-joh
the throat	la garganta	lah gar-*gan*-tah
the skin	la piel	la pee-el
the bones	los huesos	lohs hoo-*ay*-sos
the muscles	los músculos	lohs *moos*-koo-lohs
the nerves	los nervios	lohs *nayhr*-vee-ohs
the shoulder blades	las paletillas	lahs pah-lay-*tee*-jahs
the arm	el brazo	el *brah*-soh
the elbow	el codo	el *koh*-doh
the wrist	la muñeca	lah moon-*yeh*-kah
the hand	la mano	lah *mah*-noh
the chest	el pecho	el *pay*-choh

the lungs	los pulmones	lohs puhl-*moh*-nays
the heart	el corazón	el koh-rah-*son*
the ribs	las costillas	lahs kohs-*tee*-jahs
the side	el flanco	el *flahn*-koh
the back	la espalda	lay ays-*pahl*-dah
the abdomen	el abdomen	el ahb-*doh*-men
the stomach	el estómago	el ays-*toh*-mah-goh
the leg	la pierna	lah pee-ehr-nah
the thigh	el muslo	el *moos*-loh
the ankle	el tobillo	el toh-*bee*-joh
the foot	el pie	el *pee*-ay
urine	urino	u-*re*-noh

Diseases

allergy	alergia	ah-*layr*-hee-ah
anemia	anemia	ah-*nay*-mee-ah
cancer	cancer	kahn-sayr
chickenpox	varicela	vah-ree-*say*-lah
diabetes	diabetes	dee-ah-bay-tees
diphtheria	difteria	deef-*tay*-ree-ah
German measles	rubéola	roo-*bay*-oh-lah
gonorrhea	gonorrea	gun-noh-*ree*-ah
heart disease	enfermedad del corazón	ayn-*fayr*-may-*dahd* dayl koh-rah-*sohn*
high blood pressure	presión alta	pray-see-*ohn* al-ta
influenza	gripe	*gree*-pay
lead poisoning	envenenamiento con plomo	ayn-vay-nay-nah-mee-*ayn*-toh kohn *ploh*-moh
liver disease	enfermedad del hígado	ayn-*fayr*-may-dahd del *ee*-gah-doh
measles	sarampión	sah-rahm-pee-*ohn*
mumps	paperas	pah-*pay*-rahs
nervous disease	enfermedades nerviosa	ayn-fayr-may-*dahd*-days nayr-vee-oh-sah
pleurisy	pleuresía	play-oo-ray-*see*-ah
pneumonia	pulmonía	pool-moh-*nee*-ah
rheumatic fever	reumatismo (fiebre reumatica)	ray-oo-mah-*tees*-moh (fee-*ay*-bray ray-oo-*mah*-tee-kah)
scarlet fever	escarlatina	ays-kahr-lah-*tee*-nah
syphilis	sífilis	*see*-fee-lees
tuberculosis	tuberculosis	too-*bayr*-koo-lohs-sees

Signs and Symptoms

Do you have stomach cramps?	¿Tiene calambres en el estómago?	¿Tee-*ay*-nay kah-*lahm*-brays ayn el ays-*toh*-mah-goh?
chills?	escalofrios?	ays-kah-loh-*free*-ohs?
an attack of fever	un ataque de fiebre?	oon ah-*tah*-kay day fee-*ay*-bray?
hemorrhage?	hemoragia?	ay-moh-*rah*-hee-ah?
nosebleeds?	hemoragia por la nariz?	ay-moh-*rah*-hee-ah por-lah nah-rees?
unusual vaginal bleeding?	hemoragia vaginal fuera de los periodos?	ay-moh-*rah*-hee-ah *vah*-hee-nahl foo-*ay*-rah day lohs pay-ree-oh-dohs?
hoarseness?	ronquera?	rohn-*kay*-rah?
a sore throat?	le duele la garganta?	lay doo-*ay*-lay lah gahr-*gahn*-tah?

Does it hurt to swallow?	¿Le duele al respirar?	¿Lay doo-*ay*-lay ahl trah-gar?
Have you any difficulty in breathing?	¿Tiene difficultad al respirar?	¿Tee-*ay*-nay dee-fee-kool-*tahd* ahl rays-*pee*-rahr?
Does it pain you to breathe?	¿Le duele la cabeza?	¿Lay doo-*ay*-lay ahl rays-*pee*-rahr?
How does your head feel?	¿Cómo siente la cabeza?	¿*Koh*-moh see-*ayn*-tay lah kah-*bay*-sah?
Is your memory good?	¿Es buena su memoria?	¿Ays *bway*-nah soo may-*moh*-ree-ah?
Have you any pain the head?	¿Le duele al tragar?	¿Lay doo-*ay*-lay lah Kah-*bay*-sah?
Do you feel dizzy?	¿Tiene usted vértigo?	¿Tee-ay-nay ood-*stayd vehr*-tee-goh?
Are you tired?	¿Está usted cansado?	¿Ay-*stah* ood-stayd kahn-*sah*-doh?
Can you eat?	¿Puede comer?	¿*Pway*-day koh-*mer*?
Have you a good appetite?	¿Tiene usted buen apetito?	¿Tee-*ay*-nay ood-*stayd* bwayn ah-pay-*tee*-toh?
How are your stools?	¿Cómo son sus heces fecales?	¿*Kog*-moh sohn soos *bay*-says fay-*kal*-ays?
Are they regular?	¿Son regulares?	¿Sohn ray-goo-*lah*-rays?
Are you constipated?	¿Está estreñido?	¿Ay-*stah* ays-trayn-*yee*-do?
Do you have diarrhea?	¿Tiene diarrea?	¿Tee-*ay*-nay dee-ah-*ray*-ah?
Have you any difficulty passing water?	¿Tiene dificultad en orinar?	¿Tee-*ay*-nay dee-fee-kool-*tahd* ayn oh-ree-*nahr*?
Do you pass water involuntarily?	¿Orina sin querer?	¿Oh-*ree*-nah seen kay-rayr?
How long have you felt this way?	¿Desde cuándo se siente asi?	¿*Days*-day *Kwan*-doh say see-*ayn*-tay ah-see?
What diseases have you had?	¿Qué enfermedades ha tenido?	¿Kay ayn-fer-may-*dah*-days hah tay-*nee*-doh?
Do you hear voices?	¿Tiene los voces?	¿Tee-*ay*-nay los *vo*-ses?

Examination

Remove your clothing.	Quítese su ropa.	*Key*-tay-say soo *roh*-pah.
Put on this gown.	Pongáse la bata.	Phon-*gah*-say lah *bah*-tah.
We need a urine specimen.	Es necesário una muestra de su orina.	Ays nay-*say*-sar-ee-oh oo-nah moo-*ay*-strah day oh-*ree*-nah.
Be seated.	Siéntese.	See-*ayn*-tay-say.
Recline.	Acuestése.	Ah-*cways*-tay-say.
Sit up.	Siéntese.	See-*ayn*-tay-say.
Stand.	Parése.	*Pah*-ray-say.
Bend your knees.	Doble las rodíllas.	*Doh*-blay lahs roh-*dee*-yahs.
Relax your muscles.	Reláje los músculos.	Ray-*lah*-hay lohs *moos*-koo-lohs.
Try to . . .	Atente . . .	Ah-*tayn*-tay . . .
Try again.	Atente ótra vez.	Ah-*tayn*-tay *oh*-tra vays.
Do not move.	No se muéva.	Noh say moo-*ay*-vah.
Turn on (or to) your left side.	Voltese a su lado izquierdo.	Vohl-*tay*-say ah soo *lah*-doh is-key-*ayr*-doh.
Turn on (or to) your right side.	Voltése a su ládo derécho.	Vohl-*tay*-say ah soo *lah*-doh day-*ray*-choh.
Take a deep breath.	Respíra profúndo.	Ray-*speer*-rah pro-*foon*-doh.
Hold your breath.	Deténga su respiración.	Day-*tayn*-gah soo ray-speer-ah-see-*ohn*.
Don't hold your breath.	No deténga su respiración.	Noh day-tayn-gah soo ray-speer-ah-see-*ohn*.
Cough.	Tosa.	*Toh*-sah.
Open your mouth.	Abra la boca.	*Ah*-brah lah *boh*-kah.

Show me . . .	Enséñeme . . .	Ayn-*sayn*-yay-may . . .
Here?	¿Aqui?	¿Ah-*kee*?
There?	¿Allí?	¿Ah-*jee*?
Which side?	¿En qué lado?	¿Ayn kay *lah*-doh?
Let me see your hand.	Enséñeme la mano.	Ayn-*sehn*-yay-may lah *mah*-noh.
Grasp my hand.	Apriete mi mano.	Ah-*pree*-it-tay mee *mah*-noh.
Raise your arm.	Levante el brazo.	Lay-*vahn*-tay el *brah*-soh.
Raise it more.	Más alto.	Mahs *ahl*-toh.
Now the other.	Ahora el otro.	Ah-*oh*-rah el *oh*-troh.

Treatment

It is necessary.	Es necesario.	Ays neh-say-*sah*-ree-oh.
An operation is necessary.	Una operación es necesaria.	Oo-nah oh-peh-rah-see-*ohn* ays neh-say-*sah*-ree-ah.
a prescription	una receta	*oo*-na ray-say-tah
Use it regularly.	Tómelo con regularidad.	*Toh*-may-loh kohn ray-goo-*lah*-ree-dad.
Take one teaspoonful three times daily (in water).	Toma una cucharadita tres veces al dia, con agua.	*Toh*-may oo-na koo-chah-rah-*dee*-tah trays *vay*-says ahl *dee*-ah, kohn ah-gwah.
Gargle.	Haga gargaras.	*Ah*-gah gar-*gah*-rahs.
Use injection.	Use una inyección.	Oo-say oo-nah in-*yek*-see-ohn.
oral contraceptives	una pildora	*oo*-nah peel-*doh*-rah
a pill	una pastilla	*oo*-nah pahs-*tee*-yah
a powder	un polvo	oon *pohl*-voh
before meals	antes de las comidas	*ahn*-tays day lahs koh-*mee*-dahs
after meals	despues de las comidas	*days*-poo-ehs day lahs koh-mee-dahs
every day	todos los día	*toh*-dohs lohs *dee*-ah
every hour	cada hora	*kah*-dah *oh*-rah
Breathe slowly—like this (in this manner).	Respire despacio—asi.	Rays-*pee*-ray days-*pah*-see-oh—ah-*see*.
Remain on a diet.	Estar a dieta.	Ays-*tar* a dee-*ay*-tah.

General

How do you feel?	¿Cómo se siénte?	¿*Koh*-moh say see-*ayn*-tay?
Do you have pain?	¿Tiéne dolor?	¿Tee-*ay*-nay doh-*lorh*?
Where is the pain?	¿Adónde es el dolor?	¿Ah-*dohn*-day ays ayl doh-*lorh*?
Do you want medication for your pain?	¿Quiére medicación para su dolor?	¿Kay-*ay*-ray may-dee-kah see-*ohn* pak-rah soo doh-*lorh*?
Are you comfortable?	¿Está confortáble?	¿Ay-*stah* kohn-for-*tah*-blay?
Are you thirsty?	¿Tiéne sed?	¿Tee-*ay*-nay sayd?
You may not eat/drink.	No cóma/béba.	Noh *koh*-mah/bay-*bah*.
You can only drink water.	Solo puede tomar agua.	Soh-loh *pway*-day toh-mar *ah*-gwah.
Apply bandage to . . .	Ponga una vendaje a . . .	*Pohn*-gah oo-nah vehn-*dah*-hay ah . . .
Apply ointment.	Aplíquese unguento.	Ah-*plee*-kay-say oon-goo-*ayn*-toh.
Keep very quiet.	Estese muy quieto.	Ays-*tay*-say moo-ay key-*ay*-toh.
You must not speak.	No debe hablar.	Noh *day*-bay ha-*blahr*
It will be uncomfortable.	Séra incomódo.	*Say*-rah een-koh-*moh*-doh.
It will sting.	Va ardér.	Vah ahr-*dayr*.
You will feel pressure.	Vá a sentír presión.	Vah ah sayn-*teer* pray-see-*ohn*.
I am going to . . .	Voy a . . .	Voy ah . . .
Count (take) your pulse.	Tomár su púlso.	Toh-*marh* soo *pool*-soh.

Take your temperature.	Tomár su temperatúra.	Toh-*marh* soo taym-pay-rah-*too*-rah.
Take your blood pressure.	Tomar su presión.	Toh-*mahr* soo pray-see-*ohn*.
Give you pain medicine.	Dárle medicación para dolór.	*Dahr*-lay may dee-kah-see-*ohn* pah-rah doh-*lohr*.
You should (try to) . . .	Trate de . . .	*Tray*-tay day . . .
Call for help/assistance.	Llamar para asisténcia.	Yah-*marh* pah-rah ah-sees-*tayn*-see-ah.
Empty your bladder.	Orinar.	Oh-ree-*narh*.
Do you still feel very weak?	¿Se siente muy débil todavía?	¿Say see-*ayn*-tay moo-ee *day*-beel toh-dah-*vee*-ah?
It is important to . . .	Es importánte que . . .	Ays eem-por-*tahn*-tay Kay . . .
Walk (ambulate).	Caminar.	Kah-mee-*narh*.
Drink fluids.	Beber líquidos.	Bay-*bayr* *lee*-kay-dohs.

Appendix C

Two-Letter Postal ZIP Code Abbreviations

Alabama	AL	Nebraska	NE
Alaska	AK	Nevada	NV
Arizona	AZ	New Hampshire	NH
Arkansas	AR	New Jersey	NJ
American Samoa	AS	New Mexico	NM
California	CA	New York	NY
Colorado	CO	North Carolina	NC
Connecticut	CT	North Dakota	ND
Delaware	DE	Northern Mariana Islands	MP
District of Columbia	DC	Ohio	OH
Federated States of Micronesia	FM	Oklahoma	OK
Florida	FL	Oregon	OR
Georgia	GA	Palau	PW
Guam	GU	Pennsylvania	PA
Hawaii	HI	Puerto Rico	PR
Idaho	ID	Rhode Island	RI
Illinois	IL	South Carolina	SC
Indiana	IN	South Dakota	SD
Iowa	IA	Tennessee	TN
Kansas	KS	Texas	TX
Kentucky	KY	Utah	UT
Louisiana	LA	Vermont	VT
Maine	ME	Virginia	VA
Marshall Islands	MH	Virgin Islands	VI
Maryland	MD	Washington	WA
Massachusetts	MA	West Virginia	WV
Michigan	MI	Wisconsin	WI
Minnesota	MN	Wyoming	WY
Mississippi	MS	Armed Forces of the Americas	AA
Missouri	MO	Armed Forces Europe	AE
Montana	MT	Armed Forces Pacific	AP

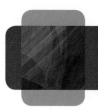

Appendix D

Abbreviations and Symbols

Abbreviations and symbols that appear in red font are considered "Dangerous Abbreviations" and should not be used.

Abbreviation or Symbol	Meaning
ā	before
A	anterior; assessment
A&P	auscultation and percussion
A&W	alive and well
AB	abortion
ABG	arterial blood gas
a.c.	before meals
ACE	angiotensin-converting enzyme
ACS	acute coronary syndrome
ACTH	adrenocorticotropic hormone
AD	right ear
ad lib.	as desired
ADH	antidiuretic hormone
ADHD	attention-deficit/hyperactivity disorder
AIDS	acquired immunodeficiency syndrome
AKA	above-knee amputation
alb	albumin
ALS	amyotrophic lateral sclerosis
ALT	alanine aminotransferase (enzyme)
a.m.	morning
amt	amount
ANS	autonomic nervous system
AP	anterior-posterior
APKD	adult polycystic kidney disease
Aq	water
AS	left ear
ASD	atrial septal defect
AST	aspartate aminotransferase (enzyme)
AU	both ears
AV	atrioventricular
Ⓑ	bilateral
BAEP	brainstem auditory evoked potential
BAER	brainstem auditory evoked response

Abbreviation or Symbol	Meaning
BCC	basal cell carcinoma
BD	bipolar disorder
b.i.d.	twice a day
BKA	below-knee amputation
BM	bowel movement
BMP	basic metabolic panel
BP	blood pressure
BPH	benign prostatic hypertrophy; benign prostatic hyperplasia
BRP	bathroom privileges
BS	blood sugar
BUN	blood urea nitrogen
Bx	biopsy
c̄	with
C	Celsius; centigrade
C&S	culture and sensitivity
CABG	coronary artery bypass graft
CAD	coronary artery disease
Cap	capsule
CAT	computed axial tomography
CBC	complete blood count
cc	cubic centimeter
CC	chief complaint
CCU	coronary (cardiac) care unit
CF	cystic fibrosis
CHF	congestive heart failure
CIN	cervical intraepithelial neoplasia
CIS	carcinoma in situ
cm	centimeter
CMP	comprehensive metabolic panel
CNS	central nervous system
c/o	complains of
CO	cardiac output
CO$_2$	carbon dioxide
COPD	chronic obstructive pulmonary disease
CP	cerebral palsy; chest pain
CPAP	continuous positive airway pressure

Abbreviation or Symbol	Meaning
CPD	cephalopelvic disproportion
CPR	cardiopulmonary resuscitation
CSF	cerebrospinal fluid
CSII	continuous subcutaneous insulin infusion
CT	computed tomography
CTA	computed tomographic angiography
cu mm or mm³	cubic millimeter
CVA	cerebrovascular accident
CVS	chorionic villus sampling
CXR	chest x-ray
d	day
D&C	dilation and curettage
D&E	dilation and evacuation
DC	discharge; discontinue; doctor of chiropractic
DDS	doctor of dental surgery
DJD	degenerative joint disease
DKA	diabetic ketoacidosis
DO	doctor of osteopathy
DPM	doctor of podiatric medicine
dr	dram
DRE	digital rectal exam
DTR	deep tendon reflex
DVT	deep vein thrombosis
Dx	diagnosis
ECG	electrocardiogram
echo	echocardiogram
ECT	electroconvulsive therapy
ECU	emergency care unit
ED	erectile dysfunction
EDC	estimated date of confinement
EDD	estimated date of delivery
EEG	electroencephalogram
EGD	esophagogastroduodenoscopy
EKG	electrocardiogram
EMG	electromyogram
ENT	ear, nose, and throat
EPS	electrophysiologic study
ER	emergency room
ERCP	endoscopic retrograde cholangiopancreatography
ESR	erythrocyte sedimentation rate
ESWL	extracorporeal shock wave lithotripsy
ETOH	ethyl alcohol
EUS	endoscopic ultrasonography
F	Fahrenheit
FBS	fasting blood sugar
Fe	iron
FH	family history
fl oz	fluid ounce

Abbreviation or Symbol	Meaning
FS	frozen section
FSH	follicle-stimulating hormone
Fx	fracture
g	gram
GAD	generalized anxiety disorder
GERD	gastroesophageal reflux disease
GH	growth hormone
GI	gastrointestinal
gm	gram
gr	grain
gt	drop
gtt	drops
GTT	glucose tolerance test
GYN	gynecology
h	hour
H&H	hemoglobin and hematocrit
H&P	history and physical
HAV	hepatitis A virus
HBV	hepatitis B virus
HCT or Hct	hematocrit
HCV	hepatitis C virus
HD	Huntington disease
HEENT	head, eyes, ears, nose, and throat
HGB or Hgb	hemoglobin
HIV	human immunodeficiency virus
hpf	high-power field
HPI	history of present illness
HPV	human papillomavirus
HRT	hormone replacement therapy
h.s.	hour of sleep
HSV-1	herpes simplex virus type 1
HSV-2	herpes simplex virus type 2
Ht	height
HTN	hypertension
Hx	history
I&D	incision and drainage
ICD	implantable cardioverter defibrillator
ICU	intensive care unit
ID	intradermal
IM	intramuscular
IMP	impression
IOL	intraocular lens
IP	inpatient
IUD	intrauterine device
I.V.	intravenous
IVP	intravenous pyelogram
IVU	intravenous urogram
JCAHO	Joint Commission on Accreditation of Healthcare Organizations
kg	kilogram

Abbreviation or Symbol	Meaning	Abbreviation or Symbol	Meaning
KUB	kidneys, ureters, bladder	O	objective
L	liter	O_2	oxygen
Ⓛ	left	OA	osteoarthritis
L&W	living and well	OB	obstetrics
LASIK	laser-assisted in situ keratomileusis	OCD	obsessive-compulsive disorder
		OCP	oral contraceptive pill
lb	pound	OD	right eye; doctor of optometry
LEEP	loop electrosurgical excision procedure	OH	occupational history
		OP	outpatient
LH	luteinizing hormone	OR	operating room
LLETZ	large-loop excision of transformation zone	ORIF	open reduction, internal fixation
LLQ	left lower quadrant	OS	left eye
LP	lumbar puncture	OU	both eyes
lpf	low-power field	oz	ounce
LTB	laryngotracheobronchitis	p̄	after
LUQ	left upper quadrant	P	plan; posterior; pulse
m	meter	PA	posterior-anterior
ⓜ	murmur	PACU	postanesthetic care unit
MCH	mean corpuscular (cell) hemoglobin	$PaCO_2$	partial pressure of carbon dioxide
MCHC	mean corpuscular (cell) hemoglobin concentration	PaO_2	partial pressure of oxygen
		Pap	Papanicolaou (smear)
MCV	mean corpuscular (cell) volume	PAR	postanesthetic recovery
MD	medical doctor; muscular dystrophy	p.c.	after meals
		PCI	percutaneous coronary intervention
mg	milligram	PD	panic disorder
MI	myocardial infarction	PDA	patent ductus arteriosus
ml or mL	milliliter	PE	physical examination; pulmonary embolism; polyethylene
mm	millimeter		
mm^3 or cu mm	cubic millimeter	PEFR	peak expiratory flow rate
MPI	myocardial perfusion image	per	by or through
MRA	magnetic resonance angiography	PERRLA	pupils equal, round, and reactive to light and accommodation
MRI	magnetic resonance imaging		
MRSA	methicillin resistant *Staphylococcus aureus*	PET	positron emission tomography
		PF	peak flow
MS	multiple sclerosis; musculoskeletal	PFT	pulmonary function testing
MSH	melanocyte-stimulating hormone	pH	potential of hydrogen
		PH	past history
MUGA	multiple-gated acquisition (scan)	PI	present illness
		PID	pelvic inflammatory disease
MVP	mitral valve prolapse	PIH	pregnancy-induced hypertension
NAD	no acute distress		
NCV	nerve conduction velocity	p.m.	after noon
NG	nasogastric	PLT	platelet
NK	natural killer (cell)	PMH	past medical history
NKA	no known allergy	PMN	polymorphonuclear (leukocyte)
NKDA	no known drug allergy	PNS	peripheral nervous system
noc.	night	p.o.	by mouth
NPO	nothing by mouth	post-op or postop	postoperative
NSAID	nonsteroidal antiinflammatory drug		
NSR	normal sinus rhythm	PPBS	postprandial blood sugar

Abbreviation or Symbol	Meaning
PR	per rectum
pre-op or preop	preoperative
p.r.n. or prn	as needed
PSA	prostate-specific antigen
PSG	polysomnography
pt	patient
PT	physical therapy; prothrombin time
PTCA	percutaneous transluminal coronary angioplasty
PTH	parathyroid hormone
PTSD	posttraumatic stress disorder
PTT	partial thromboplastin time
PUD	peptic ulcer disease
PV	per vagina
PVC	premature ventricular contraction
Px	physical examination
q	every
q.d.	every day, daily
qh	every hour
q2h	every 2 hours
q.i.d.	four times a day
q.o.d.	every other day
qt	quart
R	respiration
Ⓡ	right
RA	rheumatoid arthritis
RBC	red blood cell; red blood count
RLQ	right lower quadrant
R/O	rule out
ROM	range of motion
ROS	review of symptoms
RP	retrograde pyelogram
RRR	regular rate and rhythm
RTC	return to clinic
RTO	return to office
RUQ	right upper quadrant
Rx	recipe; prescription
$\overline{s}$	without
S	subjective
SA	sinoatrial
SAB	spontaneous abortion
SAD	seasonal affective disorder
SC	subcutaneous
SCA	sudden cardiac arrest
SCC	squamous cell carcinoma
SH	social history
Sig:	instruction to patient
SLE	systemic lupus erythematosus
SOB	shortness of breath
SPECT	single-photon emission computed tomography

Abbreviation or Symbol	Meaning
SpGr	specific gravity
SQ	subcutaneous
SR	systems review
$\overline{\overline{ss}}$	one-half
STAT	immediately
STD	sexually transmitted disease
SUI	stress urinary incontinence
suppos	suppository
SV	stroke volume
Sx	symptom
T	temperature
T_3	triiodothyronine
T_4	thyroxine
T&A	tonsillectomy and adenoidectomy
tab	tablet
TAB	therapeutic abortion
TB	tuberculosis
TEDS	thromboembolic disease stockings
TEE	transesophageal echocardiogram
TIA	transient ischemic attack
t.i.d.	three times a day
TM	tympanic membrane
TMR	transmyocardial revascularization
tPA or TPA	tissue plasminogen activator
Tr	treatment
TSH	thyroid-stimulating hormone
TURP	transurethral resection of the prostate
TV	tidal volume
Tx	treatment; traction
UA	urinalysis
UCHD	usual childhood diseases
URI	upper respiratory infection
US or U/S	ultrasound
UTI	urinary tract infection
VC	vital capacity
VCU or VCUG	voiding cystourethrogram
V/Q	ventilation/perfusion
VS	vital signs
VSD	ventricular septal defect
VT	tidal volume
w.a.	while awake
WBC	white blood cell; white blood count
WDWN	well developed, well nourished
wk	week
WNL	within normal limits
Wt	weight
x	times; for
x-ray	radiography
y.o. or y/o	year old

Abbreviation or Symbol	Meaning	Abbreviation or Symbol	Meaning
yr	year	O–	lying
♀	female	×	times; for
♂	male	>	greater than
#	number; pound	<	less than
°	degree; hour	ᵢ	one
↑	increase; above	ᵢᵢ	two
↓	decrease; below	ᵢᵢᵢ	three
✓	check	ᵢᵥ	four
Ø	none; negative	I, II, III, IV, V, VI, VII, VIII, IX, and X	uppercase Roman numerals 1–10
♀	standing		
♀	sitting		

From Willis MC. Medical Terminology: The Language of Health Care. 2nd ed. Baltimore: Lippincott Williams & Wilkins; 2006.

Appendix E

Commonly Misused Words

Because these words have similar spellings and pronunciation, they can easily be confused or misused. Watch your spelling carefully! Always proofread all business letters for accuracy and grammar.

Word	Example of Correct Use
adverse (harmful)	Some adverse reactions can be life threatening.
averse (opposed to)	I am not averse to working on Mondays.
affect (verb, to influence, change)	The protesters will not affect the outcome.
effect (noun, result)	The effect of the antibiotics has been beneficial.
already (previously)	We already tried that approach.
all ready (prepared, all set)	Are we all ready to go?
anoxia (without oxygen)	Anoxia will cause the brain cells to die quickly.
anorexia (without appetite)	Anorexia is a serious illness that affects teenagers.
aphagia (without swallowing)	A feeding tube is needed because of her aphagia.
aphasia (without speech)	Her stroke caused aphasia.
appendices (end of book)	There are five appendices at the end of the book.
appendicitis (inflammation of appendix)	The patient was treated for appendicitis.
biannual (twice a year)	Productivity reports are printed on a biannual basis.
biennial (occurring every 2 years)	Staff contracts are renewed on a biennial basis.
bite (grip with teeth)	The patient's bite is poorly aligned.
byte (character)	Buy a computer with enough bytes for future growth.
bowl (container)	The jelly beans are in the bowl.
bowel (intestines, colon)	Instruct the patient to complete the bowel preparation.
emphysema (chronic lung disease)	Smoking causes emphysema.
empyema (accumulation of pus)	Empyema most commonly occurs in the pleural cavity.
ensure (be certain)	Call the patient to ensure that he comprehends the instructions.
insure (protect against risk)	Please insure this package for $200.
assure (provide confidence)	I assure you that he is getting the correct treatment.
everyday (adjective, routine, ordinary)	Quality checks are an everyday procedure.
every day (adverbial phrase, each day)	There can be legal ramifications if this is not done every day.
except (exclude)	All antibiotics except penicillin will work.
expect (anticipate)	I expect this work to be completed by noon.
accept (agree)	I accept this challenge.
farther (greater distance)	It is 1 mile farther down the road.
further (greater degree)	The process needs further refinement.
fundus (pertains to hollow organ)	The fundus was firm after the baby's delivery.
fungus (organism that can lead to infection)	A fungus was growing under her nails.
its (possessive pronoun)	The pharmacy must protect its supply of opioids.
it's (contraction of it and is)	It's time to take a break.

Word	Example of Correct Use
lactose (type of sugar in milk)	I have a lactose allergy.
lactase (enzyme)	Lactase is responsible for dissolving lactose.
libel (written defamatory statement)	The statements about John Roberts were libel.
liable (legally responsible)	You are liable for your actions.
may be (compound verb)	Dr. Rogers may be in surgery this afternoon.
maybe (adverb, perhaps)	Maybe it will snow tomorrow.
metatarsals (bones in foot)	Crutches are often needed when the metatarsals are fractured.
metacarpals (bones in palm)	Typing is difficult for patients with a metacarpal fracture.
mucus (substance that is secreted)	The patient had a mucus plug.
mucous (membrane that secretes)	The mucous membrane secretes the mucus.
parental (pertaining to parent)	Follow parental guidelines for TV use.
parenteral (not by mouth)	Parenteral feedings will start on Monday.
postnatal (after birth)	Complications can occur in the postnatal period.
postnasal (behind nose)	Postnasal drainage can be uncomfortable.
principle (noun, law)	A key principle of economics is understanding cash flow.
principal (noun, leader; adjective, most important)	The principal's name is Tina Sefferin; her experience is the principal reason she was hired.
rubella (German measles)	You need a rubella vaccination.
rubeola (14-day measles)	There is a outbreak of rubeola at the middle school.
serum (liquid component of blood)	The patient's serum is used for various tests.
sebum (oily substance secreted by the sebaceous glands)	Sebum helps to lubricate the skin surface.
tact (behavior)	He handled his child with great tact.
tack (different direction)	A new tack may be needed for us to win that bid.
than (to show comparison)	Salaries are higher now than they were a year ago.
then (next)	Clean room 2; then go to lunch.
there (place, point)	You need to be there at 2:00 PM.
their (possessive pronoun)	Leaving their bikes on the road caused the accident.
they're (pronoun plus verb)	They're going to be late.
uvula (soft tissue at back of palate)	The patient's uvula was swollen.
vulva (external female organ)	A laceration of the vulva was noted during the gynecologic examination.
weather (climate)	The weather is unpredictable.
whether (indicating a possibility)	I wonder whether it will rain or snow.

Appendix F

Sample Medical Reports

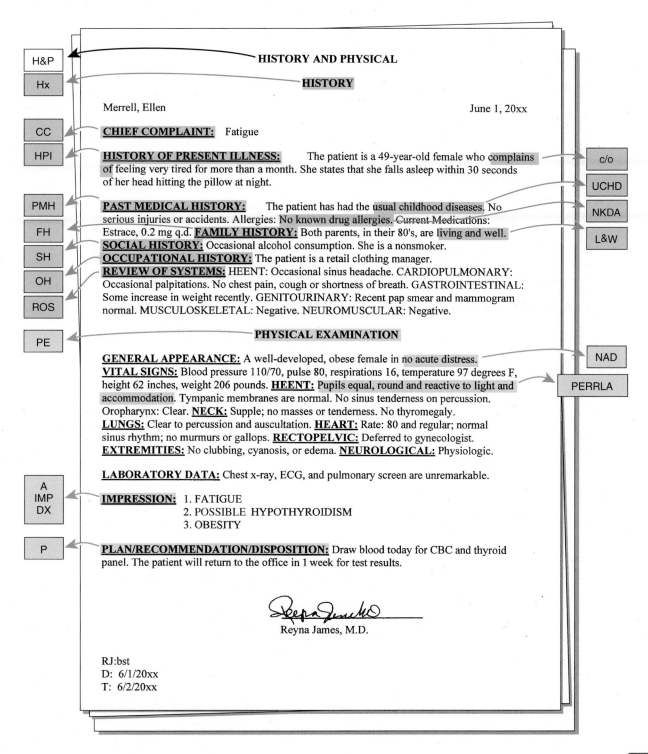

| H&P | **HISTORY AND PHYSICAL** |
| Hx | **HISTORY** |

Merrell, Ellen   June 1, 20xx

CC — **CHIEF COMPLAINT:**   Fatigue

HPI — **HISTORY OF PRESENT ILLNESS:**   The patient is a 49-year-old female who complains — **c/o**
of feeling very tired for more than a month. She states that she falls asleep within 30 seconds
of her head hitting the pillow at night.

— **UCHD**

PMH — **PAST MEDICAL HISTORY:**   The patient has had the usual childhood diseases. No
serious injuries or accidents. Allergies: No known drug allergies. Current Medications: — **NKDA**
FH — Estrace, 0.2 mg q.d. **FAMILY HISTORY:** Both parents, in their 80's, are living and well. — **L&W**
SOCIAL HISTORY: Occasional alcohol consumption. She is a nonsmoker.
SH — **OCCUPATIONAL HISTORY:** The patient is a retail clothing manager.
OH — **REVIEW OF SYSTEMS:** HEENT: Occasional sinus headache. CARDIOPULMONARY:
Occasional palpitations. No chest pain, cough or shortness of breath. GASTROINTESTINAL:
ROS — Some increase in weight recently. GENITOURINARY: Recent pap smear and mammogram
normal. MUSCULOSKELETAL: Negative. NEUROMUSCULAR: Negative.

PHYSICAL EXAMINATION

PE —

GENERAL APPEARANCE: A well-developed, obese female in no acute distress. — **NAD**
VITAL SIGNS: Blood pressure 110/70, pulse 80, respirations 16, temperature 97 degrees F,
height 62 inches, weight 206 pounds. **HEENT:** Pupils equal, round and reactive to light and — **PERRLA**
accommodation. Tympanic membranes are normal. No sinus tenderness on percussion.
Oropharynx: Clear. **NECK:** Supple; no masses or tenderness. No thyromegaly.
LUNGS: Clear to percussion and auscultation. **HEART:** Rate: 80 and regular; normal
sinus rhythm; no murmurs or gallops. **RECTOPELVIC:** Deferred to gynecologist.
EXTREMITIES: No clubbing, cyanosis, or edema. **NEUROLOGICAL:** Physiologic.

LABORATORY DATA: Chest x-ray, ECG, and pulmonary screen are unremarkable.

A
IMP — **IMPRESSION:**   1. FATIGUE
DX   2. POSSIBLE HYPOTHYROIDISM
                                                 3. OBESITY

P — **PLAN/RECOMMENDATION/DISPOSITION:** Draw blood today for CBC and thyroid
panel. The patient will return to the office in 1 week for test results.

Reyna James
Reyna James, M.D.

RJ:bst
D: 6/1/20xx
T: 6/2/20xx

CENTRAL MEDICAL CENTER

211 Medical Center Drive • Central City, US 90000-1234 • PHONE: (012) 125-6784 • FAX: (012) 125-9999

OPERATIVE REPORT

DATE OF OPERATION: June 3, 20xx.

PREOPERATIVE DIAGNOSIS: Chronic tonsillitis.

POSTOPERATIVE DIAGNOSIS: Frequent, recurrent tonsillitis.

SURGEON: Patrick Rodden, M.D.

ASSISTANT SURGEON: None

ANESTHESIOLOGIST: Robert Jung, M.D.

ANESTHESIA: General.

SURGERY PERFORMED: Tonsillectomy.

DESCRIPTION OF OPERATION: After general anesthesia induction, with intubation, the McGivor mouth gag and tongue retractor were utilized for exposure of the oropharynx. Local anesthetic consisting of 6 mL of 0.5% Xylocaine with 1:100,000 epinephrine was utilized. Tonsillectomy was carried out using dissection and air technique. The right tonsillectomy electrocoagulation Bovie suction was utilized for hemostasis. Examination of the nasopharynx was normal.

The patient tolerated the procedure well and went to the recovery room in good condition.

P. Rodden MD
PATRICK RODDEN, M.D.

JR:as
D: 6/3/20xx
T: 6/4/20xx

OPERATIVE REPORT	PT. NAME:	PERRON, CARLEEN
	ID NO:	672894017
	ROOM NO:	312
	ATT. PHYS:	PATRICK RODDEN, M.D.

CENTRAL MEDICAL CENTER

211 Medical Center Drive • Central City, US 90000-1234 • PHONE: (012) 125-6784 • FAX: (012) 125-9999

PATHOLOGY REPORT

PATIENT: PERRON, CARLEEN
            28 Y (FEMALE)

DATE RECEIVED: June 3, 20xx.   DATE REPORTED: June 4, 20xx

GROSS:

Received are two tonsils each 2.5 cm in greatest diameter.

MICROSCOPIC:

The sections show deep tonsilar crypts associated with follicular lymphoid hyperplasia. No bacterial granules are seen.

DIAGNOSIS:

CHRONIC LYMPHOID HYPERPLASIA OF RIGHT AND LEFT TONSILS.

Mary Needham MD
MARY NEEDHAM, M.D.

MN:gds

D: 6/4/20xx
T: 6/5/20xx

CENTRAL MEDICAL CENTER

211 Medical Center Drive • Central City, US 90000-1234 • PHONE: (012) 125-6784 • FAX: (012) 125-9999

DISCHARGE SUMMARY

DATE OF ADMISSION: 10/25/20xx   DATE OF DISCHARGE: 10/29/20xx

ADMITTING DIAGNOSIS:
Left ureteropelvic junction obstruction.

DISCHARGE DIAGNOSIS:
Left ureteropelvic junction obstruction.

PROCEDURE PERFORMED:
Left dismembered pyeloplasty and placement of stent.

BRIEF SUMMARY:
The patient is a 19-year-old male who was admitted to the hospital a month ago with left pyelonephritis. He was found to have a left ureteropelvic junction obstruction. The patient was brought to the hospital at this time for repair of the moderately to severely obstructed left kidney. A preoperative urine culture was sterile. The patient underwent the procedure without complication. A double-J stent was placed. The Jackson-Pratt drain was removed on the second postoperative day because of minimal drainage. The patient initially had urinary retention, but this resolved by the third postoperative day. He was doing fine at the time of discharge. His condition on discharge is good.

INSTRUCTIONS TO THE PATIENT:
1) Regular diet. 2) No heavy lifting, straining, or driving an automobile for six weeks from the day of surgery. He should also keep the incision relatively dry this week. 3) Follow up in my office in three weeks. 4) It is anticipated the stent will remain indwelling for six weeks and then will be removed cystoscopically at that time. 5) Discharge medication is Tylenol #3, 1-2 q 4 h p.r.n. pain.

L. Zlatkin, M.D.

L. Zlatkin, M.D.

LZ:mr

D: 10/29/20xx
T: 10/30/20xx

DISCHARGE SUMMARY

PT. NAME:	MERCIER, CHARLES F.
ID NO:	IP-392689
ROOM NO:	444
ATT. PHYS:	L.ZLATKIN, M.D.

CENTRAL MEDICAL CENTER

211 Medical Center Drive • Central City, US 90000-1234 • PHONE: (012) 125-6784 • FAX: (012) 125-9999

OPERATIVE REPORT

DATE: December 7, 20xx

PREOPERATIVE DIAGNOSIS: Congenital left ureteropelvic junction obstruction status post pyeloplasty. Indwelling left ureteral stent.

POSTOPERATIVE DIAGNOSIS: Congenital left ureteropelvic junction obstruction status post pyeloplasty. Indwelling left ureteral stent, removed

OPERATION: Cystoscopy, removal of left ureteral stent, and left retrograde pyelogram.

PROCEDURE: The patient was identified, was placed on the operating table, and was administered a general anesthetic. He was placed in the lithotomy position, and a KUB was obtained. The genitalia were prepped and draped in a sterile fashion. After reviewing the KUB, it was noted at this time that the position of the stent was normal. Cystoscopy was performed with a #22 French cystoscope. The stent was identified coming from the left ureteral orifice, and the end was grasped with forceps and removed through the cystoscope. A #8 French cone-tipped ureteral catheter was then placed in the left ureteral orifice and passed to 10 cm. Then, 20 cm^3 of contrast was injected into a left collecting system. A film was exposed, and this showed patency without extravasation at the left ureteropelvic junction. There was some filling of calyces and partial filling of the dilated renal pelvis. A drainage film was subsequently obtained showing complete emptying of the pelvis and partial emptying of the mid and distal ureters. Dilated calyces were noted in the kidney. The patient was allowed to awaken and was returned to the recovery room in satisfactory condition. There were no intraoperative complications. He had no bleeding. The patient did receive 1 gm Ancef one-half hour prior to the onset of the procedure.

_____
L. Zlatkin, M.D.

LZ:mr
D: 12/07/20xx
T: 12/08/20xx

OPERATIVE REPORT	PT. NAME:	MERCIER, CHARLES F.
	ID NO:	OP-912689
	ROOM NO:	ASC
	ATT. PHYS:	L.ZLATKIN, M.D.

CENTRAL MEDICAL GROUP, INC.
Department of Internal Medicine

201 Medical Center Drive • Central City, US 90000-1234 • PHONE: (012) 125-8888 • FAX: (012) 125-3434

PATIENT: COHEN, SARA E.

DATE: April 8, 20xx

HISTORY

CHIEF COMPLAINT: Epigastric distress

HISTORY OF PRESENT ILLNESS: This 33-year-old Caucasian female comes in because of excessive burping, epigastric distress and nausea for several weeks. Coffee makes it worse. She complains that it is worse at night when lying down. She gets an acid-like taste in her mouth. She has tried antacids, to no avail.

PAST MEDICAL HISTORY: The patient states that she had the usual childhood diseases. She has had no serious medical illnesses and has been involved in no accidents. Family History: There is some diabetes on her mother's side. Her mother is 52 and has hypertension. Her father, age 56, is living and well. She has a sister who is anemic and a brother who has ulcers. Social History: The patient discontinued smoking ten years ago. Drinks alcohol socially. Allergies: NKDA. Current Medications: Medications at this time consist of Entex, Guaifed, birth control pills, iron and vitamin supplements.

REVIEW OF SYSTEMS: HEENT: Chronic sinusitis. She sees an ENT specialist and an allergist. Respiratory: Negative. Cardiac: Occasional flutters. Gastrointestinal: As stated above. Genitourinary: Occasional infections. Pap smear is up-to-date and negative. She has had no mammogram at this point. Neuromuscular: Negative.

PHYSICAL EXAMINATION

GENERAL APPEARANCE: Reveals a well-developed, well-nourished female in no acute distress.

VITAL SIGNS: Blood Pressure: 120/80. Pulse: 76 and regular.

HEENT: Head normocephalic. Eyes: Pupils are equal, round, and reactive to light and accommodation. Fundi are benign. Ears, nose and throat are negative. NECK: No thyromegaly. No carotid bruits.

CHEST: Clear to percussion and auscultation. BREASTS: Reveal no masses. HEART: Normal sinus rhythm. No murmurs.

ABDOMEN: Liver, spleen and kidneys could not be felt. Femorals pulsate well, no bruits.

EXTREMITIES: No edema. Pulses are good and equal.

PELVIC & RECTAL EXAMS: Deferred to gynecologist.

NEUROLOGIC EXAM: Physiologic.

IMPRESSION: 1. PROBABLE PEPTIC ULCER DISEASE WITH GASTROESOPHAGEAL REFLUX.
2. POSSIBLE GALLBLADDER DISEASE.

PLAN: Patient started on Pepcid 40 mg, 1 at night. She is given Gaviscon tablets so she can carry them with her. Schedule routine lab work and upper GI series. If negative, schedule ultrasound of the gallbladder.

D. Everley, M.D.

DE:mc
D: 4/8/20xx
T: 4/9/20xx

CENTRAL MEDICAL GROUP, INC.
Department of Otorhinolaryngology
201 Medical Center Drive • Central City, US 90000-1234 • PHONE: (012) 125-8888 • FAX: (012) 125-3434

Patient: Perron, Carleen   DATE: February 17, 20xx

Referring Physician: C. Camarillo, M.D.

CONSULTATION

REASON FOR CONSULTATION: This 28-year-old white female presents with a one week history of upper respiratory infection (URI), sinusitis, and some periorbital headaches in recent weeks. She also has expectorated yellow-green mucus occasionally and has had a history of tonsillitis.

MEDICATIONS: None. **ALLERGIES:** No known allergies (NKA). **SURGERIES:** None. **HOSPITALIZATIONS:** None.

PAST MEDICAL HISTORY/REVIEW OF SYSTEMS: Cardiopulmonary: There is no history of angina, dyspnea, hemoptysis, emphysema, asthma, chronic obstructive pulmonary disease (COPD), hypertension, or heart murmurs. Cardiovascular: There is no history of high blood pressure. Renal: There is no history of dysuria, polyuria, nocturia, hematuria, or cystoliths. Gastrointestinal: There is no history of gallbladder disease, hepatitis, pancreatitis, or colitis. Musculoskeletal: There is no history of arthritis. Endocrine: There is no history of diabetes. Hematologic: There is no history of anemia, blood transfusion, or easy bruising. Gynecological: The patient states her menses are regular, and the start of her last menstrual cycle occurred 15 days ago.

FAMILY HISTORY: The patient states her maternal grandmother has diabetes.

SOCIAL HISTORY: The patient is single and has no children. She denies smoking tobacco. She denies drinking alcoholic beverages. She denies taking drugs.

CHILDHOOD DISEASES: The patient has had the usual childhood diseases.

OTOLARYNGOLOGIC EXAMINATION: Otoscopy: Tympanic membranes (TMs) are dull and slightly congested. Sinuses: There is maxillary fullness. Rhinoscopic examination reveals mild nasoseptal deviation (NSD). Pharynx: There is moderate inflammation; no exudates. Oropharynx: No masses. Nasopharynx: No masses. Larynx: Clear. Neck: Supple. Cervical Adenopathy: There is mild adenopathy.

IMPRESSION:
1. MAXILLARY SINUSITIS.
2. PHARYNGITIS.
3. CHRONIC TONSILLITIS.

DISPOSITION:
1. Warm salt water gargle (WSWG).
2. Ery-Tab 333, #24, 1 t.i.d. p.c.
3. Robitussin.
4. Return to office (RTO) in one week.

P. Rodden MD
PATRICK RODDEN, M.D.

JR:ti
D: 2/17/20xx
T: 2/18/20xx   9:50 a.m.

CENTRAL MEDICAL GROUP, INC.
Department of Otorhinolaryngology
201 Medical Center Drive • Central City, US 90000-1234 • PHONE: (012) 125-8888 • FAX: (012) 125-3434

PROGRESS NOTES

Patient: PERRON, CARLEEN

03/30/20xx

S: The patient presents with a sore throat × 2 weeks.

O: Sinus exam: Maxillary and frontal congestion. Hypopharynx/adenoids: No inflammation.

A: Recurrent pharyngitis/sinusitis × 2 weeks.

P: 1)   Ceftin 250 mg, #21, 1 t.i.d. p.o. p.c.

　　　2)   Entex LA, #30, 1 b.i.d. p.o.

　　　3)   Warm salt water gargle.

P Rodden MD
PATRICK RODDEN, M.D.

05/25/20xx

S: Recurrent sore throat every month.

O: Recurrent tonsillitis, cryptic tonsillitis. Sinus exam: Maxillary and frontal congestion. Neck: Supple; no masses. Hypopharynx/Adenoids: No inflammation. Paranasal Sinus X-ray: Bilateral frontal and maxillary sinusitis.

A: Recurrent tonsillitis, 8-10 times per year. Chronic maxillary and frontal sinusitis.

P: 1)   Tonsillectomy discussed with the patient. The risks of general and local anesthesia, as well as the surgical procedure, were discussed with the patient. The consent form was signed.

　　　2)   An admitting order was given to the patient for CBC, UA, and basic metabolic panel to be done one day prior to being admitted.

　　　3)   Ceftin 250 mg, #21, 1 t.i.d. p.o. p.c.

　　　4)   Entex LA, #30, 1 b.i.d. p.o.

　　　5)   Flonase nasal inhaler, 2 sprays each nostril b.i.d.

　　　6)   Warm salt water gargle.

P Rodden MD
PATRICK RODDEN, M.D.

CENTRAL MEDICAL CENTER

211 Medical Center Drive • Central City, US 90000-1234 • PHONE: (012) 125-6784 • FAX: (012) 125-9999

X-RAY REPORT

LUMBOSACRAL SPINE:
Multiple views reveal no evidence of fracture. There is slight lumbar spondylosis with slight lipping and minimal bridging. The disc spaces appear maintained except for slight narrowing at L4-L5 and L5-S1. There is also a Grade I spondylolisthesis of L5 on S1 and evidence of spondylolysis at L5 on the left. There is also slight dextroscoliosis in the lumbar region and slight increased lordosis in the lumbosacral region. The bony architecture is unremarkable except for eburnation between the articulating facets at L5-S1. The SI joints appear unremarkable. Incidentally noted are slight osteoarthritic changes involving both hips.

CONCLUSION:

1. Slight lumbar spondylosis with hypertrophic lipping and slight narrowing of the L4-L5 and L5-S1 disc spaces, rule out discogenic disease. If clinically indicated, CT of the lumbosacral spine may prove helpful in further evaluation.

2. Grade I spondylolisthesis of L5 on S1 with evidence of spondylolysis at L5 on the left.

3. Slight dextroscoliosis in the lumbar region and slight increased lordosis in the lumbosacral region.

M. Volz MD

M. Volz, M.D.

MV:ti

D: 10/19/20xx
T: 10/20/20xx

X-RAY REPORT	PT. NAME:	DORN, JAY F.
	ID NO:	RL-483091
	ATT. PHYS:	T. LIGHT, M.D.

Medical reports courtesy of Willis M. Medical Terminology: A Programmed Learning Approach to the Language of Health Care. 2nd ed. Baltimore: Lippincott Williams & Wilkins, 2007; and Willis MC. Medical Terminology: The Language of Health Care. 2nd ed. Baltimore: Lippincott Williams & Wilkins; 2006.

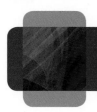

Appendix G

Metric Measurements

Unit	Abbreviation	Metric Equivalent	U.S. Equivalent
Units of Length			
kilometer	km	1000 meters	0.62 miles; 1.6 km/mile
meter*	m	100 cm; 1000 mm	39.4 inches; 1.1 yards
centimeter	cm	1/100 m; 0.01 m	0.39 inches; 2.5 cm/inch
millimeter	mm	1/1000 m; 0.001 m	0.039 inches; 25 mm/inch
micrometer	μm	1/1000 mm; 0.001 mm	
Units of Weight			
kilogram	kg	1000 g	2.2 lb
gram*	g	1000 mg	0.035 oz; 28.5 g/oz
milligram	mg	1/1000 g; 0.001 g	
microgram	μg, mcg	1/1000 mg; 0.001 mg	
Units of Volume			
liter*	L	1000 mL	1.06 qt
deciliter	dL	1/10 L; 0.1 L	
milliliter	mL	1/1000 L; 0.001 L	0.034 oz; 29.4 mL/oz
microliter	μL	1/1000 mL; 0.001 mL	

*Basic unit.

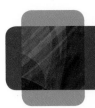
Celsius–Fahrenheit Temperature Conversion Scale

Celsius to Fahrenheit

Use the following formula to convert Celsius readings to Farenheit readings:

$$°F = 9/5 × °C + 32$$

For example, if the Celsius reading is 37°:

$$°F = (9/5 × 37) + 32$$
$$= 66.6 + 32$$
$$= 98.6°F \text{ (normal body temperature)}$$

Fahrenheit to Celsius

Use the following formula to convert Fahrenheit readings to Celsius readings:

$$°C = 5/9(°F − 32)$$

For example, if the Fahrenheit reading is 68°:

$$°C = 5/9(68 − 32)$$
$$= 5/9 × 36$$
$$= 20 °C \text{ (a nice spring day)}$$

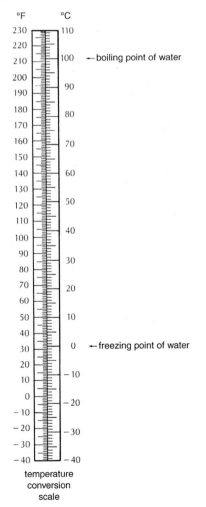

temperature
conversion
scale

From Memmler RL, Cohen BJ, Wood, DL. The Human Body in Health and Disease. 10th ed. Baltimore: Lippincott Williams & Wilkins; 2005.

Glossary

A

abandonment   withdrawal by a physician from a contractual relationship with a patient without proper notification while the patient still needs treatment.

accounting cycle   a consecutive 12-month period for financial record keeping following either a fiscal year (starting on a specified date) or the calendar year (January to December).

accounts payable   a record of all monies owed.

accounts receivable   a record of all monies due.

accreditation   a nongovernmental professional peer review process that provides technical assistance and evaluates educational programs for quality based on pre-established academic and administrative standards.

administrative   pertaining to administration (e.g., office procedures and nonclinical tasks that a medical assistant will perform).

advance beneficiary notice   document that informs covered patients that Medicare may not cover a certain service and the patient will be responsible for the bill.

advance directive   a statement of a patient's wishes regarding health care prior to a critical medical event.

affiliation   to connect or associate with, as a medical site would associate with a school to assist in completion of student training.

agenda   a brief outline of the topics to be discussed at a meeting.

aging schedule   a form used to track outstanding balances.

allergen   any substance that causes manifestations of an allergy, usually a protein to which the body has built antibodies.

allergy   acquired abnormal response to a substance (allergen) that does not ordinarily cause a reaction.

alphabetic filing   arranging of names or titles according to the sequence of letters in the alphabet.

alternative   an option or substitute to the standard medical treatment plan, e.g. herbal therapies, acupuncture, hypnosis.

American Association of Medical Assistants (AAMA)   professional organization for medical assistants.

Americans with Disabilities Act (ADA)   a law designed to meet the needs of people with physical and mental challenges.

annotation   the process of reading, highlighting, and summarizing a document for another person.

antiseptic   any substance that inhibits the growth of bacteria; used on skin before any procedure that breaks the integumentary barrier.

appeal   process by which a higher court reviews the decision of a lower court.

assault   an attempt or threat to touch another person without his or her consent.

assessment   process of gathering information about the patient and the presenting condition.

assignment of benefits   transfer of the patient's legal right to collect third-party benefits for medical expenses to the provider of the services.

astigmatism   unfocused refraction of light rays on the retina.

atraumatic   without injury; may pertain to treatments or instruments that are not likely to cause further damage.

attitude   a state of mind; how a person feels about a given subject or at a given time.

attribute   a characteristic or quality of a person; usually considered a positive feature.

audit   a review of an account; inspection of records to determine compliance and to detect fraud.

autoclave   appliance used to sterilize medical instruments with steam under pressure.

autonomic   self-controlling, spontaneous.

autonomous   existing or functioning independently.

B

back-up   *noun*, a duplicate file made to a separate disk to protect information; *verb*, to make a duplicate file.

bactericidal   substance that kills or destroys bacteria.

bacteriology   the science and study of bacteria.

balance   equality between the debit and credit sides of an accounting equation; that which is left over after additions and subtractions have been made to an account; remainder; amount due.

balance billing   billing the patient for the balance or difference between the physician's charges and the Medicare-approved charges; prohibited by most managed care contracts.

battery   actual touching of a person without his or her consent.

beliefs   ideas that are held to be true.

bench trial   trial in which the judge hears the case and renders a verdict; no jury is present.

benign   not cancerous or malignant.

bias   formation of an opinion without foundation or reason; prejudice.

BiCaps   words or phrases with unusual capitalization.

bioethics   moral issues and concerns that affect a person's life.

biohazard   biological agent that has the capacity to harm humans.

biohazard symbol   icon on the label for specimens containing potential biological agents.

biohazardous   describing a substance that is a risk to the health of living organisms.

biohazardous waste   infectious waste or biomedical waste; any waste containing infectious materials or potentially infectious substances such as blood.

biological agent   bacteria, viruses, fungi, other microorganisms, and their toxins.

bioterrorism intentional release of a biologic agent with the intent to harm individuals.

birthday rule determination of which policyholder's insurance is the first to pay when a patient is covered by two policies. The policyholder whose birth month and day comes first in the calendar is primary.

bloodborne pathogens viruses that can be spread through direct contact with blood or body fluids from an infected person.

body fluids any of the fluids that accumulate in the compartments of the body, such as the blood plasma, and the intracellular and extracellular spaces.

body mass index (BMI) a measurement of an individual's ratio of fat to lean body mass. It is calculated by using the following formula: [weight (pounds) ÷ height (inches)^2] × 703. A BMI over 30 is considered obese.

body mechanics using the correct muscles and posture to complete a task safely and efficiently.

bookkeeping organized and accurate record keeping for financial transactions.

boot to start up the computer.

bore diameter of the interior of a needle.

breach an infraction, such as breach of contract, in which the agreed-on terms are violated.

budget financial planning tool that helps an organization estimate its anticipated expenditures and revenues.

buffer extra time to accommodate emergencies, walk-ins, and other demands on the provider's daily time schedule that are not considered direct patient care.

buffer system system that guards against sudden shifts in acidity and alkalinity depending on the body's own naturally occurring weak acids and weak bases.

C

caduceus a symbol using a wand or staff with two serpents coiled around it; sometimes used as the sign of the medical profession (the more appropriate symbol has only one snake).

capitation managed care plan that pays a certain amount to a provider over a specific time for caring for the patients in the plan regardless of what or how many services are performed.

carrier person infected with a microorganism but without signs of disease; a company that assumes the risk of an insurance company.

cassette light-proof holder in which x-ray film is exposed.

Centers for Disease Control and Prevention (CDC) U.S. federal agency under the Department of Health and Human Services that works to protect public health and safety. CDC provides information to enhance health decisions.

Centers for Medicare and Medicaid Services (CMS) government department that mandates the use of panels defined by the American Medical Association (AMA) for national standardization of nomenclature and testing.

central processing unit (CPU) circuitry imprinted on a silicon chip that processes information; the "brain" of the computer.

Certificate of Waiver (CW) one of four types of certificates issued under CLIA; certifies the laboratory to perform waived testing.

certification voluntary process that involves a testing procedure to prove an individual's baseline competency in a particular area.

chain-of-custody procedure accurate written record to track the possession, handling, and location of chain-of-custody samples and data from collection through reporting.

charge slip a preprinted three-part form that can be placed on a daysheet to record the patient's charges and payments along with other information in an encounter form.

check register place to record checks that have been written.

check stub indicates to whom a check was issued, in what amount, and on what date.

chief complaint main reason for the visit to the medical office.

chronic long-standing.

chronological order placing in the order of time; usually the most recent is placed foremost.

civil law a branch of law that focuses on issues between private citizens.

claims requests to an insurance company for reimbursement of costs.

claims administrator an individual who manages the third-party reimbursement policies for a medical practice.

clarification explanation; removal of confusion or uncertainty.

clearinghouse a company that receives, reviews, sends, and manages insurance claims for physicians.

CLIA certification required by any group that performs even one test, including a waived test on materials derived from the human body for the purpose of providing information for the diagnosis, prevention, or treatment of any disease or impairment of, or the assessment of the health of, human beings to meet certain federal requirements. See *Clinical Laboratory Improvement Amendments*.

clinical diagnosis a diagnosis based only on the patient's clinical symptoms.

Clinical Laboratory Improvement Amendments (CLIA) guidelines established by Congress in 1988 to standardize and improve laboratory testing.

Clinical and Laboratory Standards Institute (CLSI) a committee appointed to establish rules to ensure the safety, standards, and integrity of all testing performed on human specimens.

cloning genetically identical replication of cells, an organ, or an organism in the laboratory.

closed captioning printed words displayed on a television screen to help people with hearing disabilities or impairments.

closing a one- to two-word phrase that precedes the sender's signature and indicates the end of the letter.

clustering grouping patients with similar problems or needs.

coagulate change from a liquid to a solid or semi-solid mass.

coinsurance the agreed-upon amount paid to the provider by a policyholder. Also called *copayment*.

collection a process of acquiring funds that are due.

Commission on Office Laboratory Accreditation (COLA) works to support the health care industry by providing knowledge and resources for maintaining quality laboratory operations.

common law traditional laws that were established by the English legal system.

comparative negligence a percentage of damage awards based on the contribution of negligence between two parties.

competency assessment evaluation of a person's ability to perform a test and to use a testing device.

compliance willingness of a patient to follow a prescribed course of treatment.

compliance officer person charged with ensuring that a facility follows laws, policies, and protocols.

concierge medicine is a new type of medicine in which a patient pays an annual fee or retainer in exchange for enhanced care by the primary care physician.

computed tomography (CT) a diagnostic procedure that uses x-rays to produce cross-sectional views of internal body structures.

concussion injury to the brain due to trauma.

confidentiality protection of patient data from unauthorized personnel.

consent an agreement between a patient and physician to do a given medical procedure.

constellation of symptoms a group of clinical signs indicating a particular disease process.

consultation request for assistance from one physician to another.

continuing education units (CEUs) credits awarded for attendance at approved local and state AAMA meetings and seminars, completion of guided study courses, and journal articles designed to submit a posttest for CEU credit.

contract an agreement between two or more parties for a given act.

contracture abnormal shortening of muscles around a joint caused by atrophy of the muscles and resulting in flexion and fixation.

contraindication situation or condition that prohibits the prescribing or administering of a drug or medication.

contrast medium substance ingested or injected into the body to facilitate imaging of internal structures.

contributory negligence a defense strategy in which the defendant admits to negligence but claims that the plaintiff assisted in promoting the damages.

control a device or solution used to monitor the test to ensure correct test results.

contusion collection of blood in tissues after an injury; a bruise.

conventions general notes, symbols, typeface, format, and punctuation that direct and guide the coder to the most complete and accurate ICD-9 code.

cookies tiny files that are left on your computer's hard drive by a website without your permission.

coordination of benefits the method of designating the order in which multiple carriers pay benefits to avoid duplication of payment.

copayments that part of an insured service the patient must pay.

coping mechanisms unconscious methods of alleviating intense stressors.

coronary artery bypass graft surgical procedure that increases the blood flow to the heart by bypassing the occluded or blocked vessel with a graft.

covered entity anyone required to follow the Health Insurance Portability and Accountability Act's requirements. Health care providers, insurance companies, and insurance clearinghouses are covered entities.

credit balance in one's favor on an account; promise to pay a bill at a later date; record of a payment received.

criteria the standard, rule, or test by which something or someone can be judged.

critical values considered to be life-threatening test results.

crossover claim a claim that crosses over automatically from one coverage to another for payment.

cross-reference notation in a file telling that a record is stored elsewhere and giving the reference; verification to another source; checking the tabular list against the alphabetic list in ICD-9 coding.

Current Procedural Terminology a comprehensive list of codes used by physicians to bill for procedures and services.

cursor flashing line on the monitor indicating where data input will occur.

cytology Study of the microscopic structure of cells.

D

DACUM a code of educational standards for medical assisting students developed by the American Association of Medical Assistants.

damages the resulting injury or suffering that resulted from negligence.

data information that is stored and processed by the computer.

database accumulation of files on the computer

daysheet/daily journal a daily business record of charges and payments.

debit a charge or money owed on an account.

decibel (db) unit of intensity of sound.

deductible a specified amount paid by the policyholder before the carrier begins paying.

defamation of character making false or malicious statements about a person's character or reputation.

defendant the party that is accused.

degenerative joint disease (DJD) also known as *osteoarthritis*; arthritis characterized by degeneration of the bony structure of the joints, usually noninflammatory.

demeanor the way a person looks, behaves, and conducts himself or herself.

dementia progressive organic mental deterioration with loss of intellectual function.

demographic relating to the statistical characteristics of populations.

denial saying that something is not true; refusing to acknowledge.

dental cavities holes in the teeth.

Department of Health and Human Services (HHS) U.S. government's agency for protecting the health of all Americans and providing essential human services.

dependent spouse, children, and sometimes other individuals designated by the insured who are covered under a health care plan.

deposition a process in which one party questions another party under oath.

descriptor description of a service listed with its code number.

diagnosis identification of a disease or condition by evaluating physical signs and symptoms, health history, and laboratory tests; a disease or condition identified in a person.

diagnostic test medical test performed to aid in the diagnosis or detection of disease.

diagnostic-related group (DRG) categories used to determine hospital and physician reimbursement for Medicare patients' inpatient services.

diaphoresis profuse sweating.

diction the style of speaking and enunciating words.

differential diagnosis a diagnosis made by comparing the patient's symptoms to two or more diseases that have similar symptoms.

diplomacy the art of handling people with tact and genuine concern.

directory a "table of contents" of a file system.

discrimination making a difference in favor of or against someone.

disease definite pathologic process having a distinctive set of symptoms and course of progression.

disinfectant a chemical that can be applied to objects to destroy microorganisms; will not destroy bacterial spores.

disinfection killing or rendering inert most but not all pathogenic microorganisms.

disk drive a device that gets information on and off a floppy disk.

dissemination the process of distributing information on community resources.

distal away from the origin.

documentation the process of recording patient information.

donor one who contributes something to another.

double booking the practice of booking two patients for the same period with the same physician

downloading transferring information from an outside location to your computer.

dressing a covering applied directly to a wound to apply pressure, give support, absorb secretions, protect from trauma or microorganisms, stop or slow bleeding, or hide disfigurement.

drug any substance that may modify one or more of the functions of an organism.

due process a formal proceeding in which the accused is considered not guilty until a verdict is reached.

durable power of attorney a legal document giving another person the authority to act on one's behalf.

duress the act of compelling or forcing someone to do something that they do not want to do.

E

E-codes codes indicating the external cause or reason for an injury or illness.

ecchymosis characteristic black and blue mark that results from blood as it accumulates under the skin.

electrocardiography procedure that produces a record of the electrical activity of the heart.

electroencephalogram (EEG) tracing of the electrical activity of the brain.

electronic health records information about patients that is recorded and stored on computer.

element a substance that cannot be separated or broken down into substances with properties other than its own; a primary substance.

eligibility the determination of an insured's right to receive benefits from a third-party payer based on such criteria as payment of premiums and date of start of coverage.

emancipated minor a patient under the age of majority but who is legally considered to be an adult.

emergency medical services (EMS) a group of health care providers working as a team to care for sick or injured patients before they arrive at the hospital.

empathy the ability to understand or to some extent share what someone else is feeling.

employee a person hired to perform given duties in return for financial compensation.

enclosure indication for the reader that an item is accompanying the letter.

encounter form a preprinted statement that lists codes for basic office charges and has sections to record charges incurred in an office visit, the patient's current balance, and next appointment.

encryption scrambling e-mail messages as they leave one site and unscrambling them when they arrive at the designated address.

endemic a disease that occurs continuously in a particular population but has a low mortality; used in contrast to epidemic.

endocarditis inflammation of the inner lining of the heart.

endocrine system of glands which secrete a type of hormone directly into the bloodstream to regulate the body.

endocrinologist a physician who specializes in disorders of the endocrine system.

endorphins chemicals that are often called the body's "natural painkillers" that tend to produce a euphoria, or "good feeling." Release of endorphins is often caused by physical movement or exercise.

eponym word derived from a personal name, e.g., *Alzheimer* disease.

ergonomic describes a workstation designed to prevent work-related injuries and to promote work efficiency.

ergonomics the study of human physical characteristics and their environment to minimize the risk for injury through the use of appropriate adaptive equipment.

erythema redness of the skin.

ethernet system that allows the computer to be connected to a cable or DSL system.

ethics guidelines for moral behavior that are enforced by peer groups.

etiology cause of disease.

euphoria a feeling of well-being.

euthanasia allowing a patient to die with minimal medical interventions.

evaluation the process of indicating how well the patient or person is progressing toward a particular goal; to appraise; to determine the worth or quality of something or someone.

expected threshold a numerical goal.

expert witness a professional who testifies on the standard of care in a trial.

explanation of benefits (EOB) a statement that accompanies a payment from an insurance carrier and outlines which dates and services are being paid.

exposure control plan written plan required by the Occupational Safety and Health Administration that outlines an employer's system for preventing infection.

exposure risk factors conditions that tend to put employees at risk for contact with biohazardous agents such as bloodborne pathogens.

express consent a statement of approval from the patient for the physician to perform a given procedure after the patient has been educated about the risks and benefits of the particular procedure; also referred to as informed consent.

express contracts formal agreements between two or more people.

expulsion formal discharge from a professional organization.

externship an educational course that allows the student to obtain hands-on experience. Also referred to as practicum.

extracellular outside of the cell.

eyewashes used to irrigate and flush the eyes following a hazardous exposure.

F

familial referring to a disorder that tends to occur more often in a family than would be anticipated solely by chance.

Family and Medical Leave Act a law designed to allow an employee up to 12 weeks of unpaid leave from his or her job to meet family needs.

febrile having an above-normal body temperature.

Federal Insurance Contributions Act (FICA) the law that established Social Security and that mandates Social Security tax payments and benefits.

Federal Register official daily publication of the federal government; includes rules, proposed rules, notices of federal agencies and organizations, executive orders and other presidential documents.

federal unemployment tax tax used to finance all administrative expenses of the federal/state unemployment insurance system and the federal costs involved in extended benefits.

fee-for-service an established set of fees charged for specific services and paid by the patient or insurance carrier.

fee schedule a list of pre-established fee allowances set for specific services and procedures performed by a provider.

fee splitting sharing of fees between physicians for patient referrals.

feedback in communication, the response to input from another.

file grouping of data that is given a name for easy access.

filing system a method for organizing records so that they can be found when needed.

film raw material on which x-rays are projected through the body; prior to processing, it does not contain a visible image (similar to photographic film).

fixative a chemical substance used to bind, fix, or stabilize specimens of tissue to slides for later examination.

floppy disk thin magnetic film on which to store data.

flow sheet color-coded sheets that allow information to be recorded in graphic or tabular form for easy retrieval; form that gathers all the important data regarding a patient's condition and stays in the patient's chart as a reminder of care and a record of whether care expectations have been met.

font a typeface; affects the way written messages look.

Food and Drug Administration (FDA) responsible for protecting and promoting public health through the regulation and supervision of blood transfusions, medical devices, and other medically and nonmedically related products.

fraud a deceitful act with the intention to conceal the truth.

full block a type of letter format in which all letter components are justified left.

full-thickness burn burn that has destroyed all skin layers.

G

gait manner or style of walking.

generic name official name given to a drug whose patent has expired.

germicide chemical that kills most pathogenic microorganisms; disinfectant.

gerontologist specialist who studies aging.

grief great sadness caused by loss.

gross income the amount of money earned by an employee before taxes are withheld.

group member a policyholder who is a member of a group and covered by the group's insurance carrier.

H

hard drive a place where the computer stores programs and data files.

hardware equipment on the computer system, e.g., keyboard, disk drive, monitor, printer.

Hashimoto thyroiditis diffuse infiltration of the thyroid gland with lymphocytes, resulting in diffuse goiter and hypothyroidism.

HCFA *see* Health Care Financing Administration.

HCPCS *see* Health Care Financing Administration Common Procedures Coding System.

Healthcare Common Procedure Coding System American Medical Association's coding system based on CPT-4. Assigns alphabetic and numeric codes to items such as ambulance service, wheelchairs, and injections.

Health Care Financing Administration (HCFA) a federal agency that regulates health care financing and the procedural classification (Volume 3 of the ICD-9-CM coding book).

Health Care Financing Administration Common Procedures Coding System (HCPCS) a numerical system used by HCFA for services not covered by the CPT coding system.

health care savings accounts (HSAs) a benefit offered by some employers that allows employees to save money through payroll deduction to accounts that can only be used for medical care.

health insurance a policy that promises to pay some or all of a customer's medical bills.

Health Insurance Portability and Accountability Act (HIPAA) federal law, originally passed as the Kassebaum-Kennedy Act, that requires all health care settings to ensure privacy and security of patient information. Also requires health insurance to be accessible for working Americans and available when changing employment.

health maintenance organization (HMO) an organization that provides a wide range of services through a contract with a specified group at a predetermined payment.

heat cramps type of hyperthermia that causes muscle cramping resulting from high-sodium heat exhaustion; hyperthermia resulting from physical exertion in heat without adequate fluid replacement.

heat exhaustion a type of hyperthermia that causes an altered mental status due to inadequate fluid replacement.

heat stroke most serious type of hyperthermia; body is no longer able to compensate for elevated temperature.

hereditary referring to traits or disorders that are transmitted from parent to offspring.

HIPAA *see* Health Insurance Portability and Accountability Act.

Hippocratic Oath a code of ethics written by Hippocrates.

histology study of the microscopic structure of tissue.

homeopathic referring to an alternative type of medicine in which patients are treated with small doses of substances that produce similar symptoms and use the body's own healing abilities.

homeostasis maintaining a constant internal environment by balancing positive and negative feedback.

human immunodeficiency virus (HIV) virus that causes acquired immunodeficiency syndrome (AIDS); the immune system begins to fail, leading to life-threatening opportunistic infections.

hyperventilation a respiratory rate that greatly exceeds the body's oxygen demands.

I

iatrogenic a condition caused by treatment or medical procedures.

idiopathic unknown etiology.

immunity lack of susceptibility to a disease.

immunization act or process of rendering an individual immune to specific disease.

immunodeficiency parts of the immune system fail to provide an adequate response.

immunology the study of antigen–antibody reactions.

implementation the process of initiating and carrying out an action such as a teaching plan or patient treatment.

implied consent an informal agreement of approval from the patient to perform a given task.

implied contracts contracts between physician and patient not written but assumed by the actions of the parties.

incident report a form used by an organization to document an unusual occurrence to a patient, visitor, or employee.

independent practice association (IPA) several independently practicing physicians contracted with a health maintenance organization to provide services to health maintenance organization members.

infection invasion by disease-producing microorganisms.

informed consent a statement of approval from the patient for the physician to perform a given procedure after the patient has been educated about the risks and benefits of the procedure; also referred to as expressed consent.

inpatient a medical setting in which patients are admitted for diagnostic, radiographic, or treatment purposes.

inspection visual examination.

installment partial payment of a bill.

institutional review board internal committee that reviews ethical issues.

insured an individual who owns a policy that promises to pay some or all of his or her medical bills.

interaction effects, positive or negative, of two or more drugs taken by a patient.

intercaps words or phrases with unusual capitalization.

intermittent occurring at intervals.

internal control control built into the testing device.

Internal Revenue Service (IRS) a federal agency that regulates and enforces various taxes.

International Classification of Diseases, Ninth Revision, Clinical Modification a system for transforming verbal descriptions of disease, injuries, conditions, and procedures to numeric codes.

Internet global system used to connect one computer to another.

intranet a private network system of computers.

invoice a statement of debt owed; a bill.

isolate separate from any other microorganisms present.

J

job description a statement that informs an employee about the duties and expectations for a given job.

Joint Commission, The a voluntary organization that sets and evaluates the standards of care for health care institutions (formerly Joint Commission on Accreditation of Healthcare Organizations); based on The Joint Commission evaluation, an accreditation title will be given to the organization.

K

key components the criteria or factors on which the selection of a CPT-4 evaluation and management is based.

kinesics a form of nonverbal communication including gestures, body movements, and facial expressions.

kit a packaged set containing test devices, instructions, reagents, and supplies needed to perform a test and generate results.

L

laboratory a place where research, investigation, or scientific testing takes place.

laboratory procedure manual Clinical Laboratory Improvement Amendments regulations require each laboratory to have its own procedure manual describing how to perform every test in the laboratory.

late effects conditions that result from another condition. For example, left-sided paralysis may be a *late effect* of a stroke.

learning objectives steps that need to be achieved to accomplish the learning goal.

learning goal an agreed upon outcome of the teaching process.

ledger card a record of the patient's financial activities; a continuous record of business transactions with debits and credits.

legally required disclosure reporting of certain events to governmental agencies without the patient's consent.

liabilities amounts the practice owes.

libel written statements that defame a person's reputation or character.

licensure granting of a license or legal permission to perform a certain profession.

literary search finding professional journal articles on a given subject.

litigation process of filing or contesting a lawsuit.

locum tenens a substitute physician.

login use of a password to gain access to the computer.

lordosis abnormally deep ventral curve at the lumbar flexure of the spine; also known as *swayback*.

M

magnetic resonance imaging imaging technique that uses a strong magnetic field.

main terms words in a multiple-word diagnosis that a coder should locate in the alphabetic listing. They represent the condition (not the location) to be coded.

mainframe central computer to which individual computers are connected; used in large institutions.

malignant cancerous.

malpractice a tort in which the patient is harmed by the actions of a health care worker.

managed care the practice of third-party payers to control costs by requiring physicians to adhere to specific rules as a condition of payment.

manipulation skillful use of the hands in diagnostic procedures.

margin the blank space around the edges of a piece of paper, such as a letter or page of a book.

material safety data sheet (MSDS) a detailed record of all characteristics and protection required from a hazardous substance.

matrix a system for blocking off unavailable patient appointment times.

medical asepsis removal or destruction of microorganisms.

medical assistant a multiskilled health professional who performs a variety of clinical and administrative tasks in a medical setting.

medical history record containing information about a patient's past and present health status.

medical necessity a determination made by a third party that a certain service or procedure was necessary based on sound medical practice.

medical setting a place that is designed to meet the health care needs of patients; may be inpatient or outpatient.

Medicare Social Security–established health insurance for the elderly.

megabyte one million bytes; a way to measure the quantity of computer information that a particular device can hold.

memorandum a type of written documentation used for interoffice communication.

message words sent from one person to another; information sent through spoken, written, or body language.

methicillin-resistant *Staphylococcus aureus* a strain of *Staphylococcus aureus* bacteria that is resistant to many antibiotics used to treat *Staphylococcus* skin infections. Commonly abbreviated MRSA.

metric system system of measurement that uses grams, liters, and meters.

microfiche sheets of microfilm.

microfilm photographs of records in a reduced size.

microorganisms microscopic living organisms.

microprocessor a chip that allows the computer to function.

mission statement a statement describing the goals of the medical office and those it serves.

modem (modulator/demodulator) a communication device that connects a computer to the standard telephone system, allowing information exchange with other computers off site.

modifiers letters or numbers added to a code to clarify the service or procedure.

morphology description of the structural characteristics of blood cells.

motherboard fiberglass board that contains the central processing unit (CPU), memory, and other pieces of circuitry.

mourning to demonstrate signs of grief; grieving.

multidisciplinary involving many disciplines; a group of health care professionals from various specialties brought together to meet the patient's needs.

multimedia various forms of communication available on the computer, e.g., stereophonic sound, animation, full-motion video, photographs.

multipara woman who has given birth to more than one viable fetus.

multiskilled health professional an individual with versatile training in the health care field.

mycology the science and study of fungi.

myocardial infarction (MI) death of cardiac muscle due to lack of blood flow to the muscle; also known as *heart attack*.

N

narrative a paragraph indicating the contact with the patient, what was done for the patient, and the outcome of any action.

negative feedback a decrease in function in response to a stimulus.

negative stress stress that does not allow for relaxation periods.

negligence performance of an act that a reasonable health care worker would not have done or the omission of an act that a reasonable person would have done.

neonatologist physician who specializes in the care and treatment of newborns.

neoplasm abnormal growth of new tissue; tumor.

net pay the amount of money an employee is paid after all taxes are withheld.

networking a system of personal and professional relationships through which to share information.

neurogenic shock shock that results from dysfunction of nervous system following spinal cord injury.

neuron a nerve cell.

nocturia excessive urination at night.

non compos mentis mental incompetence.

noncompliance the patient's inability or refusal to follow prescribed orders.

non–insulin-dependent diabetes mellitus (NIDDM) a type of diabetes in which patients do not require insulin to control the blood sugar.

nonlanguage not expressed in spoken language, e.g., laughing, sobbing, grunting, sighing.

nonwaived testing complex tests that do not meet the Clinical Laboratory Improvements Amendments' criteria for waiver and require training and specific quality measures to ensure the accuracy and reliability of test results.

NPO patient must have nothing by mouth after midnight until the procedure is done; patient cannot have water.

nuclear medicine branch of medicine that uses radioactive isotopes to diagnose and treat disease.

nulligravida a woman who has never been pregnant.

numeric filing arranging files by a numbered order.

nutrition the study of food and how it is used for growth, nourishment, and repair.

O

obligate to require; a parasite that has no choice but to attach to a living organism.

Occupational Safety and Health Administration (OSHA) the federal agency that oversees working conditions, with the mission to protect employees from work-related hazards.

oncology the medical treatment of cancer.

online direct link to off-site computers.

operating system the program that tells the computer how to interface with hardware and software.

ophthalmic describing medication instilled into the eye.

ophthalmologist physician who specializes in treatment of disorders of the eyes.

ophthalmoscope lighted instrument used to examine the inner surfaces of the eye.

opportunistic infection infection resulting from a defective immune system that cannot defend against pathogens normally found in the environment.

optician specialist who grinds lenses to correct errors of refraction according to prescriptions written by optometrists or ophthalmologists.

optometrist specialist who can measure for errors of refraction and prescribe lenses but who cannot treat diseases of the eye or perform surgery.

organizational chart a flow sheet depicting the members of a team in a structured or hierarchical manner.

OSHA *see* Occupational Safety and Health Administration.

otolaryngologist physician who specializes in treatment of diseases and disorders of the ears, nose, and throat.

otoscope instrument used for visual examination of the ear canal and tympanic membrane.

outlier a patient whose hospital stay is longer than allowed by the DRG.

outpatient a medical setting in which patients receive care but are not admitted.

overdraft protection protection against having insufficient funds to cover checks.

over-the-counter (OTC) available without a prescription; includes herbal and vitamin supplements.

P

packing slip a document that accompanies a supply order and lists the enclosed items.

palliative easing symptoms without curing.

palmar the palm surface of the hand.

palpate to examine by feeling or pressing, used in diagnostic procedures such as vein location for phlebotomy.

palpation technique in which the examiner feels the texture, size, consistency, and location of parts of the body with the hands.

palpitations feeling of an increased heart rate or pounding heart that may be felt during an emotional response or a cardiac disorder.

Papanicolaou (Pap) test or smear smear of tissue cells examined for abnormalities including cancer, especially of the cervix; named for George N. Papanicolaou, a physician, anatomist, and cytologist.

paralanguage factors connected with, but not essentially part of, language, e.g., tone of voice, volume, pitch.

parameters values used to describe or measure a set of data representing a physiologic function or system.

paraphrasing restating what you heard using your own words.

parasite organism that derives nourishment and protection from other living organisms known as *hosts*.

parasitology the science and study of parasites.

parasympathetic the part of the autonomic nervous system involved in periods free from stress.

parenteral describing medication administered by any method other than orally.

participating providers those who agree to participate with managed care contracts and other third-party payers in exchange for building a solid patient base.

passive range of motion assisted range-of-motion movements.

pathogens disease-causing microorganisms.

patient copayment the part of an insured service that the patient must pay.

patient education active participation of the patient in a process that will yield a change in behavior.

pediatrician physician who specializes in the care of infants, children, and adolescents.

pediatrics specialty of medicine that deals with the care of infants, children, and adolescents.

pediculosis infestation with parasitic lice.

peer review organization of a group of physicians and specialists that conducts a review of a disputed case and makes a final recommendation.

percussion striking with the hands to evaluate the size, borders, consistency, and presence of fluid or air.

PERRLA abbreviation used in documentation to denote pupils equal, round, reactive to light, and accommodation if all findings are normal; refers to the size and shape of the pupils, their reaction to light, and their ability to adjust to distance.

personal protective equipment (PPE) equipment used to protect a person from exposure to blood or other body fluids.

pharmacodynamics study of how drugs act within the body.

pharmacokinetics study of the action of drugs within the body from administration to excretion.

pharmacology study of drugs and their origins, natures, properties, and effects upon living organisms.

physician hospital organization a coalition of physicians and a hospital contracting with large employers, insurance carriers, and other benefits groups to provide discounted health services.

physician office laboratory (POL) laboratory in a medical office.

physiology the study of the function of the body.

placebo an inert substance given as a medicine for its suggestive effect; an inert compound identical in appearance to material being tested in experimental research, which may or may not be known to the physician and/or patient, administered to distinguish between drug action and suggestive effect of the material under study.

plaintiff   the party who initiates a lawsuit.

plan maximum   the highest amount paid by a third-party payer for any given service.

planes   a point of reference made by a straight cut through the body at any given angle.

planning   the process of using information gathered during the assessment phase to organize learning or patient care objectives in order to accomplish the specific learning or treatment goal.

policy   a statement that reflects the organization's rules on a given topic.

portfolio   a portable case containing documents.

positive feedback   an increase in function in response to a stimulus.

positive stress   stress that allows a person to perform at peak levels and then relax afterward.

positron emission tomography (PET)   computerized radiography using radioactive substances to assess metabolic or physiologic functions within the body rather than anatomic structures.

postexposure testing   laboratory tests that may be performed after a person comes into contact with a biohazard.

posting   listing financial transactions in a ledger.

postural hypotension   sudden drop in blood pressure upon standing.

practicum   an educational course that allows the student to obtain hands-on experience; also referred to as externship.

precedents   the use of previous court decisions as a legal foundation.

preceptor   a teacher; one who gives direction, as in a technical matter.

precertification   approved documentation prior to referrals to specialists and other facilities.

precision   test results are similar when test is repeated.

preexisting condition   medical problem treated by a physician before an insurance plan's effective date. A third-party payer may exclude coverage for preexisting conditions.

preferred provider organization (PPO)   an organization whose purpose is to contract with providers and then lease this network of contracted providers to health care plans.

presbyacusis   (also: presbycusis) loss of hearing associated with aging.

presbyopia   vision change (farsightedness) associated with aging.

present illness   a specific account of the chief complaint, including time frames and characteristics.

primary diagnosis   the condition or chief complaint that brings a person to a medical facility for treatment.

primary survey   an initial assessment of an emergency patient for life-threatening problems.

problem-oriented medical record (POMR)   a common method of compiling information that lists each problem of the patient, usually at the beginning of the folder, and references each problem with a number throughout the folder.

procedure   a series of steps required to perform a given task; a medical service or test that is coded for reimbursement.

procedure manual   handbook that contains test methods and other information needed to perform testing, is suggested by the United States Department of Health and Human Services (HHS) and the Centers for Disease Control and Prevention (CDC) as a valuable resource for Certificate of Waiver sites.

product insert   written product information usually supplied by the manufacturer with each test kit or test system containing instructions and critical details for performing the test; also referred to as the package insert.

professional courtesy   a discount fee given to health care professionals.

proficiency testing   program to assess tests and the testers' performance by providing challenge samples to test as if they were patient specimens.

profit-and-loss statement   statement of income and expenditures; shows whether, in a given period, a business made or lost money and how much.

proofreading   the part of editing a document in which the writer reads the draft for accuracy and clarity and corrects errors.

prophylaxis   prevention of development of a disease or condition.

proprietary   private school with preset curricula.

protected health information (PHI)   individually identifiable personal health information as defined by the Health Insurance Portability and Accountability Act. Information that can be linked to a particular individual by name, code, or number is PHI.

protocol   a code of proper conduct; a treatment plan.

provider   a health care worker who delivers medical care.

psychogenic   of psychological origin.

psychomotor   describes a physical task.

psychosocial   relating to mental and emotional aspects of social encounters.

purchase order   a document that lists the required items to be purchased.

purulent   describes drainage that is white, green, or yellow; characteristic of an infection.

pyrexia   body temperature of 102°F or higher rectally or 101°F or higher orally.

Q

quadrants   a division of the abdomen into four equal parts by one horizontal and one vertical line dissecting at the umbilicus.

qualitative   has positive or negative results; not a specified amount.

quality assessment   plan for ensuring the quality of all areas of the laboratory's technical and support functions.

quality assurance (QA)   an evaluation of health care services as compared to accepted standards.

quality control (QC)   method to evaluate the proper performance of testing procedures, supplies, or equipment in a laboratory.

quality improvement   a plan that allows an organization to scientifically measure the quality of its product and service.

quantitative test   quantity measured and reported in a number value.

R

radiograph   processed film that contains a visible image.

radiographer   technical specialist who works to assist the radiologist in the performance of procedures and who is responsible for producing routine examination images for the radiologist to interpret.

radiography   art and science of producing diagnostic images with x-rays.

radiologist   physician who specializes in radiology; performs some procedures and interprets images to provide diagnostic information.

radiology   branch of medicine including diagnostic and therapeutic applications of x-rays.

random access memory (RAM)   temporary memory; data is lost when the computer is turned off if it is not backed up on disk.

range of motion (ROM)   range in degrees of angle through which a joint can be extended and flexed.

read only memory (ROM)   permanent memory inside the computer.

receptionist   a person who greets patients as they arrive at a medical office and performs various administrative tasks.

recertification   certification renewed either by taking the examination again or by completing a specified number of continuing education units in a 5-year period.

recommended dietary allowance (RDA)   the amount of a nutrient most people need each day to stay healthy.

reconstitution   adding water to bring a material back to its liquid state.

referral   instruction to transfer a patient's care to a specialist.

referral laboratory   a large facility in which thousands of tests of various types are performed each day.

reflecting   repeat what one heard using open-ended questions.

registration   enrollment in a particular professional entity that endorses one's skills and abilities.

requisition   an order form for laboratory tests; must accompany each sample submitted to the laboratory.

res ipsa loquitur   "the thing speaks for itself."

res judicata   "the thing has been decided."

resident flora   microorganisms normally found in the body; also known as *normal flora*.

resistance   body's immune response to prevent infections by invading pathogenic microorganisms.

resistant   describes organisms that grow even in the presence of an antimicrobial agent.

Resource-Based Relative Value Scale (RBRVS)   a value scale designed to decrease Medicare Part B costs and establish national standards for coding and payment.

respondant superior   "let the master answer."

restrain   control or confine movement.

résumé   document summarizing individual's work experience or professional qualifications.

returned check fee   amount of money a bank or business charges for a check written with insufficient funds.

reverse chronological order   items placed with oldest first.

risk factors   any issue that possesses a safety or liability concern for an organization.

role delineation chart   a list of the areas of competence expected of the graduate.

S

salutation   an introductory phrase that greets the reader of a letter.

sanitation   maintenance of a healthful, disease-free environment.

sanitization   processes used to lower the number of microorganisms on a surface by cleansing with soap or detergent, water, and manual friction.

sanitize   reduce the number of microorganisms on a surface by use of low-level disinfectant practices.

scanner   a piece of office equipment that transfers a written document into a computer.

scope of practice   the procedures, actions, and processes that are permitted for a particular health care profession.

screening   a preliminary procedure, such as a test or exam, to detect the more characteristic signs of a disorder.

search engine   program that allows you to find information on the Internet rapidly and effectively.

secondary survey   an assessment of an emergency victim for head to toe injuries.

self boundaries   the limits set on the relationships between health care professionals and their patients

semi-block   a type of letter format that is styled the same as block, except the first sentence of each paragraph is indented five spaces.

senility   general mental deterioration associated with aging.

sentinel event   an unexpected death or serious physical or psychological injury to a patient in a health care facility.

service   medical interventions completed by a provider.

service charge   a charge by a bank for various services.

sharps container   a rigid, leak-proof, plastic container used to discard disposable sharp devices in a manner to reduce needlesticks.

shift   a situation in which quality control results make an obvious change in performance levels.

shock   lack of oxygen to individual cells of the body.

sick-child visit   a pediatric visit for the treatment of illness or injury.

signs   objective indications of disease or bodily dysfunction as observed or measured by the health care professional.

slander   oral statements that defame a person's reputation or character.

SOAP   a style of charting that includes subjective, objective, assessment, and planning notes.

software   application programs that direct the hardware to perform given tasks.

sound   long instrument for exploring or dilating body cavities or searching cavities for foreign bodies.

specialty   a subcategory of medicine, such as pediatrics, studied after completion of medical school.

specificity   relating to a definite result.

specimen   a small portion of anything used to evaluate the nature of the whole; samples, such as blood or urine, used to evaluate a patient's condition.

spore   bacterial life form that resists destruction by heat, drying, or chemicals. Spore-producing bacteria include botulism and tetanus.

staff privileges   hospital approval for a physician to admit patients for treatment.

standard precautions   usual steps to prevent injury or disease.

staphylococci spherical microorganism found in grapelike clusters.

stare decisis "the previous decision stands."

STAT immediately.

statute of limitations a legal time limit; e.g., the length of time in which a patient may file a lawsuit.

statutes laws that are written by federal, state, or local legislators.

stereotyping to place in a fixed mold, without consideration of differences.

sterilization process, act, or technique for destroying microorganisms using heat, water, chemicals, or gases.

streaming a method of allotting time for appointments based on the needs of the individual patient to minimize gaps in time and backups.

Streptococcus genus of bacteria commonly implicated in infections of the skin.

stress a factor that induces body tension; can be positive or negative.

subject filing arranging files according to their title, grouping similar subjects together.

subpoena a court order requiring an individual to appear at court at a given date and time.

subpoena duces tecum a court order requiring medical records to be submitted to the court at a given date and time.

summarizing briefly reviewing the information discussed to determine the patient's comprehension.

summation report any report that provides a summary of activities, such as a payroll report or a profit-and-loss statement.

superbill preprinted patient bill that lists a variety of procedures.

superficial describes fungal infections limited to skin, hair, and nails.

superficial burn burn limited to the epidermis.

surfing navigating the Internet.

surgical asepsis destruction of organisms before they enter the body.

surgical pathology the primary subspecialty of anatomic pathology. Studies are performed on tissue and body fluid specimens from aspirations, autopsies, biopsies, organ removal, and other procedures to identify or evaluate the effects of cancer and other diseases.

suspension temporary removal of privileges.

sustained fever fever that is constant or not fluctuating.

sympathy feeling sorry for or pitying someone.

symptoms subjective indications of disease or bodily dysfunction as sensed by the patient.

syncope sudden fall in blood pressure or cerebral hypoxia resulting in loss of consciousness.

system a collection of organs that perform a certain function.

systemic describes an infection of the internal organs.

T

tactile pertaining to the sense of touch.

task force a group of employees that works together to solve a given problem.

tax withholding the amount of tax that is withheld from a paycheck.

teleradiology use of computed imaging and information systems to transmit diagnostic images to distant locations.

teletypewriter (TTY) a special machine that allows communication on a telephone with a hearing-impaired person.

template a skeleton of a letter or document with preset and prespaced elements.

therapeutic having to do with treating or curing disease; curative.

therapeutic phlebotomy phlebotomy done as part of the patient's treatment for certain blood disorders.

third-party administrator administrator who processes claims for the sponsor of self-funded benefit planning.

threshold the least amount of something that produces a response.

titer measure of the amount of an antibody in serum.

tort the righting of wrongs or injuries suffered by someone because of another person's wrongdoing.

toxicology the study of the presence and measurement of drugs in the blood.

toxoid toxin treated to destroy its toxicity but still capable of inducing formation of antibodies.

trade name name given to a medication by the company that owns the patent.

transcription the process of typing a dictated message.

transient flora microorganisms that do not normally reside in a given area; transient flora may or may not produce disease.

traumatic causing or relating to tissue damage.

trend when control results progressively increase or decrease over time.

triage sorting of patients into categories based on their level of sickness or injury to ensure that life-threatening medical conditions are treated immediately.

tympanic thermometer device for measuring the temperature using the blood flow through the tympanic membrane, or eardrum.

U

ultrasound imaging technique that uses sound waves to diagnose or monitor various body structures.

unbundling the practice of submitting a claim with several separate procedure codes rather than a single code that represents the services performed.

unemployment tax federal tax paid by the employer based on each employee's gross income.

unit each part of a name or title that is used in indexing; a quantity of a standard measurement.

universal precautions controlling infection by treating all human blood and certain human body fluids as if known to be infectious for HIV, hepatitis B virus, hepatitis C virus, and other bloodborne pathogens.

upcoding billing more for a patient care service than it is worth by selecting a code that is higher on the coding scale; this is an illegal practice.

usual, customary, and reasonable (UCR) the basis of a physician's fee schedule, the usual and customary cost of the same service or procedure in a similar geographic area and under the same or similar circumstances.

utilization review an analysis of individual cases by a committee to make sure services and procedures being billed to a third-party payer are medically necessary and to ensure compliance with its rules and regulations regarding reimbursement.

V

V-codes codes assigned to patients who receive service but have no illness, injury, or disorder, e.g., a vaccination or a screening mammogram.

vaccine suspension of infectious agents or some part of them; given to establish resistance to an infectious disease.

values established ideals of life, conduct, customs, etc., of an individual person or members of a society.

virtual a paperless system or chart on your computer.

virulent highly pathogenic and disease-producing; describes a microorganism.

virus a harmful invader that can damage your computer.

visualization a relaxation technique that allows the mind to wander and the imagination to run free and focus on positive and relaxing situations.

W

waived test determined by Clinical Laboratory Improvement Amendments to be so simple that there is little risk of error.

wave scheduling system a flexible scheduling method that allows time for procedures of varying lengths and the addition of unscheduled patients, as needed.

well-child visit visit to the medical office for administration of immunizations and evaluation of growth and development.

withdrawing the act of terminating a medical treatment that has already been initiated.

withholding not initiating certain medical treatments.

workers' compensation employer insurance for treatment of an employee's injury or illness related to the job.

write-off cancellation of an unpaid debt.

X

x-rays invisible electromagnetic radiation waves used in diagnosis and treatment of various disorders.

Index

Page numbers in *italics* denote figures; those followed by a t denote tables.

developing material, 87–88
disseminating information, 88
selecting and adapting material, 86–87
Telecommunication device for the deaf (TDD), 64
Telecommunication relay systems (TRS), 111
Telephone
auto-attendant, 111
cellular, 111
collecting a debt, 238
equipment and services, 111, 113
etiquette, 108
importance in medical office, 105
incoming calls
appointments, 107
billing inquiries, 107
challenging, 108–109
irate patients, 108
medical emergencies, 108–109
from other physicians, 107
personal calls, 107
prescription refills, 107
progress reports, 107
taking messages, 109
test results, reports from laboratories, 107
test results request from patients, 107
triaging, 105–106
unidentified callers, 105
medical record documentation of
communication, 169–170
multiple lines, 111
outgoing calls
emergency medical services, *110,*
110–111
general guidelines, 109–110
long distance, 109
reminders, 123–124, *124*
Spanish terminology, 112
telecommunication relay systems (TRS), 111
use guidelines
courtesy, 106, *106*
diction, 105
expression, 106
listening, 106
pronunciation, 105
Telephone numbers, in written communications,
140, 147
Teletypewriter (TTY), 111
Television
closed captioning, 102
as teaching tool, 102
in waiting room, 102
Temperature
Celsius-Fahrenheit temperature conversion
scale, 373
Template, letterhead, 141
Terminally ill patients
communicating with, 67
hospice, 67
Terminating employees, 206–207
Termination or withdrawal of contract,
30–31, *31*
Text messaging, 111
Text telephone (TTY), 64
Thank you letter, *343*
Therapeutic touch, 57, *57*
Third-party administrator (TPA), 276

Tickler file, 211
Time, in written communication, 140
Time sheet, externship, *331*
Tort law, 28, 37
Tort of outrage, 39
Torts
defined, 37
intentional
assault and battery, 38
defamation of character, 39
duress, 38
fraud, 39
invasion of privacy, 38
tort of outrage, 39
undue influence, 39
unintentional, 37–38
damage, 38
dereliction of duty, 38
direct cause, 38
duty, 38
jury awards, 38
malpractice, 37
negligence, 37
Touch, therapeutic, 57, *57*
Toys, waiting room, 103
TPA (*see* Third-party administrator (TPA))
Training
computer, 194
Translation, Web sites, 188
Traveler's check, 254
Trial, 39
TRICARE, 278–279
TRS (telecommunication relay systems), 111
Truth-in-lending form, 236, *237*
TTY (Teletypewriter), 111

U
Undue influence, 39
Uniform Anatomical Gift Act, 48
Unintentional torts, 37–38
United States Postal Service (USPS), 148–149
Universal serial bus (USB), 182
Upcoding, 319
USB (universal serial bus), 182
USDA (United States Department of
Agriculture), 185
USP (United States Pharmacopeia) label, 83
USPS (United States Postal Service), 148–149
Usual, customary, and reasonable (UCR), 287
Utilization management, 279
Utilization review, 279

V
V-codes, 294
Vaccine side effects, 32
Verbal communication, 55–56
Verified Internet Pharmacy Practice Site
(VIPPS), 189
Vesalius, Andreas, *5*
Violent injuries, reporting of, 35
VIPPS (Verified Internet Pharmacy Practice
Site), 189
Virus, computer, 185
Visualization, 86

Vital statistics, 33
Voice mail systems, 100

W
Waiting time, managing, 101
Web browser, 184, 185
White-out, 258
Withdrawal (defense mechanisms), 85t
Withdrawing treatment, 48
Withholding treatment, 48
Witness, expert, 37–38
Women in medicine, 6
Word processing, 141
Workers' compensation, 282
Workers' compensation records, 170
World Health Organization (WHO), 291
World Wide Web (WWW) (*see* Internet)
Write-off, 236
Written communications, 134–153
agendas, 146, *146*
annotation, 150
guidelines for document production
abbreviations and symbols, 139–140
accuracy, 137–138
capitalization, 138–139
grammar and punctuation, 134–137
numbers, 140
plural and possessive, 140
spelling, 135, 137–138
incoming mail, 150
letters
components of, 141–143, *141*–*143*
composition, 144, 151
editing, 144–145
formats, *142,* 143, *143*
how to start writing, 144
preparation, 143
types of, 145
memorandum, 145–146, *146*
minutes, 146–147
opening and sorting, 150, 152
overview, 135
sending, 147–150
addressing envelopes, 148, *148*
electronic mail, 148
facsimile machines, *147,* 147–148
mailing options, 149
postage, 149
special services, 149, *149*
United States Postal Service, 148–149
via delivery services, 150
Spanish terminology, 150

X
X-ray report, 371
X-rays
discovery of, 6

Y
Yanagimachi, Rvuzo, 6
Yoga, 82

Z
Zip code Abbreviations, 355